Cancer and the Kidney
The frontier of nephrology and oncology

SECOND EDITION

Edited by

Eric P. Cohen

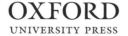

OXFORD
UNIVERSITY PRESS

OXFORD

UNIVERSITY PRESS

Great Clarendon Street, Oxford OX2 6DP

Oxford University Press is a department of the University of Oxford.
It furthers the University's objective of excellence in research, scholarship,
and education by publishing worldwide in

Oxford New York

Auckland Cape Town Dar es Salaam Hong Kong Karachi
Kuala Lumpur Madrid Melbourne Mexico City Nairobi
New Delhi Shanghai Taipei Toronto

With offices in

Argentina Austria Brazil Chile Czech Republic France Greece
Guatemala Hungary Italy Japan Poland Portugal Singapore
South Korea Switzerland Thailand Turkey Ukraine Vietnam

Oxford is a registered trade mark of Oxford University Press
in the UK and in certain other countries

Published in the United States
by Oxford University Press Inc., New York

© Oxford University Press, 2011

The moral rights of the author have been asserted

Database right Oxford University Press (maker)

First edition published 2005
Second edition published 2011

British Library Cataloging in Publication Data

Data available

Library of Congress Cataloging in Publication Data

Data available

Typeset in Minion by Glyph International, Bangalore, India
Printed in Great Britain
on acid-free paper by
CPI Antony Rowe, Chippenham, Wiltshire

ISBN 978–0–19–958019–4

10 9 8 7 6 5 4 3 2 1

Foreword

The impact of cancer in its different forms on clinical nephrology continues to expand, and the second addition of this compact and useful textbook is once again timely. The first edition provided a niche monograph and easily accessible resource for the busy clinician, and interested non-clinical scientist, on 'cancer and the kidney' in all its forms and clinical consequences. It did this by adopting a combined approach to the subject, bringing together physiology, cancer biology, nephrology, oncology, and urology in a series of distinct—yet complementary—chapters, each introduced by a brief clinical vignette, to put a topic in its clinical context, which proves a helpful literary device.

This book still stands alone in its succinct coverage of the subject and in its target readership. The second edition has been significantly revised and updated, adding almost 60 pages to the original text. While many of the original chapter headings remain the same, the number has increased from 11 to 13, to include more on new cancer therapies and the effects of cancer on renal function. The overall format is much the same, but in addition to the chapter headings, subheadings are now included, which aid the reader in finding his or her way around the book, and in making it easier to 'dip into' the text as a useful day-to-day reference source.

There have been important developments in cancer biology and cancer treatments since the last edition, and while new side effects of some novel treatments are beginning to emerge, patients are living longer, and in many cases can be considered as 'cured'. However, one of the important developments in adult nephrology in recent years is a much greater awareness of, and involvement in, the consequences of these novel forms of therapy on kidney function, especially the late effects of chemotherapy or radiation given in childhood or adolescence, something this book helps to highlight. Since cancer treatment will continue to advance and treatment protocols will continue to change, it is particularly important for the clinical nephrologist to be kept abreast of these developments and how they might impact on nephrology practice; so a third and future edition will, I'm sure, be necessary in due course.

Finally, adapting a quotation attributed to the father of bedside medicine Sir William Osler ('In science the credit goes to the man who convinces the world, not to the man to whom the idea first occurs'), it should be said of this book that credit is certainly due to the editor, Eric Cohen, in successfully communicating a valuable and complex set of ideas on an important subject to a wider audience, as much as it is to each of the contributing authors.

Professor Robert J Unwin
Centre for Nephrology
UCL Medical School
University College London
London, UK

Preface

This book addresses the area at the difficult frontier of nephrology and oncology. Cancer patients may develop kidney problems, and people with kidney disease may develop cancer. Neither nephrologist nor oncologist is apt to be comfortable in the other's field. This book aims to relieve that discomfort by supplying facts and advice.

I came to this overlap area by two pathways. The first was my recognition and study of the problem of acquired cysts and cancers in native kidneys of subjects with renal failure. Cysts form in failing kidneys, which are usually only a benign curiosity. But sometimes cancers form in those kidneys, and may be lethal. As is carefully detailed by Dr. Ishikawa in chapter 11 of this book, these native kidney cancers can happen before the start of dialysis, when a patient is on long-term dialysis, or in a kidney transplant patient. Mechanisms of formation of these native kidney cancers are not known. The roles of the VHL gene or jade-1, and perhaps the role of chronic hypoxia in the failing kidney are clear candidates for study.

The second pathway was my experience with and study of the problem of kidney disease after hematopoietic stem cell transplantation ('bone marrow transplant', HSCT or BMT). The clinical problem of acute renal failure after HSCT is well known to HSCT/BMT units. What is less clear is the problem of chronic kidney disease, a complication that occurs in long-term survivors of HSCT. At the Medical College of Wisconsin, we have shown that radiation injury is an important cause of chronic kidney disease (CKD) after HSCT. Our laboratory and clinical work has shown that this injury can be treated and mitigated. Yet other causes of CKD after HSCT can occur, including drug toxicities, injury from graft versus host disease, and others, as are clearly described by Dr. Humphreys in chapter 8 of this book. People whose cancer is cured by HSCT are at risk for CKD, so their long-term follow-up is essential for proper recognition and treatment, should kidney disease develop.

These two specific interests became a more general one, which led to the first and now second edition of this book. The topics that we address are real, everyday ones, yet pose their own intellectual challenges for further study. The second edition is different from the first because each chapter has been updated, and two chapters have been added. The chapter on CKD after HSCT has already been mentioned. The new chapter on biologics is a key addition because of the increasing use of non-traditional agents in cancer treatment, including specific antibodies and agents with novel targets, as alternatives to traditional chemotherapy.

Our editors at Oxford University Press have provided excellent support. Helen Liepman and Susan Crowhurst have my particular thanks. This book will be useful for all who care for people with cancer who develop kidney problems, or for those with kidney disease who develop cancer.

Contents

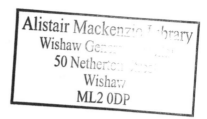

Contributors

Bahar Bastani
Division of Nephrology
Saint Louis University School of
Medicine
St. Louis, USA

Joseph F. Buell
Tulane Abdominal Transplant
Institute
Tulane University
New Orleans, USA

Eric P. Cohen
Medical College of Wisconsin
Milwaukee, USA

Roger B. Cohen
Hospital of the University of
Pennsylvania
Division of Hematology–Oncology
Philadelphia, USA

Carlos D. Flombaum
Memorial Sloan-Kettering
Cancer Center
New York City, USA

Ilya G. Glezerman
Renal Service, Department of
Medicine
Memorial Sloan-Kettering
Cancer Center
New York City, USA

Lee A. Hebert
Ohio State University Medical
Center
Columbus, USA

Benjamin D. Humphreys
Renal Division, Brigham and
Women's Hospital and Dana Farber
Cancer Institute,
Boston, USA

Isao Ishikawa
Division of Nephrology
Asanogawa General Hospital
Kanazawa, Ishikawa, Japan

Jean-Marie Krzesinski
Université de Liège
Liège, Belgium

Sheron Latcha
Renal Service, Department of
Medicine
Memorial Sloan-Kettering Cancer
Center
New York City, USA

Vincent Launay-Vacher
Department of Nephrology
Hôpital Pitie-Salpetriere
Paris, France

Martine Leblanc
Nephrology and Critical Care
Maisonneuve-Rosemont Hospital
University of Montreal
Montreal, Canada

Jasmin Levallois
Nephrology and Critical Care
Maisonneuve-Rosemont Hospital
University of Montreal
Montreal, Canada

Michael Marvin
Jewish Hospital Transplant Center
Louisville, USA

John E. Moulder
Medical College of Wisconsin
Milwaukee, USA

Marie Philipneri
Division of Nephrology
Saint Louis University School of
Medicine
St. Louis, USA

Elizabeth R. Plimack
Fox Chase Cancer Center
Philadelphia, USA

Kadiyala V. Ravindra
Jewish Hospital Transplant Center
Louisville, USA

Christopher Valentine
Ohio State University Medical
Center
Columbus, USA

Robin G. Woolfson
Transplantation and
Immunology Division
Royal Free Hospital
London, UK

Abbreviations

2,3-DRG	2,3-diphosphoglycerate
ABV	doxorubicin, bleomycin, and vincristine
ACD	acquired cystic disease
ACDK	acquired cystic disease of the kidney
ACE	angiotensin-converting-enzyme
ACEI	ACE inhibitor therapy
ACTH	adrenocorticotropic hormone
ADH	anti-diuretic hormone
ADQI	Acute Dialysis Quality Initiative group
AIDS	acquired immunodeficiency syndrome
AKI	acute kidney injury
AKIN	Acute Kidney Injury Network
ALT	alanine aminotransferase
AMACR	alpha-methylacyl-CoA racemase
aMDRD	abbreviated modification of diet in renal disease
ANCA	antineutrophil cytoplasmic antigen
ARB	angiotensin receptor blockers
ARF	acute renal failure
ASO	American Society of Oncology
AST	aspartate aminotransferase
ATN	acute tubular necrosis
ATP	adenosine phosphate
AUC	area under the plasma concentration–time curve
AVP	arginine vasopressin
bFGF	basic fibroblast growth factor
β-FGF	fibroblast growth factor beta
BMSC	bone marrow stromal cell
BMT	bone marrow transplantation
BP	blood pressure
BUN	blood urea nitrogen
CAPD	continuous ambulatory peritoneal dialysis
CaSR	calcium sensing receptor
CBC	complete blood count
CCRCC	clear cell renal cell carcinoma
CD38	cluster of differentiation 38 (glycoprotein)
CDI	central diabetes insipidus

CDR	complementarity-determining region
CEA	carcinoembryonic antigen
CGN	crescentic GN
cGVHD	chronic GVHD
CHOP	cyclophosphamide, doxorubicin, vincristine, and prednisone
CK7	cytokeratin 7
CKD	chronic kidney disease
CNI	calcineurin inhibitor
COPD	chronic obstructive pulmonary disease
COX-2	cyclooxigenase-2
CMV	cytomegalovirus.
CNS	central nervous system
CRC	colorectal cancer
CrCl	creatinine clearance
CRP	C-reactive protein
CRRT	continuous renal replacement therapy
CSF1R	colony-stimulating factor 1 receptor
CT	computed tomography
CTL	cytotoxic T-lymphocyte
DCIS	ductal carcinoma in situ
dFdU	difluorodeoxyuridine
DOTATOC	dota-D-phe-tyr-octreotide
DRE	digital rectal examination
EBV	Epstein–Barr virus
EC	extracellular space
ECOG	Eastern Cooperative Group Oncology
EGFR	epidermal growth factor receptor
eGFR	estimated glomerular filtration rate
EMA	European Medicines Agency
EORTC	European Organisation for the Research and Treatment of Cancer
EPO	erythropoietin
ERA-EDTA	European Renal Association-European Dialysis and Transplant Association
ERK	extracellular-signal-regulated kinase
ESRD	end-stage renal disease
ETOH	alcohol
FBAL	α-fluoro-β-alanine
FDA	United States Food and Drug Administration
FEK	fractional excretion of potassium
FENa	fractional excretion of sodium
FGF	fibroblast growth factor
FGF23	fibroblast growth factor 23
FHIT	fragile histidine triad

FLC	free serum light chain
FLT1	fms-related tyrosine kinase 1
FLT3	fms-related tyrosine kinase 3
FSGS	focal segmental glomerulosclerosis
GBM	glioblastoma multiforme
GFR	glomerular filtration rate
GI	gastro-intestinal
Global ARCC	Global Advanced Renal Cell Carcinoma
GN	glomerulonephritis
GVHD	graft vs. host disease
HBV	hepatitis B virus
HCDD	heavy chain deposition disease
HCM	hypercalcemia of malignancy
HCV	hepatitis C virus
HER-2	human epidermal growth factor receptor 2
HGF	hepatocyte growth factor/scatter factor
HHM	humoral hypercalcemia of malignancy
HHV8	human herpes virus 8
HIF	hypoxia induced factor
HIV	human immunodeficiency virus
HPRCC	hereditary papillary RCC
HSCT	hematopoietic stem cell transplantation (HSCT)
HTLV-1	human T-cell lymphotropic virus type 1
HTN	arterial hypertension
HUS	hemolytic uremic syndrome
IC	intracellular
ICAM-1	intracellular adhesion molecule-1
IFN	interferon
IFNγ	interferon-gamma
IgA	immunoglobulin A
IgA N	IgA nephritis
IGF	insulin-like growth factor
IgG	immunoglobulin G
IgM	immunoglobulin M
IL-1β	interleukin-1 beta
IL-6	interleukin-6
IL-12	interleukin-12
IPITTR	Israel Penn International Transplant Tumor Registry
ISR	immunosuppression reduction
IV	intravenously
IVP	intravenous pyelogram
JVP	jugular venous pulse

KS	Kaposi's sarcoma
LCDD	light chain deposition disease
LCIS	lobular carcinoma in situ
LDH	lactic acid dehydrogenase
LHCDD	light and heavy chain deposition disease
LMW	low molecular weight
L-NAME	N(omega)-nitro-L-arginine methyl ester
LOH	loss of heterozygosity
MAHA	microangiopathic hemolytic anemia
MCD	Minimal Change Disease
MDRD	Modification of Diet in Renal Disease
MEK	MEK
MESNA	mercaptoethanesulfonate
MGUS	monoclonal gammopathy of unknown significance
MIDD	monoclonal immunoglobulin deposition disease
MMC	mitomycin C
MMF	mycophenolate mofetil
MN	membranous nephropathy
MPGN	Membranoproliferative glomerulonephritis
MRI	magnetic resonance imaging
MSKCC	Memorial Sloan-Kettering Cancer Center
NCI	National Cancer Institute
NDI	nephrogenic diabetes insipidus
NF-kB	nuclear factor-kB
NMSC	non-melanoma skin cancer
NSAID	non-steroidal anti-inflammatory drug
OPG	osteoprotegerin
OPTN	Organ Procurement and Transplantation Network
OS	overall survival
PAS	periodic acid-Schiff
PDGF	platelet derived growth factor
PDGFR	platelet derived growth factor receptor
PDGFR-β	platelet derived growth factor receptor-
PET	positron emission tomography
pI	isoelectric points
POEMS	polyenuropathy, organomegaly, endocrinopathy, m-band and skin changes
PSA	prostatic-specific antigen
PT	proximal renal tubule
PTH	parathyroid hormone
PTHrP	parathyroid hormone related peptide/protein
PTLD	post-transplant proliferative disease
Pu	proteinuria

QALY	quality-adjusted life year
QTc	QT interval corrected
RA	rheumatoid arthritis
RANKL	receptor activator nuclear factor-κ ligand
RBC	red blood cell
RCC	renal cell carcinoma
RECIST	response evaluation criteria in solid tumors
RF	renal failure
RFA	radiofrequency ablation
RFS	refeeding syndrome
RI	renal impairment
RIFLE	risk-injury-failure-loss-ESRD
RR	relative risk
RRT	renal replacement therapy
RTA	renal tubular acidosis
SA-A	serum amyloid A
SAP	serum amyloid-P component
SCC	squamous cell cancer
SCr	serum creatinine
SEER	surveillance, epidemiology, and end results
SG	specific gravity
SIADH	syndrome of inappropriate ADH secretion
SIR	standardized incidence ratio
SLE	systemic lupus erythematosus
SPS	Sodium Polystyrene Sulfonate
SQ	subcutaneous
SWOG	South West Oncology Group
TAL LOH	thick ascending limb of the loop of Henle
TBI	total body irradiation
TCC	transitional cell carcinoma
T-DM1	trastuzumab-DM1
TGF-β	transforming growth factor-beta
THP	Tamm--Horsfall mucoprotein
TKI	tyrosine kinase inhibitor
TLS	tumor lysis syndrome
TMA	thrombotic microangiopathy
TmP/GFR	tubular maximum phosphate reabsorption per glomerular filtration rate
TNF	tumor necrosis factor
TNF-α	tumor necrosis factor-alpha
TRICC	transfusion requirements in critical care
TSC	uberous sclerosis complex

TTKG	transtubular potassium gradient
TTP	thrombotic thrombocytopenic purpura
UNOS	United Network for Organ Sharing
UPJ	uretero-pelvic junction
US FDA	United States Food and Drug Administration
USRDS	United States Renal Data System
UVJ	ureterovesical junction
VCAM-1	vascular cell adhesion molecule-1
VEGF	vascular endothelial cell growth factor
VEGF-A	VEGF antibody
VEGFR	VEGF receptors
VHL	Von Hippel–Lindau
VIII/vWF	Von Willebrand's Factor VIII
VOD	veno-occlusive disease
WBC	white blood cell

Chapter 1

The assessment of kidney function

Eric P. Cohen and Jean-Marie Krzesinski

Case report

A 36-year-old woman was admitted to the medical ward for left Herpes Zoster opthalmicus. She had developed breast cancer one year before, and had been treated by surgery, radiotherapy, and chemotherapy. The last treatment was three months before the current admission.

Her physical exam showed the ocular Herpes Zoster and the right mastectomy. She was thin. Her weight was 43 kg, and her height was 163 cm. Her blood pressure was 110/60 mmHg.

The serum chemistries showed a serum creatinine of 100 µmol/L (1.1 mg/dL) by the enzymatic IDMS traceable creatinine measurement. The estimated glomerular filtration rate (eGFR) reported by the hospital laboratory, according to the MDRD equation, was 56 mL/min/1.73 m2. The blood urea was 8 mmol/L (BUN = 22 mg/dL). Acyclovir was given intravenously at the dose of 10 mg/kg three times a day for seven days, the usual dose for immunosuppressed subjects because she had been recently treated by chemotherapy.

After three days, she became confused and had hallucinations. There was an increase in serum creatinine and urea levels, to115 µmol/L and 12.5 mmol/L, respectively. The urinalysis was unremarkable.

Encephalitis was ruled out. The antiviral treatment was temporarily stopped because acyclovir toxicity was felt to be the cause of the confused mental state.

The renal function returned to the initial value 36 hours after stopping acyclovir. It was started again orally at the dose of 800 mg twice daily for the next three days.

A 24-hour urine collection had only 450 mg of creatinine. The creatinine clearance was 28 mL/min, when the serum creatinine was 1.1 mg/dL. The urea clearance was also decreased, being 20 mL/min.

By using the Cockcroft formula, for the same serum creatinine, the creatinine clearance was 48 mL/min. By the Wright formula, the eGFR was 56 mL/min.

All these different values are summarized in Table 1.1.

This case shows the difficulty of accurately determining the GFR in patients with low body weight. This patient had low body weight and low muscle mass, as shown by the low total amount of creatinine in her 24-hour urine collection. This accounts for her low serum creatinine. Her GFR could also be estimated as the average of the creatinine and urea clearances, being 24 mL/min, instead of 56 as reported on the automatic lab report.

This patient's actual GFR was probably closest to the value given by the 24-hour urine studies, and not by any formula. That is also based on her adverse response to the acyclovir.

Table 1.1 Glomerular filtration rate (GFR) according to the method used, and for a serum creatinine of 1.1 mg/dL

Method for GFR	result
MDRD formula	56 mL/min/1.73m^2
Cockcroft-Gault formula	48 mL/min
Wright formula	56 mL/min
24-hour urine creatinine clearance	28 mL/min

In patients with low muscle mass due to cachexia or severe illness, a 24-hour urine collection may be better to calculate the creatinine clearance rather than estimating the GFR from a formula derived from the plasma creatinine concentration alone. One could also use a reference technique for GFR determination such as iohexol, EDTA, or iothalamate. The European Medicines Agency (EMEA) recommends these latter techniques for the evaluation of new medicines in subjects with reduced kidney function. The expense of these tests may be well worthwhile, because that expense may avoid the morbidity of medication toxicity.

Introduction

This case illustrates the use of the serum creatinine and the equations dependent on its value to estimate the glomerular filtration rate (GFR). It shows clearly the difficulty in the assessment and management of reduced kidney function in subjects with cancer. In them, as in this patient, a low body and muscle mass will reduce the creatinine production, and what appears to be a normal serum creatinine will instead indicate a reduced GFR. The formula-based estimates of GFR appear in this case to have been overestimates, whereas the 24-hour urine studies indicated a GFR of about 25 mL/min. That latter value is consistent with her adverse response to the intravenous acyclovir.

The level, or amount, of kidney function is often conflated with the GFR, or even more commonly, with the level of the serum creatinine. While this approximation is useful for day-to-day management, it has some inaccuracies and it ignores some of the other aspects of kidney function, including proteinuria and the differentiation of tubular from glomerular injury. This chapter will discuss the assessment of kidney function by history and physical exam, urinalysis, testing the GFR, assessment of proteinuria and testing the renal tubular function.

History and physical exam

Past and family history may indicate a predisposition to kidney disease, for instance from diabetes or polycystic kidney disease, but these do not indicate the level of kidney function.

Features of the history include the exposure to potential nephrotoxins in sufficient amounts and with an appropriate chronology. The use of radiocontrast, for example, may cause acute renal failure within days of its use, but renal failure several weeks after its use is not due to radiocontrast. Knowledge of cancers that may involve the urinary tract should be sought in the history, such as lymphomas, or treatments that may affect kidney function, such as cis-platinum.

The timing of the onset of edema is usually straightforward. But in the absence of this symptom, the onset of kidney disease may be insidious. The degree of edema is not a good marker of the degree of kidney function loss. A loss of urine concentrating ability, which can occur at a GFR of 60 mL/min or less, may result in nocturia.

Hypertension may occur because of kidney disease, but is often asymptomatic and thus not a reliable feature of the history. A documented new onset of hypertension may be useful in timing the onset of kidney disease. The degree of blood pressure elevation is not a good marker of the level of kidney function.

A patient may provide information on a change in urine output or its color, which may help in identifying the timing of kidney disease.

Symptoms of renal failure, such as decreased appetite, may be noticed when the GFR is less than 20 mL/min, but nausea or vomiting are a later manifestations of renal failure, occurring when the GFR is 10 mL/min or less.

The physical exam is non-specific until over half of the normal kidney function is lost. Anemia, for instance, occurs in direct relation to the serum creatinine, but this relationship is imprecise and other causes for anemia may exist in a cancer patient. Muscle cramps may occur when the kidney function is down to 25% of normal, sometimes in association with hypocalcemia. A sallow 'dirty-yellow' hue to the skin may be apparent in a subject with chronic renal failure whose kidney function is less than 10% of normal. Itching also occurs in severe chronic kidney failure, generally when the serum creatinine has reached 400 μmol/L or higher, and scratch marks can be seen on the skin. But itching is not a feature of acute renal failure. Another skin finding is the occurrence of blotchy subepidermal hemorrhages, generally on the dorsum of the forearms. This can occur when the GFR is less than 25% of normal, and is related to the reduction in the platelet function in subjects with renal impairment.

Abnormalities of tubular function may cause symptoms and signs but these are even less specific than those of renal failure. A renal tubular acidosis caused by amphotericin could cause weakness, either related to acidosis or the hypokalemia. Deep tendon reflexes could even be lost at severe degrees of hypokalemia, i.e. less than 2 mmol/L. Similarly, hypophosphatemia could result in weakness, but its cause would only be apparent upon lab testing.

The assessment of a patient's extracellular volume status, by evaluating changes in body weight or blood pressure (BP), may be important in establishing the cause of renal failure. For instance, an increase in pulse of greater than 30 beats/min and a drop in BP of more than 20 mmHg on changing from the lying down to the standing up position may indicate extracellular volume depletion, which can cause pre-renal azotemia. However, those changes of the pulse and BP do not tell us the level of kidney function. In addition, these signs are not always present in a subject with volume depletion (1). A patient with reduced kidney function may have signs of fluid overload such as hypertension, edema, increased of jugular venous pressure, a cardiac gallop, or pulmonary crackles. Here again, these features do not tell us what is the level of kidney function.

Urinalysis

For this purpose, 10 mL of freshly voided urine should be centrifuged at 2500 rpm for 5 min. The supernatant should be tested chemically and the sediment placed on a slide using a Pasteur pipette.

The use of analytical 'dipsticks' and the conventional light microscopy are the standard tools for urine analysis that are easily available and very informative. Table 1.2 shows some features of the urinalysis that are useful in diagnosis. Fig. 1.1 shows muddy brown casts, which are seen in the urine sediment of patients with acute tubular necrosis, caused by sepsis and hypotension. Fig. 1.2 shows multiple uric acid crystals in a urine sediment, as might be seen in acute hyperuricemic nephropathy that could complicate the treatment of a rapidly growing lymphoma.

A 'benign' urinalysis (i.e. one without proteinuria or formed elements in the sediment) can also be informative inasmuch as it may suggest causes of renal failure outside the kidneys, such as urinary tract obstruction or pre-renal azotemia.

Table 1.2 Urinalysis features and associated conditions

Feature	Site of injury	Example
Proteinuria, 2+ or more	Glomerulus	Amyloidosis
Red cell cast	Glomerulus	Crescentic glomerulonephritis
Urine pH >6.5	Tubule	Renal tubular acidosis
Muddy brown casts	Tubule	Acute tubular necrosis
Uric acid crystals	Tubule	Hyperuricemic nephropathy

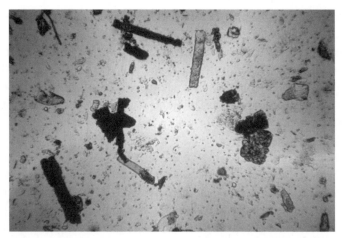

Fig. 1.1 A photomicrograph of muddy-brown casts seen in an unstained urine sediment. These are typical of acute tubular necrosis, as might be seen after use of radiocontrast dye or in a hypotensive septic patient.

Proteinuria

In health, urine contains little or no protein. An injury to the glomeruli or the tubules could result in proteinuria. The albumin contained in the serum, normally at 40 g/L concentration, traverses the glomerular filtration barrier in only scant amounts. Thus, the glomerular filtrate contains albumin, but only at a concentration of 3.5 mg/L (2). The majority of this filtered albumin is

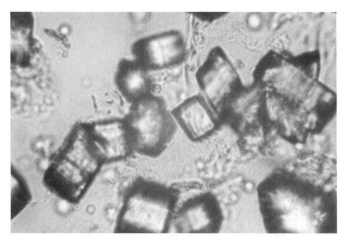

Fig. 1.2 Photomicrograph of uric acid crystals seen in an unstained urine sediment. The typical rhomboid shape is apparent. Such abundant uric acid crystals might be seen after cell lysis, as might occur subsequent to chemotherapy for Burkitt lymphoma.

reabsorbed by the tubules, by a receptor-dependent endocytosis, and normal urine contains no more than 30 mg of albumin per day, and no more than 100 mg of protein per day. That amount is below the detection limit of the standard dipstick test for proteinuria, and will also not be detected by the sulfosalicylic acid test. Microalbuminuria, which is urinary albumin between 30 and 300 mg per day, is important in the management of subjects with diabetes and nascent diabetic nephropathy, but has little importance in cancer patients.

With a normal GFR of 120 mL/min (2 mL/s or ~ 150 L/day), there are thus about 500 mg of albumin in the daily total glomerular ultrafiltrate. Urinary albumin in quantities greater than this suggests glomerular injury. Alterations in the charge and the pore-size characteristics of the glomeruli may permit greater amounts of serum protein to traverse the glomeruli, including albumin as well as globulins. But globulins, specifically light chains, may reach the urinary space without the requirement for a change in the glomerular filtration barrier. An analysis of urinary protein by use of electrophoresis will differentiate these circumstances (Fig. 1.3). Albuminuria greater than 3 g per day may result from the nephrotic syndrome, whereas light chain proteinuria indicates a paraproteinemia. These are discussed in Chapters 2 and 5, respectively.

The quantification of proteinuria has historically been made by urinalysis followed by 24-hour urine collections. The use of a single, 'spot' urine specimen to assess proteinuria is well established as a reliable way to quantify urine protein (3). This test yields a ratio that is closely correlated to the 24-hour urine protein. A urine protein-to-creatinine ratio of less than 0.1 is normal, i.e. shows no excess urinary protein, while a ratio of 2 g/g suggests nephrotic range proteinuria, i.e. greater than 3 g of urinary protein excreted per day.

Glomerular filtration rate

Clinical use of the serum creatinine concentration for assessment of the kidney function is over 75 years old (4). Its elevation beyond 3 mg/dL (~250 μmol/L) was an acknowledged correlate of uremia. By 1954, the elevation of the serum creatinine to 2 mg/dL (180 μmol/L) or more was deemed abnormal (5). Since creatinine is freely filtered by the glomeruli, and because its tubular secretion is quantitatively a lot less than its filtration, its clearance from the body approximates the actual GFR (Fig. 1.4). It varies inversely with GFR. Twelve- or 24-hour urine collections are used for the calculation of the creatinine clearance, in mL/min, using the clearance formula, clearance = U × V/S. In this equation, U is the urinary creatinine, V is the urinary volume per minute, and S is the serum creatinine. Mass units or Système international (SI) units can be

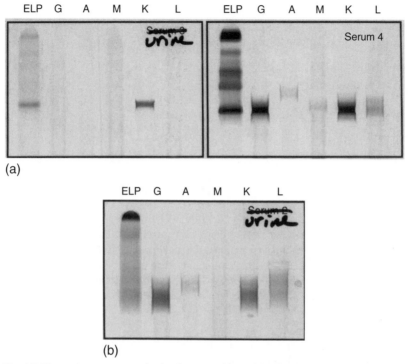

Fig. 1.3 These show serum and urine immunoelectrophoretic patterns. Fig. 1.3a shows the serum and urine immunoelectrophoretic pattern in a subject with an IgG kappa paraproteinuria. The right panel shows the dense band of the monoclonal IgG paraprotein in the serum. The left panel shows the corresponding dense band of the free monoclonal kappa chains in the urine. Fig. 1.3b shows the urine immunoelectrophoresis in a subject with non-selective proteinuria. Albumin and globulin are present and there is no monoclonal band. These images were provided by Dr. Carl Becker, Medical College of Wisconsin, Milwaukee, Wisconsin, USA.

used, as long as they are the same in the numerator and denominator. A timed urine collection begins at a specified time, at which the voided urine is discarded. All of the subsequent voided urine is collected, up to and including the ending time of the collection. A simultaneous blood sample is taken for serum creatinine. The amount of creatinine excreted is directly proportional to muscle mass because creatinine is a non-enzymatic breakdown product of the muscle creatine. The amount of creatinine excreted in 24 h provides an indication of the completeness of the urine collection, it being 15–20 mg/kg body weight in women and 20–25 mg/kg in men. These normal values might be less in a cancer patient who has lost muscle mass. Such a patient might have a lower than expected serum creatinine level, yet have a normal, or even reduced

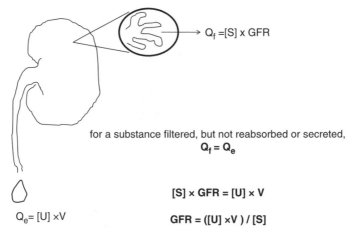

$$Q_f = [S] \times GFR$$

for a substance filtered, but not reabsorbed or secreted,

$$Q_f = Q_e$$

$$Q_e = [U] \times V$$

$$[S] \times GFR = [U] \times V$$

$$GFR = ([U] \times V) / [S]$$

Fig. 1.4 A schematic representation of the clearance concept. For a substance that is filtered but not re-absorbed or secreted, the quantity filtered (Qf) will equal the quantity excreted (Qe). The serum concentration of that substance [S] times the glomerular filtration rate (GFR) will equal Qf. The quantity excreted will equal the urinary concentration of the substance [U] times the urinary volume (V). Thus, GFR = ($U \times V$)S.

GFR. This is shown by the case for this chapter, in which the 24-hour urine creatinine was only 10 mg/kg, a value which shows a low creatinine production. Her initial serum creatinine was near the normal range for the hospital laboratory but her GFR was very much reduced.

The studies of Rehberg (6) established the correlation of creatinine clearance to the glomerular filtration rate (GFR). Further studies confirmed the close correlation of creatinine clearance to the GFR, the latter being measured by inulin clearance (7) (Fig. 1.5). This correlation of creatinine clearance to the GFR depends on a steady state of creatinine production, its complete glomerular filtration, and a lack of significant tubular secretion of creatinine. Inulin clearance is a reliable, albeit a cumbersome method for the calculation of the GFR, because inulin, a 5000 dalton polysaccharide, is filtered at the glomeruli, but not reabsorbed or secreted by the tubules. No matter what the substance used, clearance calculations cannot be relied on when subjects are not in a steady state, as might occur with rapidly changing renal function. Abrupt increases in creatinine production, as in rhabdomyolysis, could cause the serum creatinine to rise before the kidneys were damaged by the myoglobinuria, which would invalidate the measured clearance. Certain drugs, including trimethoprim and cimetidine, block creatinine secretion, thus raising the serum creatinine level by about 20 to 25% without affecting the glomerular creatinine clearance.

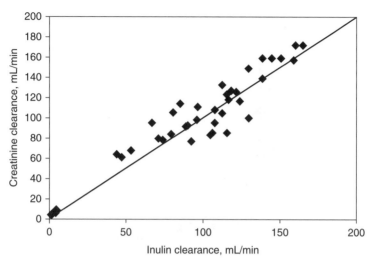

Fig. 1.5 This shows the excellent correlation between endogenous creatinine clearance and inulin clearance, the data points being derived from the studies of Steinitz and Jürkand (7). The line of identity is drawn.

A good correlation exists between the GFR and the average of the creatinine and urea clearances (8). The urea clearance is normally less than the GFR, because of the tubular reabsorption of urea. The creatinine clearance is a bit higher than the GFR, because of tubular secretion of creatinine. The calculation of the urea clearance uses the familiar $U \times V/S$ formula, where U is the urinary concentration of urea nitrogen, V is the urinary volume per minute, and S is the blood urea nitrogen (BUN). Mass units or Système international (SI) units can be used, as long as they are the same in the numerator and denominator.

Of more immediate use is the correlation of serum creatinine to creatinine clearance. This inverse relationship is predictable based on the clearance equation, but like all inverse relationships, it is not intuitive for easy clinical use. When the serum creatinine rises from 1–2 mg/dL, one has lost 50% of the normal GFR, which is more than the loss of function than when the serum creatinine rises from 2–10 mg/dL.

The correlation of serum (or plasma) creatinine to the GFR is imperfect. Recent studies show that this correlation is particularly imprecise in the GFR range of 60–20 mL/min (Fig. 1.6). Some authors state that the serum creatinine level might be 1.5 mg/dL for a GFR of 60 mL/min and also be at this level for a GFR of 40 mL/min. In practice, this imprecision is an inter-subject rather than an intra-subject problem. Thus, if the serum creatinine is 1.5 mg/dL at a GFR of 60 mL/min, a further decline in the GFR to 40 mL/min is

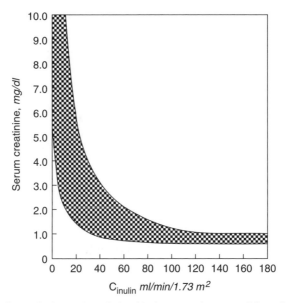

Fig. 1.6 This shows the imprecise relationship between the serum (plasma) creatinine and the simultaneously measured inulin clearance. These cross-sectional data show that at an inulin clearance of 60 mL/min, for instance, the serum creatinine could be in the normal range, at 1 mg/dL, or it could be above that, at 1.5 mg/dL. But, importantly, this cross-sectional variability does not mean that the serum creatinine will remain deceptively stable in a subject whose kidney function declines. Thus, serial measurements of the simple serum creatinine level retain their utility in an individual. From Ovadia Shemesh, Helen Golbetz , Joseph P Kriss and Bryan D Myers (1985). Limitations of creatinine as a filtration marker in glomerulopathic patients. *Kidney International*, **28**:830-8. Reprinted by permission from Macmillan Publishers Ltd.

accompanied by an increase in the serum creatinine level, perhaps to 2 mg/dL. Thus, serial monitoring of the serum creatinine or the derivative values, such as the 100/serum creatinine quotient, remain valid in clinical patient care such as in a cancer patient treated repetitively with potential nephrotoxins such as cis-platinum, ifosfamide, or amphotericin.

There are potential problems with the method of testing for creatinine. Ketones could cause a modest increase in the creatinine level as tested by the picric acid assay, the so-called Jaffé reaction. There is also an enzymatic assay for creatinine, with creatininase, creatinase, sarcosine oxidase, and an imine dye colorimetric endpoint (Roche®). The enzymatic assays for serum creatinine using the Ektachem analyzer may be falsely elevated in the presence of flucytosine (9). There has been much recent discussion of the method for creatinine measurement. The 'gold standard' is the isotope dilution mass spectrometry method (IDMS). Other methods can be calibrated or adjusted to yield values consistent with this method. The method of testing the serum creatinine affects the form of the MDRD equation. Even with use of the most precise method, some analytical and biological variability remains, such that formula-based measurements of the GFR may yield values that differ by 10–15 mL/min from the true value (10). In the case at the beginning of this chapter, there was a much greater difference between the formula-based estimate of the GFR and the measured kidney function because of the cancer -related loss of muscle mass.

Because the serum level of creatinine depends on its constant release from the creatine in the muscle, and because children have a lesser muscle mass compared to adults, the expected normal serum creatinine ranges are lower in children as compared to adults. These are shown in Fig. 1.7.

Conversion of the serum creatinine to its reciprocal, 1/serum creatinine, converts a non-linear indicator of the GFR to a linear one. Multiplication of 1/serum creatinine times 100 yields a number that approximates the GFR in absolute numbers, when the serum creatinine is expressed in mg/dL. This is valid for adults, but not for children, because their lesser absolute value of serum creatinine does not correspond to a higher-than-adult GFR. When the serum creatinine is expressed in μmol/L, one can create a similar quotient, as 1000/serum creatinine. One can graph the 100/serum creatinine quotient vs. time to gauge the pace of decline of kidney function, to test whether an intervention has changed the course of renal failure, or to predict the occurrence and timing of an end-stage renal disease, i.e. terminal renal failure. Fig. 1.8 shows the progressive loss of kidney function as 100/s creatinine vs. time in a patient who was treated with cis-platinum and ifosfamide, a combination that can be particularly nephrotoxic.

The correlation of the level of function with symptoms and signs is a useful concept. It is unlikely, for instance, that a patient with a serum creatinine of

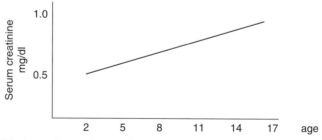

Fig. 1.7 This shows the usual range for the serum or plasma creatinine levels in mg/dL, depending on age, in children. A progressive increase is seen in the value corresponding to normal kidney function, which is the consequence of increasing muscle mass with age (multiply values by 88 for S.I. units).

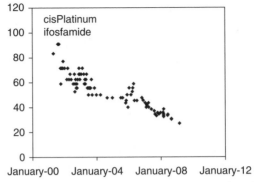

Fig. 1.8 The evolution of kidney function in a recent case, as a function of time. This is graphed as 100/serum creatinine, latter in mg/dl, vs time. The steady decline of kidney function is shown, since the use of cisplatinum and ifosfamide. No other cause for chronic renal failure has been found in this case.

1.5 mg/dL would be anemic because of an impaired kidney function. So, too, would it be very unlikely for a patient with a serum creatinine of 1.5 mg/dL to have itching related to an impaired kidney function. Fig. 1.9 shows the approximate correspondence of symptoms and signs to the serum creatinine level and to the approximate corresponding GFR. These levels and their correlations are valid for adults.

A number of formulas have been created to estimate the GFR without using a urine collection. The best known are the Cockcroft–Gault and the MDRD formulas in adults, and the Schwartz formula in children (11–13) (Table 1.3). The correlations of these formulas with the 'gold-standard' measurements of the GFR are very good. None of these formulas are valid in acute renal failure, however.

For the purposes of clinical follow-up, the simple serum creatinine or its reciprocal are important and useful indicators of the GFR. Formula-derived estimates of the GFR, such as the Cockcroft–Gault formula or the MDRD formula, are also useful. There are websites that permit the rapid calculation of the formula-based GFR estimates, such as www.hdcn.com. It is not established what is the best way to adjust drug doses for the actual GFR. In practice, the Cockcroft–Gault formula is often used to guide dose adjustments. The Food and Drug Administration (FDA) uses this formula to guide drug dosing. The Cockcroft–Gault formula is more immediately useful than the MDRD formula, because it can be quickly derived on a pocket calculator. Besides, there are over 30 years of experience with the Cockcroft–Gault formula and it is useful and accurate in cancer patients, for instance in the dose adjustment of carboplatin (14). The Wright formula has been developed for use in cancer patients (15). It is GFR = {[6580 – (38*age)] *BSA* [1–(0.168*0 if male)]}/S

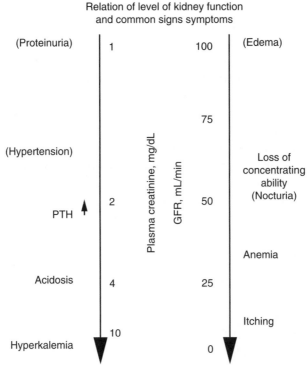

Fig. 1.9 Scheme of the relationship between the level of kidney function and common signs and symptoms. Features that may be absent are in parentheses. Kidney function is shown as the serum, or plasma, creatinine, in mg/dL, and as the approximate corresponding glomerular filtration rate in mL/min (GFR). The downward directed arrows display the progressive nature of many kidney diseases.

creat, in μmol/L. This formula requires knowledge of the body surface area (BSA) and is thus not easy to use. Statistical analysis suggests that the MDRD formula may have a slight advantage over the Cockcroft–Gault formula for adjusting drug dosages according to the GFR, but this analysis did not use patient outcome data (16).

Table 1.3 Equations to estimate the glomerular filtration rate (GFR)

Formula name	Formula
Cockcroft-Gault creatinine clearance	[(140-age)(wt, kg)]/[72*Screat(mg/dl)] times 0.85 in women
MDRD GFR	175*(Screat(mg/dl) $^{(-1.154)}$)*(age, years) $^{(-0.203)}$ times 1.21 for blacks times 0.742 for women
Schwartz GFR/1.73 m^2	kL/serum creatinine(mg/dl), when L is body length in cm and k is 0.7 in teenage boys and 0.55 in children and teenage girls

Note: MDRD expressed for serum creatinine measurement made by or traceable to IDMS method

The perceived shortcomings of the use of serum creatinine or the formula-dependent ways of estimating the GFR have prompted the study of alternative markers of the GFR. In recent years, cystatin C, a 13 kD endogenous protease inhibitor, has been studied as such a marker. There may indeed be a modest gain in sensitivity of detection for renal insufficiency when using cystatin C levels compared to those of creatinine (17–18). The elevation of serum cystatin C levels may begin at lesser degrees of reduction in the GFR than is the case for serum creatinine. But the measurement of cystatin C is four times as expensive as measuring serum (or plasma) creatinine. Thus, its greater sensitivity may not be cost beneficial. Finally, there are reports that the cystatin C levels may be increased in cancer patients in the presence of normal creatinine clearance (19). Thus, cystatin C measurements are not recommended for the assessment of kidney function in cancer patients.

Tubular function

The normal tubules, proximal and distal, act to reabsorb much of the glomerular filtrate, to achieve electrolyte and acid-base balance, and to adjust water excretion to maintain body tonicity. Abnormalities of the tubular function may be evident as changes in tubular excretion of normally reabsorbed substances, abnormalities of urine pH or acid excretion, or abnormalities of body tonicity.

Tests of β-2-microglobulin levels in blood or urine may be useful. This protein of 12 kD size, is freely filtered by the glomeruli, then almost completely reabsorbed by the proximal tubules (20). Its normal serum concentration is 1–2 mg/L, which may be raised in patients with multiple myeloma, without there being a change in kidney function. It is not surprising that this may occur because β-2-microgobulin is a component of the class I major HLA complex on the surface of all nucleated cells. The increased numbers of the malignant plasma cells would be directly responsible for higher blood levels of β-2-microglobulin. Increased urinary β-2-microglobulin, over its expected amount of less than 500 mg/24 h, may occur in a variety of disorders including aminoglycoside, cis-platinum, or radiocontrast nephrotoxicity, as well as, interstitial nephritis. This could occur because of the failure of tubular reabsorptive function.

The evaluation of the excretion of various *cations and anions* may be helpful in the evaluation and management of subjects with altered kidney function (3).

In health, 99% of the filtered *sodium* is reabsorbed by the tubules, such that the normal fractional excretion of sodium (FENa) is 0.01 or 1%, when expressed as a percentage. The FENa is the clearance of sodium divided by that of creatinine, which may also be written as $[(UNa \times Screat)/(Ucreat \times SNa)]$. This number is multiplied times 100 to express it as a percentage. The FENa rises in chronic renal failure, such that the lesser nephron numbers can proportionally excrete more sodium, thus tending the body towards sodium balance. In the steady state, in chronic renal failure, the FENa, as a percentage, approximates the serum creatinine, in mg/dL.

The FENa also rises in acute renal failure, because the damaged tubular epithelium reabsorbs less of the filtered sodium. The FENa is below its expected value when there is under-perfusion of the kidneys, so-called pre-renal azotemia. This occurs because under-perfusion of the kidneys, as might occur in hemorrhage, is accompanied by activation of sodium-conserving mechanisms, including renal nerves and the renin-angiotensin system.

A significant adjunct to the calculation of the fractional excretion of sodium is the calculation of the fractional excretion of urea (21). Both creatinine and urea are filtered at the glomeruli, but urea is also reabsorbed in the distal nephron, in part to play a role in establishing a medullary concentrating gradient for the reabsorption of water. Thus, the normal urea clearance is only about 60 mL/min, in contrast to that of creatinine, which is 100 mL/min or more. The fractional excretion of urea is thus normally about 0.6, or 60%. It is calculated as $[(Urine\ urea\ nitrogen \times Screat)/(Ucreat \times BUN)]$, which is multiplied times 100 for its expression as a percentage. In states of hypotension or volume depletion, the reduction in urinary flow and the release of vasopressin cause enhanced urea reabsorption, thus reducing its fractional excretion. When the FEurea is 35% or lower, there is evidence of pre-renal azotemia. The calculation of the FEurea is useful if a patient is using diuretics, because diuretics will raise the FENa but they will not raise the FEurea.

Potassium is also freely filtered by the glomeruli, but in effect only 90% reabsorbed by the tubules. Thus in health, the FEK as a percentage is about 10%.

The FEK rises in chronic renal failure, such that its value, in percent, approximates 10 times the serum creatinine in mg/dL. In a subject with hyperkalemia caused by kidney diseases or by drugs, such as ACE inhibitors or non-steroidal anti-inflammatory agents, the FEK would be lower than expected.

In the assessment of potassium excretion, the transtubular potassium gradient (TTKG) has been used. This is the potassium (K) clearance divided by the osmolar clearance, and gives an insight into the activity of the distal nephron, where K excretion takes place (22). There are, however, less data for the TTKG than there are for the FEK, and it is less easily understood.

Calcium excretion depends on its dietary intake, filtration of its diffusable fraction, the action of parathyroid hormone (PTH), and the sodium balance. In health, the total daily urinary calcium excretion should not exceed 4 mg/kg in men and 3 mg/kg in women. The normal fractional excretion of calcium, is 0.02 and that calculation should use the diffusable, or the ionizable calcium, in the formula [(UCa × Screat)/(Ucreat × SCa)] × 100. With moderate renal insufficiency, the FECa falls below 0.02 (or 2%, when expressed as a percentage) and does not rise above that level until the GFR is 10 mL/min or less (23). In hypercalcemia of malignancy, the FECa could be higher than normal because of a high filtered load, or, if mediated by PTH-related-peptide, could be lower (24). In a series of 31 subjects with solid cancers and hypercalcemia, 29 had low urinary calcium excretion, suggesting the role of a PTH-like substance in humoral hypercalcemia of malignancy (25).

The urinary excretion of *phosphorus*, as phosphate, is also dependent on its dietary intake, and also on parathyroid hormone. The fractional excretion of phosphorus is 15% in normal subjects, and rises in a linear fashion to over 50% in severe renal failure, with a GFR of 10 mL/min or less (23). Both the PTH and the PTH-related peptide will cause phosphaturia, i.e. elevation of the fractional excretion of phosphorus. In the rare syndrome of oncogenic osteomalacia, hyperphosphaturia, hypophosphatemia, and osteomalacia may occur in association with mesenchymal tumors and a humoral factor, now identified as the fibroblast growth factor 23 (26). This syndrome, and the tubular phosphate leak, should resolve on resection of the tumor. Hypophosphatemia, and a higher than normal fractional excretion of phosphate, was also reported as a side effect of imatinib therapy (27).

Urinary acidification

The excretion of the fixed acid of daily metabolism is achieved by tubular reclamation of filtered bicarbonate, by ammoniagenesis, and by excretion of titratable acid. The achievement of an acidic urine pH in itself is only a minor player in urinary acidification, given that the [H+] in urine is 100 micro-equivalents at a pH = 4. The urine ammonium excretion, NH4+, which is in milli-equivalents per liter, may be estimated by use of the urine anion gap, UNa + UK − UCl, which will have a greater negative value with greater amounts of urinary NH4+ (28). As a consequence of renal insufficiency per se, acidosis does not occur until the GFR is reduced to 25% of normal, i.e. less than 30 mL/min. That is because the renal tubular epithelium can increase ammoniagenesis fourfold. A greater than fourfold reduction in the renal tubular mass is thus required before there would be acidosis resulting from insufficient overall renal function. In a subject with acidosis, i.e. serum bicarbonate of 15 mmol/L or less, a urine pH greater than 6 would suggest a tubular acidification defect, as would a urine anion gap having a positive value.

Urinary concentrating ability

The maintenance of body tonicity, expressed as osmolarity, is ensured by the sensation of thirst and the regulation of water excretion. In health, urinary osmolarity may vary from 50 to 1000 mOsm/L, depending on the requirements for water excretion or water conservation by the kidneys. The urinary osmolarity can be measured by freezing point depression, or it can be estimated using the urinary specific gravity. The absolute value of the hundredths and the thousandths digit of the specific gravity may be multiplied 30 times as an estimate of a urinary osmolarity. For instance, a urinary specific gravity of 1.015 corresponds to an osmolarity of 450 mOsm/L.

Hyponatremia may occur as a manifestation of cancer (see Chapter 3). When that is mediated by an inappropriate and an unregulated secretion of vasopressin (anti-diuretic hormone), the urine osmolarity is inappropriately elevated, often higher than the osmolarity of the serum. It is not necessary to measure the vasopressin levels to make the diagnosis of the syndrome of inappropriate anti-diuretic hormone secretion (SIADH). That is because most cases of hyponatremia depend on increased vasopressin levels. Their confirmation does not indicate the cause of the hyponatremia. The diagnosis of the SIADH, in particular, depends on the clinical exclusion of other causes of excess vasopressin. Mere extra-cellular volume depletion may cause a stimulation of vasopressin secretion and thereby cause water retention with subsequent hyponatremia. Such a problem may be identified by a urine sodium concentration of less than 30 mmol/L (29).

References

1 McGee S, Abernethy WB, Simel DL (1999). The rational clinical examination. Is this patient hypovolemic? *J Am Med Assoc* **281**: 1022–9.

2 Norden AG, Lapsley M, Lee PJ, et al. (2001). Glomerular protein sieving and implications for renal failure in Fanconi syndrome. *Kidney Int* **60**: 1885–92.

3 Cohen EP, Lemann J (1991). The role of the laboratory in evaluation of kidney function. *Clin Chem* **37**: 785–96.

4 Patch FS and Rabinowitch IM (1929). Urea and creatinine contents of the blood in renal disease. *J Am Med Assoc* **90**: 1092–5.

5 Fishberg AM (1954). Azotemia. In: Hypertension and nephritis (ed. AM Fishberg), p. 60. Lea & Febiger, Philadelphia.

6 Rehberg PB (1926). Studies on kidney function. The rate of filtration and reabsorption in the human kidney. *Biochem J* **20**: 447–60.

7 Steinitz K, Jürkand H (1940). The determination of the glomerular filtration by the endogenous creatinine clearance. *J Clin Invest* **19**: 285–98.

8 Lavender S, Hilton PJ, Jones NF (1969). The measurement of glomerular filtration-rate in renal disease. *Lancet* **2**: 1216–18.

9 Mitchell EK (1984). Flucytosine and false elevation of serum creatinine level. *Ann Intern Med* **101**: 278.

10 Delanaye P, Cohen EP (2008) Formula-based estimates of the GFR: equations variable and uncertain. *Nephron Clin Pract* **110**: c48–c54.

11 Cockcroft DW, Gault, MH (1976). Prediction of creatinine clearance from serum creatinine. *Nephron* **16**: 31–41.

12 Levey AS, Bosch JP, Breyer Lewis J, Greene T, Rogers N, Roth D (1999). A more accurate method to estimate glomerular filtration rate from serum creatinine: A new prediction equation. *Ann Intern Med* **130**: 461–70.

13 Springate JE, Christensen SL, and Feld LG (1992). Serum creatinine level and renal function in children. *Am J Dis Child* **146**: 1232–5.

14 Okamoto H, Nagatomo A, Kuniton H, et al. (1998). Prediction of carboplatin clearance calculated by patient characteristics or 24-hour creatinine clearance: a comparison of the performance of three formulae. *Cancer Chemoth Pharmacol* **42**: 307–12.

15 Wright JG, Boddy AV, Highley M, et al. (2001). Estimation of glomerular filtration rate in cancer patients. *Brit J Cancer* **84**: 452–9.

16 Stevens LA, Nolin TD, Richardson MM, et al. (2009). Comparison of drug dosing recommendations based on measured GFR and kidney function estimating equations. *Am J Kidney Dis* **54**: 33–42.

17 Coll E, Botey A, Alvarez L, et al. (2000). Serum cystatin C as a new marker for noninvasive estimation of glomerular filtration rate and as a marker for early renal impairment. *Am J Kidney Dis* **36**: 29–34.

18 Page, MK, Bukki J, Luppa P, Neumeier D (2000). Clinical value of cystatin C determination. *Clin Chim Acta* **297**: 67–72.

19 Nakai K, Kikuchi M, Fujimoto K, et al (2008). Serum levels of cystatin C in patients with malignancy. *Clin Exper Nephrol* **12**: 132–9.

20 Schardijn GH, Statius van Eps, LW (1987). Beta 2-microglobulin: its significance in the evaluation of renal function. *Kidney Int* **32**: 635–41.

21 Carvounis CP, Nisar S, Guro-Razuman S (2002). Significance of the fractional excretion of urea in the differential diagnosis of acute renal failure. *Kidney Int* **62**: 2223–9.

22 Ethier JH, Kamel KS, Magner PO, Lemann J, Halperin ML (1990). The transtubular potassium concentration in patients with hypokalemia and hyperkalemia. *Am J Kidney Dis* **15**: 309–15.

23 Popovtzer MM, Schainuck LI, Massry SG, Kleeman CR (1970). Divalent ion excretion in chronic kidney disease: relation to degree of renal insufficiency. *Clin Sci* **38**: 297–307.

24 Syed MA, Horwitz MJ, Tedesco MB, Garcia-Ocana W, Wisniewski SR, Stewart AF (2001). Parathyroid hormone-related protein-(1–36) stimulates renal tubular calcium reabsorption in normal human volunteers: implications for the pathogenesis of humoral hypercalcemia of malignancy. *J Clin Endocrinol Metab* **86**: 1525–31.

25 Ralston SH, Fogelman I, Gardner MD, Dryburgh FJ, Cowan RA, Boyle IT (1984). Hypercalcaemia of malignancy: evidence for a nonparathyroid humoral agent with an effect on renal tubular handling of calcium. *Clin Sci* **66**: 187–91.

26 Fukumoto S, Yamashita T (2002). Fibroblast growth factor 23 is the phosphaturic factor in tumor-induced osteomalacia and may be phosphotonin. *Curr Opin Nephrol Hypertens* **11**: 385–9.

27 Berman E, Nicolaides M, Maki RG, et al. (2006). Altered bone and mineral metabolism in patients receiving imatinib mesylate. *N Engl J Med* **354**: 2006–13.

28 Batlle DC, Hizon M, Cohen E, Gutterman C, Gupta R (1988). The use of the urinary anion gap in the diagnosis of hyperchloremic metabolic acidosis. *N Engl J Med* **318**: 594–9.

29 Chung HM, Kluge R, Schrier RW, Anderson RJ (1987). Clinical assessment of extracellular fluid volume in hyponatremia. *Am J Med* **83**, 905–8.

Chapter 2

Fluid and electrolyte disorders associated with cancer

Ilya G. Glezerman and Sheron Latcha

Calcium disorders

Hypercalcemia

Case report

A 54-year-old female with history of HTLV-1 associated T-cell lymphoma presented to the emergency room with lethargy, confusion, and poor oral intake. Two weeks prior to presentation patient was noted to have calcium level of 3.05 (2.12–2.62) mmol/L. Positron emission tomography scan obtained at that time revealed multiple skeletal sites of disease. She received pamidronate 60 mg intravenously (IV) and her serum calcium normalized. In the emergency room she had normal vital signs, was in no acute distress and able to void 240 mL of clear urine. The laboratory investigation revealed a calcium level of 4.87 mmol/L; creatinine 176.8 (53.04–114.92) μmol/L; albumin 43 (40 – 52) gm/L; parathyroid hormone (PTH) 6 (12 – 65) ng/L; parathyroid hormone related peptide (PTHrP) <1.5 (≤4.7) ng/L; 25-hydroxyvitamin D (25(OH) Vit D) 18.4 (22.5–93.8) nmol/L and 1,25-dihydroxyvitamin D (1,25(OH)$_2$ Vit D) 18.2 (57.2–174.2) pmol/L. Patient was started on aggressive hydration and received another dose of pamidronate 60 mg IV. Her calcium level returned to normal on day 2 of hospitalization. However, on day 8 she was noted to have worsening hypercalcemia and received another dose of pamidronate 60 mg IV. Thereafter, patient required monthly administration of IV bisphosphonate to maintain normocalcemia. She died three months later from progression of disease.

Hypercalcemia of malignancy (HCM) is a serious complication of cancer and carries a poor prognosis. It occurs in 20–30% of patients with malignancies at some point during their illness (1). Patients with renal cell cancer have highest incidence of severe HCM (>3 mmol/L) followed by non small cell lung cancer, multiple myeloma, leukemia, and breast cancer (2). In 126 consecutive patients with HCM 34% had squamous lung tumors, 17% breast cancer, 12% genitourinary malignancies, 11% lung cancer other then squamous, 8% unknown primary adenocarcinoma, and 6% in multiple myeloma. Patients with lymphoma, head and neck malignancies, liver cancer, and pancreatic cancer each represented less then 5% of the total (3). HCM is rare in colorectal and prostate cancer (4). The survival in patients with HCM is poor, with a median life expectancy of 29–35 days (4). It has not changed significantly because median survival is 64 days in patients with HCM on bisphosphonate therapy (5).

HCM affects nervous, gastrointestinal, cardiovascular, and renal systems. The symptoms usually are non-specific and may be confused with manifestations of progression of disease or side effects of chemotherapy. Patients commonly develop thirst, polyuria, nausea, anorexia, constipation as well as drowsiness and lethargy. Electrocardiogram may show shortened QTc interval but significant rhythm disturbances are rare (6). In the kidneys HCM impairs urinary concentrating ability via its action on the calcium sensing receptor (CaSR). High serum calcium level activates the CaSR leading to decreased transport of sodium chloride in the thick portion of the loop of Henle causing impairment of the countercurrent mechanism and reduced concentrating ability. Additionally, activation of the CaSR blunts the response to antidiuretic hormone in the collecting ducts. The resulting diuresis and volume contraction may lead to acute decrease in glomerular filtration rate (GFR), acute renal insufficiency and a further decrease in calcium excretion. High calcium may also directly affect GFR via renal smooth muscle cell vasoconstriction (7).

Three distinct pathophysiologic mechanisms of HCM have been described to date. First is replacement of normal bone structure by metastatic malignant cells. The bone matrix is degraded due to the release of various cytokines such as interleukin-1, interleukin-6 and tumor necrosis factor alpha which in turn stimulate osteoclastic activity. This process is common in breast cancer and multiple myeloma. The second mechanism is also known as humoral hypercalcemia of malignancy and is caused by a release of PTHrP by malignant cells. PTHrP is a peptide with substantial homology to a biologically active portion of PTH. It binds to the PTH receptor in kidney and bone and has similar effects such as increased bone resorption, calcium reabsorption and phosphate excretion in kidney and $1,25(OH)_2$ Vit D synthesis. In the bone PTHrP stimulates secretion of receptor activator nuclear factor-κ ligand (RANKL) by osteoblasts which in turn activated osteoclast precursors leading to bone resorption and elevated extracellular calcium levels (8). This mechanism occurs in squamous cell carcinoma of the lung, head and neck, and renal cell cancers as well as HTLV associated lymphoproliferative disorders. Interestingly, in our case report metastatic bone disease was presumed to be the cause of HCM given that the PTHrP level was low. Finally, all types of lymphoma cells have been described to secrete $1,25(OH)_2$ Vit D leading to the increased intestinal absorption of calcium and the development of HCM (9). A few rare cases of ectopic

PTH producing tumors have been described in the literature. It also should be noted that primary hyperparathyroidism can occur in patients with cancer and hypercalcemia. In one series eight out of 133 patients were found to have primary hyperparathyroidism (1).

Since a significant portion of the circulating calcium is bound to serum albumin hypoalbuminemia may cause decrease in serum calcium level without affecting the concentration of biologically active ionized calcium fraction. While methods to calculate 'corrected' calcium levels exist they are not precise and it may be beneficial to measure the ionized calcium level (10). Additionally, in rare cases of multiple myeloma, calcium binding immunoglobulins are produced resulting in pseudohypercalcemia. These patients have no symptoms of hypercalcemia and have normal ionized calcium levels (1). In cancer patients with hypercalcemia, a PTH level should be obtained to test for primary hyperparathyroidism. Measurement of PTHrP is not always necessary as diagnosis of HCM can be made on clinical grounds once primary hyperthyroidism is excluded via suppressed PTH level. Bone imaging studies may be obtained to assess the skeletal burden of disease. $1,25(OH)_2$ Vit D levels should be obtained in patients with lymphoma and hypercalcemia. Finally, 25(OH)-Vit D measurement may be helpful to determine vitamin D intoxication (11).

The therapeutic approach to the hypercalcemia is usually two-pronged. Initially, treatment is geared towards acutely reducing the calcium level to improve the symptoms. However, this needs to be followed by therapy directed at underlying cancer to achieve a durable effect. Since most patients with HCM are volume depleted the first step is restoration of intravascular volume with normal saline to improve GFR and calcium excretion. The use of loop diuretics is somewhat controversial as they may worsen volume depletion and hypercalcemia (12). Nonetheless, loop diuretics have a calciuretic effect in the loop of Henle and can be used once intravascular volume is restored (1, 9).

Treatment with intravenous bisphosphonates has become a cornerstone of management of HCM. Bisphosphonates act by inhibiting osteoclastic activity in the bones. Pamidronate and zoledronate are approved in the United States for treatment of HCM. Ibandronate is also available but not approved for HCM use. The bisphosphonate therapy should be initiated as soon as HCM has been discovered since the onset of action of these agents does not occur until 2–4 days after initial dose and the calcium nadir occurs in 4–7 days. Between 60% and 90% of patients achieve normocalcemia and this effect lasts one to three weeks (1). While pamidronate has been associated with nephrotic syndrome and collapsing focal segmental glomerulosclerosis after prolonged use (13) it appears to be safe in patients with chronic kidney disease and hypercalcemia (14).

Zoledronate on the other hand has been associated with toxic acute tubular necrosis. Ibandronte has not been associated with renal toxicity presumably due to its protein binding and the shorter renal half-life of this drug (13). The American Society of Oncology guidelines recommend that for patients with mild to moderate renal impairment (creatinine clearance (CrCl) 30–60 mL/min), the dose of zoledronate is reduced; the pamidronate dose does not require adjustment. For patients with severe renal impairment (CrCl<30 mL/min) zoledronate is contraindicated and pamidronate infusion time should increase to 4–6 hr with a reduction in dose. Although bisphosphonates should be withheld should the patients develop otherwise unexplained increase in serum creatinine (SCr), they may be re-challenged once SCr returns to within 10% of the pre-treatment baseline (13).

Although gallium, calcitonin, and mitramycin have been used in treatment of HCM in the past, they have all been abandoned in favor of bisphosphonates, either due to their overall transient effect on HCM or their unfavorable toxicity profile. Corticosteroids are still used when HCM is suspected to be due to $1,25(OH)_2$ Vit D production by lymphoma cells (1).

Novel therapies are being developed now for treatment of HCM. These are based on mechanisms of HCM described above. Denosumab, a fully humanized antibody directed against RANKL, has shown early and sustained decrease in bone resorption. Osteoprotegerin (OPG) is a tumor necrosis factor family member which binds RANKL and inhibits its activity. Recombinant OPG has been shown to be effective in murine models of PTHrP-dependent HCM. Humanized antibody against PTHrP has been effective in animal models of PTHrP-dependent HCM in achieving normocalcemia (9). Finally, cinacalcet, a CaSR agonist, has been used effectively in patients with parathyroid cancer and hypercalcemia whose HCM is due to PTH production. Cinacalcet binds to CaSR expressed in tumor cells and downregulates PTH synthesis leading to decrease in calcium levels (15).

In patients who cannot tolerate intravenous hydration due to congestive heart failure and in oliguric patients with evidence of acute kidney injury hemodialysis can be used successfully for treatment of hypercalcemia. The recommended dialysate calcium concentration is 1.25mmol/L. Using lower concentrations may result in overly rapid correction of ionized serum calcium leading to tetany and seizures (16).

Hypocalcemia

As with hypercalcemia, in hypocalcemia, knowing the serum albumin concentration can be important. It is best to measure ionized calcium concentration, as calculated 'corrected' levels of serum calcium are not always reliable (10).

Historically, the incidence of hypocalcemia has been reported to be 1.6% in unselected cancer patients and as high as 16% in patients with bone metastases (17). In a study of patients with bone metastases treated with zoledronate the incidence was as high as 38.8% (18). Since extracellular calcium is important in maintenance of normal function of muscles and nerves, symptoms of hypocalcemia are related to neuromuscular hyperexcitability. Patients may initially present with muscle twitching, spasms, tingling and numbness progressing to tetany, seizures, and cardiac dysrhythmias with prolonged QTc interval. In asymptomatic patients, signs of hyperexcitability can be elicited by the signs of Chvostek (tapping parotid gland over the facial nerve) or Trousseau (carpopedal spasm induced by inflation of blood pressure cuff to greater than the systolic blood pressure for three minutes) (19).

Osteoblastic metastatic bone disease has been long recognized as a major cause of hypocalcemia in cancer patients. Prostate cancer is the most common etiology followed by breast and lung malignancies. Calcium balance studies in these patients showed excessive accretion of calcium into the bone. Hypomagnesemia and hypophosphatemia are also associated with this condition, presumably due to sequestration of these ions into the bone as well. PTH levels may be inappropriately normal, possibly due to hypomagnesemia. Of note, correction of hypomagnesemia does not lead to improvement in hypocalcemia in this group of patients (17).

Tumor lysis syndrome (TLS) is another common cause of hypocalcemia in patients with malignancy treated with chemotherapy. It is more common in hematologic cancers but rarely may arise in solid tumors. It also causes hyperphosphatemia and is associated with precipitation of calcium phosphate in tissues which may explain the hypocalcemia (17, 20).

Hypomagnesemia can cause hypocalcemia by inducing functional hypoparathyroidism either by decreasing PTH secretion or increased tissue resistance to PTH. The incidence of combined hypomagnesemia and hypocalcemia in one series of cancer patients was 28% (21). Cisplatin is most commonly reported to cause hypomagnesemia resulting in hypocalcemia. Recently, Cetuximab has been associated with hypomagnesemia and hypocalcemia (22–3).

Hypocalcemia is one of major side effects of bisphosphonates. The incidence of hypocalcemia may vary depending on underlying disease. In one trial of patients with breast cancer treated with zoledronate, hypocalcemia was seen in 39% of patients versus 7% in the placebo arm (24). The onset of symptomatic hypocalcemia varies from a few days after initial treatment to several months after repeated infusion. Although patients may present with classic symptoms of hypocalcemia, commonly only lethargy, shakiness, and tingling are seen at presentation. Some patients remain asymptomatic despite marked hypocalcemia.

Vitamin D deficiency is common in cancer patients treated with bisphosphonates (25) and is a risk factor for hypocalcemia. Other risk factors for the development of hypocalcemia include hypoparathyroidism and hypomagnesemia. Concurrent administration of aminoglycoside antibiotics and interferon alfa also predispose to hypocalcemia via inhibition of osteoclastic activity by these agents. Finally, in patients with osteoblastic metastasis treated with bisphosphonates, hypocalcemia is more likely to occur via avid uptake of calcium in the bone (24).

Acquired hypoparathyroidism and hypocalcemia may develop in patients after thyroidectomy, parathyroidectomy, or neck dissection due to inadvertant removal or damage to parathyroid glands. The incidence of hypoparathyroidism after thyroidectomy ranges from 0.5% to 6.6%. The risk factors include the surgeon's experience, extent of resection, and nodal dissection. The risk is also greater in re-operations or when one or more parathyroid glands are not identified intraoperatively. Given that one parathyroid gland is sufficient to maintain normal calcium homeostasis, extensive damage must occur before development of hypoparathyroidism in these patients. Rarely, metastatic disease to the parathyroid glands or neck radiation can also result in hypocalcemia with low PTH levels (26).

Finally, Fanconi syndrome with generalized proximal tubular dysfunction may result in urinary calcium wasting and hypocalcemia as well as decreased synthesis of $1,25(OH)_2$ Vit D. Multiple myeloma and ifosfamide therapy are most commonly associated with Fanconi syndrome (27–8).

The treatment of hypocalcemia depends on severity and acuity of symptoms and underlying cause. Any medications associated with hypocalcemia should be discontinued. Acute symptomatic hypocalcemia should be treated with intravenous infusion of calcium gluconate. Based on clinical experience and expert recommendations, asymptomatic patients with corrected calcium of less than 1.9 mmol/L should be considered for intravenous therapy as they are at risk for the development of serious complications of hypocalcemia (19); however asymptomatic patients with TLS should not be treated, because calcium supplementation can precipitate malignant calcifications when there is hyperphosphatemia (20). In patients with hypocalcemia due to underlying hypomagnesemia, magnesium stores have to be restored before hypocalcemia may be corrected. Patients with milder asymptomatic hypocalcemia should receive oral calcium supplementation. Empiric vitamin D administration is also recommended, particularly in patients receiving bisphosphonate therapy. Pre-existing hypocalcemia, particularly in patients with osteoblastic metastases, should be treated prior to initiation of bisphosphonates (29). After normalization of calcium level, patients may be re-challenged with bisphosphonates with careful monitoring of electrolyte levels but recurrent hypocalcemia has been reported despite aggressive calcium and vitamin D supplementation (24).

Phosphate disorders

Hypophosphatemia

Close to 0.4% of hospitalized patients develop severe hypophosphatemia (<0.32 mmol/L) (30). Approximately 6% of hypophosphatemic patients have cancer (31). Even though severe hypophosphatemia is associated with significant risk of mortality, it commonly goes unrecognized and inappropriately treated (30).

Symptoms of hypophosphatemia generally occur at levels <0.32 mmol/L. Phosphorus is mostly an intracellular mineral and exists in organic phosphate compounds such as creatine phosphate, adenosine phosphate (ATP) and 2,3-diphosphoglycerate (2,3-DRG) and in the bone in inorganic hydroxyapatite. Reduced ATP and 2,3-DPG account for most symptoms of hypophosphatemia because ATP is the reservoir for cellular energy and 2,3-DPG influences oxygen delivery by hemoglobin. Myocardial dysfunction, respiratory failure, rhabdomyolysis, and hemolysis have been described in hypophosphatemic patients presumably due to ATP deficiency. Seizures, coma, severe neuropathy, and paresthesias have also been reported. Chronic phosphate deficiency results in proximal muscle weakness and bone pain (32).

Hypophosphatemia may be caused by decreased intestinal reabsorption, redistribution between extracellular and intracellular compartments, and increased renal excretion of phosphate. It is rare for decreased dietary intake to cause hypophosphatemia unless there is a concurrent intake of phosphate binders (33).

Hypophosphatemia due to redistribution of phosphorus is most commonly caused by respiratory alkalosis and refeeding syndrome (RFS). Respiratory alkalosis enhances phosphorus uptake by muscle. This is caused by stimulation of glycolysis and increased production of sugar phosphates leading to intracellular phosphate entry. Hypophosphatemia is associated with conditions leading to respiratory alkalosis such as sepsis, heat stroke, and liver disease (33). RFS is acute development of electrolyte deficiencies in malnourished patients upon administration of either enteral or intravenous nutrition. It is caused by a shift of phosphorus due to increased intracellular requirements during tissue anabolism. Cancer patients are at risk for malnutrition due to various mechanisms including disease related anorexia, treatment associated nausea, gastrointestinal toxicity, and mucositis. This leads to loss of lean body mass and phosphorus stores. RFS typically manifests 48–72 hours after initiation of nutritional support and may result in profound, life-threatening hypophosphatemia (34). Similarly, hypophosphatemia due to increased anabolism and intracellular influx is observed in patients with hematopoietic reconstitution after allogeneic stem cell transplantation and in leukemia patients with rapid tumor cell proliferation (33).

Several chemotherapy agents can lead to renal phosphate wasting. To distinguish between renal losses and gastrointestinal losses or redistribution syndrome, renal threshold phosphate concentration (TmP/GFR) can be derived using the nomogram (Fig. 2.1) (33, 35). In hypophosphatemia that is not caused by renal losses, TmP/GFR should be <2.5 mg (0.08 mmol) per 100 mL. Ifosfamide is associated with proximal tubular toxicity leading to Fanconi syndrome. It is usually reversible; however, permanent renal damage and hypophosphatemia may persist in 25–44% of patients. Risk factors include a cumulative dose of >50 mg/m^2, preexisting renal disease or nephrectomy, younger age at treatment (<5-year-olds most at risk), Wilm's tumor, and prior

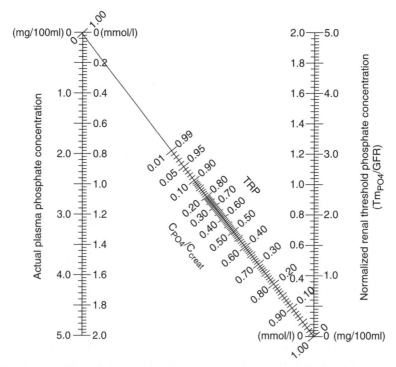

Fig. 2.1 Evaluating the patient with hypernatremia. Cpo$_4$-phosphate clearance; Ccr-creatinine clearance; TRP-tubular reabsorption of phosphate (1-Cpo$_4$/Ccr). Reproduced with permission from Pollack M, Yu A. Clinical Disturbances of Calcium, Magnesium, and Phosphate Metabolism. In: Brenner B, editor. Brenner and Rector's the Kidney. 7 ed. Philadelphia: Saunders; 2004. p.1041–76.

treatment with cisplatin. While the mechanism of tubular injury is not completely understood there is a concern that 2-Mercaptoethanesulfonate Sodium (MESNA-administered for prevention of hemorrhagic cystitis) may contribute to proximal damage (27). Additionally, cisplatin, carmustine, azacitidine, pamidronate, lenalidomide, and imatinib have been reported to cause Fanconi syndrome (27, 36–8). Monoclonal gammopathies can also cause Fanconi syndrome and hypophosphatemia due to deposition of light chains resistant to lysosomal degradation in the proximal tubules (28). Besides Fanconi syndrome, imatinib, a multi-target tyrosine kinase inhibitor, may also induce hypophosphatemia, presumably due to inhibition of platelet-derived growth factor receptor expressed on osteoclasts with subsequent decreased bone resorption, decreased calcium, and phosphate egress from the bone leading to elevated PTH levels and further renal phosphate wasting (39). Sunitinib and sorafenib, two other multi-target tyrosine kinase inhibitors, have also been associated with hypophosphatemia (40). Finally, in clinical trials of intravenous bisphosphonates severe hypophosphatemia approached 50% and was most common in patients treated for HCM (24).

Tumor-induced or oncogenic osteomalacia is a rare disorder of renal phosphate wasting, abnormal vitamin D metabolism and osteomalacia. This condition is associated with tumors of mesenchymal origin, the majority localized in the craniofacial area and the long bones. Oncogenic osteomalacia is associated with high levels of fibroblast growth factor 23 (FGF23). The hypophosphatemia resolves after the removal of the tumor and normalization of FGF23 levels.

It is recommended that patients with severe hypophosphatemia <0.32 mmol/L are treated to avoid complications. The safest mode of replacement is an oral route, and cow's milk is a good source of exogenous phosphorus (6.4 mmol or 200 mg of elemental phosphate per 200 mL) in patients who can tolerate an oral diet. Potassium and sodium phosphate oral preparations are also commercially available. In critically ill patients unable to tolerate oral diet, intravenous supplementation is given as sodium or potassium phosphate at a rate of 0.08 or 0.16 mmol/kg over six hours depending on the severity of the deficit. Infusion of 20 mmol/h of potassium phosphate for either one or two hours was also found to be safe and effective (32).

Hyperphosphatemia

Hyperphosphatemia is defined as a serum phosphate level >1.61 mmol/L. Children and infants have higher levels of serum phosphate and consequently higher upper normal phosphate levels (41). The most common cause of hyperphosphatemia is renal insufficiency. In cancer patients hyperphosphatemia is most commonly encountered in patients with TLS, when a large amount of phosphate is released from intracellular space due to the cytotoxic effect of the chemotherapy. Electrolyte abnormalities usually develop 24–28 hours after initiation of therapy (20). Most important clinical manifestations of hyperphosphatemia are due to concurrent hypocalcemia from calcium phosphate precipitation in tissues. The manifestations of hypocalcemia were described earlier in the chapter. In the kidneys, calcium phosphate precipitation may lead to intrarenal calcification, nephrocalcinosis, nephrolithiasis, and acute obstructive uropathy (20, 41). Since calcium infusions can worsen metastatic calcifications in the setting of hyperphosphatemia, this treatment should be reserved only for patients with symptomatic hypocalcemia. Treatment of acute hyperphosphatemia includes administration of oral phosphate binding agents to decrease phosphate absorption in the gut as well as infusion of hypertonic dextrose and insulin in an attempt to induce intracellular phosphate shift (42). Continuous peritoneal dialysis, continuous veno-venous hemofiltration, and hemodialysis have been successfully employed in treatment of TLS-associated acute hyperphosphatemia (20).

It is important to note that pseudohyperphosphatemia has been reported in patients with paraproteinemias as a result of interference between abnormal proteins and laboratory assay (41). A similar problem was reported in patients receiving high dose liposomal amphotericin B for treatment of severe fungal infections. The phosphate levels were reported to be as high as 4.75 mmol/L. The falsely elevated phosphate readings were obtained only on Synchron LX20 analyzer (Beckman Coulter Inc., Brea, CA) and were corrected by the ultrafiltration of the specimen (43).

Sodium disorders

Serum sodium, with its associated anions, is the major serum osmole. Dysnatremias produce changes in serum osmolality, which is normally tightly maintained between 280–290 mOsm/L, and within 1–2% in a particular individual (44). Small increases in serum osmolality above 280 mOsm/L will stimulate vasopressin (AVP) release, and thirst will occur at yet higher values of serum osmolarity. AVP binds V2 receptors on the basolateral membrane of cells in the collecting ducts to increase resorption of solute free water to produce concentrated urine. Thirst stimulates water intake. Small decreases in serum osmolarity below a threshold value will cause excretion of a dilute urine and dissipate thirst. Disorders of sodium balance are best thought of as disorders of water balance.

Hyponatremia

Case report

We evaluated a 24-year-old male for hyponatremia five days after receiving cisplatin and ifosfamide for treatment of a nonseminomatous germ cell tumor. At the time of evaluation, the patient had postural hypotension after receiving 5 L of IV 0.9% NS; his weight was 4.6 kg lower than the admission weight, and he was febrile, 38.8°C. The patient was awake and alert, complained of fatigue and anorexia, but denied nausea, vomiting, or diarrhea. Lab data were: serum sodium 131 mmol/L; urine sodium 36 mmol/L; serum osmolality 266 mmol/kg; urine osmolality 340 mmol/kg; serum creatinine 123.8μmol/L; TSH 0.62 mcUnits/mL; and AM cortisol 562.8nmol/L. The patient was diagnosed with salt wasting nephropathy due to cisplatin and possibly ifosfamide exposure. He received 0.9% NS at 250 cc/hr in addition to NaCl tabs 5.4 gm/day and fludrocortisone acetate 0.1 mg daily. The postural hypotension and hyponatremia resolved and he was discharged six days later on salt tablets and fludrocortisone.

When approaching the patient with hyponatremia, the answer to three questions will clarify the etiology in most cases: 1) Are there osmotically active particles, other than sodium, that are pulling water out of the intracellular space? 2) What is the volume status of the patient? 3) Is the AVP level appropriate or inappropriate given the patient's volume status? The relevance of each question in cancer patients is explained.

Presence of osmotically active particles

The first step in evaluating hyponatremia is to identify hyperosmolar hyponatremia and pseudohyponatremia. Osmotically active particles like mannitol and glycine cause translocation of water from the intracellular to extracellular compartment, decreasing serum sodium, with no change in total body sodium. Large volumes of nonconductive flushing solutions containing mannitol and glycine used during transurethral resection of the prostate, bladder tumor, or during a hysteroscopy, can be rapidly absorbed during these procedures. Hyperglycemia will also produce a similar osmotic effect. An osmolal gap (normal gap 5–10 mOsmol/kg) will be present in these circumstances. The osmolal gap (Posm) is calculated using the formula:

$$\text{Osmolar gap} = \text{measured Posm} - \text{calculated Posm, where}$$

$$\text{Calculated Posm} = 2 \times \text{plasma [Na]} + [\text{glucose}]/18 + [\text{BUN}]/2.8$$

The presence of excessive amounts of proteins in patients with multiple myeloma and other paraproteinemias can lower the measured serum sodium if the flame photometry method is used. This is referred to as pseudohyponatremia since the serum osmolarity is within the normal range. The ion specific electrode method obviates this miscalculation.

Assessment of the patient's volume status

Fig. 2.2 offers an algorithm for delineating the etiology of hypo osmolar hyponatremia based on assessment of the patient's volume status. If it is physically possible, all patients with hypo osmolar hyponatremia should have orthostatic blood pressure readings performed. This involves checking blood pressure and pulse readings with the patient in the supine, sitting, and standing position. Orthostatic hypotension is diagnosed if any of the following is observed as the patient moves from the supine to standing position: 1) symptoms of hypoperfusion (dizziness, lightheadedness, blurry vision); 2) a decrease in systolic blood pressure of at least 20 mm Hg; or 3) a decrease in diastolic blood pressure of at least 10 mm Hg. The presence of edema does not exclude intravascular volume depletion in cancer patients since this finding can be associated with other conditions found in this population, including severe hypoalbuminemia, lower extremity deep venous thrombosis, lymphatic obstruction from pelvic lymphadenopathy, and hepatorenal syndrome from metastatic

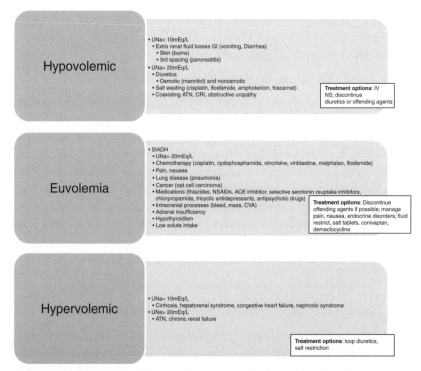

Fig. 2.2 Approach to the patient with hypo osmolar hyponatremia based on volume status. (Categories are shown by dark shading; causes in light shading, and treatments in white boxes.)

disease to the liver. An assessment of extracellular volume status informs about the level of total body sodium. Hypovolemic hyponatremia suggests decreased total body sodium and water, with relatively more water than sodium. Hypervolemic hyponatremia implies increased levels of sodium and water, with relatively more water than sodium. The patient who has euvolemic hyponatremia also has relatively more body water relative to sodium, but edema is not present on exam because two-thirds of total body water is in the intracellular space (45).

Hyponatremia in cancer patients can result from poor solute intake and malnutrition, which in turn, will impair free water clearance. If normal protein turnover results in a solute excretion of 600 mmol/kg, then with minimally concentrated urine of 60 mmol/kg, the maximum urine output will be 10L/day. On a sustained low solute intake, if solute excretion is halved to 300 mmol/kg, and the urine is minimally concentrated, then the maximal urine output will only be 5L.

Is the AVP level appropriate in light of the patient's volume status?

A hypovolemic patient should appropriately secrete AVP, and if their kidney function is normal, will generate a concentrated urine with a low urinary sodium (<10 mmol/L) and high urine osmolality and high urine specific gravity (SG). The edematous patient with congestive heart failure can also avidly resorb sodium in the distal tubule and have a UNa <10 mmol/L. Therefore, the urinary sodium, in the absence of volume assessment, provides inadequate information about the etiology of hyponatremia.

Interpreting urinary indices

The solute concentration of urine can be estimated by measuring the urine Na, urine osmolality and the urine specific gravity. The urine specific gravity is less accurate than the urine osmolarity, since the former is dependent on the size as well as the number of solute particles in urine. For example, glucosuria can produce a high urine specific gravity. Calculating the fractional excretion of sodium (FeNa) also provides information of the volume status of the patient. The FeNa is calculated using the equation:

$$FeNa\% = UNa \times Pcr/PNa \times Ucr \times 100$$

$$UNa = \text{urine sodium; } PNa = \text{plasma sodium}$$

$$UCr = \text{urine creatinine; } PCr = \text{plasma creatinine}$$

A FeNa of <1% and a urine Na <10 mmol/L indicates intravascular volume depletion. Exposure to intravenous contrast will also produce a FeNa of <1%.

In the presence of hypervolemia and hyposmolarity, AVP release will be abolished, resulting in dilute urine. The urine osmolality and urine specific gravity are expected to be low (below 200 mmole/kg and 1.010, respectively).

The UNa can be >20 mmol/L. In the setting of hypovolemia or hyperosmolarity, AVP is released, resulting in more concentrated urine. The urine osmolarity and urine specific gravity are generally greater than 600 mmole/kg and 1.020, respectively. The urine Na is expected to <10 mmol/(46).

Importantly, these indices only hold true when renal tubular function is intact and when the tubules are able to respond appropriately to AVP. These urinary indices become unreliable in the setting of acute tubular injury (ATN), chronic renal failure, obstructive uropathy, and with the use of osmotic and non-osmotic diuretics. Salt wasting is another clinical scenario which can produce confusion between what the volume status of the patient is and what the urinary indices suggest. Commonly used chemotherapeutic agents (cisplatin, ifosfamide) and anti-infective agents (amphotericin and foscarnet) can cause injury to the renal tubules, resulting in salt wasting. Renal tubular salt wasting will produce intravascular volume depletion and hypotension. Because sodium is lost in the urine, the urine osmolality, urine specific gravity, and urine sodium will all be elevated, and the FeNa is >1%.

Syndrome of Inappropriate ADH secretion (SIADH)

While hypovolemia and hyperosmolality are appropriate stimuli for vasopressin secretion, the syndrome of inappropriate vasopressin secretion, SIADH, occurs in cancer patients for a number of reasons. At one cancer center, SIADH accounted for one-third of all etiologies of hyponatremia (47). Common etiologies for SIADH include chemotherapy (cisplatin, cyclophosphamide, vincristine, vinblastine, melphalan, ifosfamide) (48); oat cell c arcinoma; pulmonary disease; pain; nausea; intracranial lesions (49, 50–1); adrenal insufficiency (from adrenal masses or long-term steroid exposure), and hypothyroidism (52). Since the urine osmolality in SIADH can be identical to that of a patient with appropriate vasopressin secretion due to volume depletion, careful volume assessment will often yield the correct diagnosis.

Importantly, appropriate vasopressin secretion from volume contraction can coexist in a patient with underlying SIADH from pain or chemotherapy. In these patients, the volume stimulus for vasopressin secretion should be corrected until they are no longer orthostatic and, if hyponatremia persists, the patient should then be managed with fluid restriction or as otherwise clinically appropriate for the underlying SIADH state. In this setting, the sodium will initially increase with 0.9% NS; and when the patient is no longer volume depleted, the sodium will decrease if the IV fluids are continued. This is because renal sodium handling is normal in patients with SIADH but free water excretion is impaired.

Management

Hyponatremia produces cerebral edema and can manifest clinically as anorexia, nausea, lethargy, abnormal sensorium, and seizures. Regardless of the patient's volume status, symptomatic hyponatremia should be managed in the intensive care unit setting with 3% saline. The goal is to prevent seizures. Because the solution contains more sodium than free water, the patient will gain more sodium than free water, regardless of the initial relative concentrations of salt and water in their serum. The sodium deficit is measured with the equation:

$$\text{Na deficit} = [\text{Body weight (kg)} \times 0.5] \times [\text{desired Na (mmol/L)} - \text{initial Na (mmol/L)}]$$

The goal is to correct no more than 8 mmol/L in a 24-hour period. Each 1 L of 0.9% NS contains 154 mmol of NaCl and each 1 L of 3% saline contains 513 mmol, or roughly 0.5 mmol of NaCl per each cc.

The asymptomatic patient can be treated as indicated by their volume status. The edematous patient is treated with loop diuretics and salt restriction. Thiazide diuretics can worsen hyponatremia because they affect the diluting segment of the nephron and impair free water clearance. The hypovolemic patient can receive 0.9% NS until euvolemic.

In patients with SIADH, anti-emetics and pain medications can be used if indicated to decrease these stimuli for vasopressin secretion. Culprit medications (listed in Fig. 2.2) should also be eliminated, if possible. For the inpatient, the V2 receptor antagonist (conivaptan 20 mg infused over 30 minutes as a loading dose, followed by a continuous infusion of 20 mg over 24 hours) will, in most cases, predictably increase serum sodium by 8 mEq/L over a 24-hour infusion (53). Options for inpatients and outpatients with SIADH include demeclocycline (600–900 mg/day, divided every 6–8 hours), loop diuretics with salt tablets (1–2 gms/day) and fluid restriction (1 L/day). Any one therapy can be used alone or combined with one another. For example, fluid restriction can be combined with demeclocycline or with a loop diuretic and salt tablet. Therapy can be selected based on patient tolerance (54).

Hypernatremia

Hypernatremia can be approached in the same manner as hyponatremia. That is to say, the central questions are 1) what is the concentration of salt relative water in the serum, and 2) what is the volume status of the patient? When the serum osmolality increases above 280 mmol/kg, vasopressin release acts in the renal tubules to effect water conservation and a return of serum osmolality to a normal range. The osmotic threshold for thirst is 10 mosm/kg higher than that for vasopressin release. Therefore, thirst is stimulated when serum hyperosmolarity surpasses the protective effect of the kidney (55). Consequently, as long as the thirst mechanism is intact, the individual can 'drink themselves down' to a normal serum osmolarity. Hyperosmolarity and hypernatremia primarily presents in individuals with impaired thirst due to hypothalamic lesions, and those who cannot access free water due to decreased mentation or immobilization. Its occurrence depends on the combination of impaired renal water conservation and impaired thirst.

Hypernatremia is an excess of sodium relative to water. The volume-expanded patient has excess total body sodium from exogenous sodium chloride (IV normal saline or hypertonic saline, oral sodium chloride tablets, oral or intravenous sodium bicarbonate, hypertonic dialysate solutions) or from excessive renal tubular sodium absorption (mineralocorticoid excess states). In hypovolemic or euvolemic patients, a thorough history can uncover the source of free water losses from the kidney (diuretics, mannitol, hyperglycemia), respiratory tract (ventilated patients), insensible losses from the skin (high fevers, excessive sweating), and volume loss from the GI tract (diarrhea, vasoactive intestinal peptide producing tumors, VIPomas). VIPomas secrete vasoactive intestinal peptide, resulting in a secretory diarrhea, hypokalemia, and stool volumes of up to 7 L per day (56).

The presence, of polyuria, arbitrarily defined as a urine output of greater than 3 L/day, in the absence of diuretic use, signals a defect in AVP synthesis or release from the pituitary (central diabetes insipidus, CDI), or renal tubule unresponsiveness to AVP (nephrogenic DI). Most patients with CDI or NDI will have a normal thirst mechanism and will also present with polydipsia. The most common etiologies of CDI are neurosurgery, trauma, primary or metastatic tumors, and infiltrative diseases (57). CDI from leukemic infiltration of the pituitary stalk in patients with acute leukemias has also been reported (58–9). In adults, the most common causes of NDI are chronic lithium use, hypokalemia and hypercalcemia (57). Obstructive uropathy from bladder neck or ureteral obstruction can also cause ADH unresponsiveness (60). Amyloid deposition along the basement membrane of medullary collecting ducts has been associated with unresponsiveness to AVP (61). Chemotherapeutic agents, and medications commonly used for the management of infectious complications from chemotherapy and bone marrow transplantation are also associated with NDI (cidofovir, indinavir, tenofovir, foscarnet, amphotericin, ifosfamide, cyclophosphamide, methotrexate, ofloxacin) (62–6). A water deprivation test can help to distinguish CDI from NDI. Details of the test and interpretation of the results are outlined in Fig. 2.4. A more detailed explanation for interpreting the results is discussed elsewhere (57).

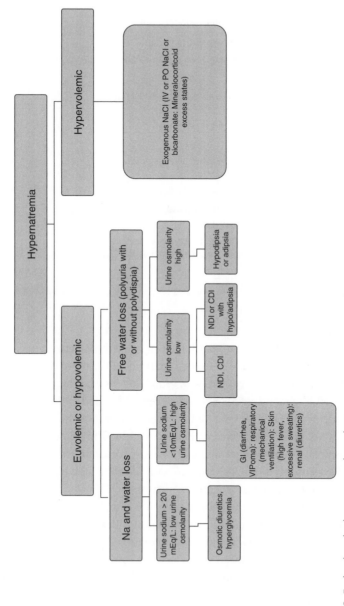

Fig. 2.3 Evaluating the hypernatremic patient.

1) Begin test in the AM.

2) Every hour - obtain patient weight, urine osmolality, urine specific gravity, and urine volume.

3) Every 2 hours—obtain serum osmolality and serum sodium.

4) Continue the test until any of the following occurs:

    a. Serum osmolarity is above 295 mmol/kg

    b.Urinary concentration does not increase further in sequential urine specimens

    c.Hypotension occurs

    d.Urine osmolarity normalizes, generally 600mmol/kg.

Interpreting the results:

Complete nephrogenic DI—no elevation in urine osmolality

Partial nephrogenic DI—up to 45% rise in urine osmolality

Complete central DI—100% rise in urine osmolality

Partial central DI—15–50% rise in urine osmolality

Distinguishing partial NDI from partial CDI

In general, patients with partial CDI will be able to achieve a urine osmolality > or = 300mosmol/kg while patients with partial CDI will continue to have a dilute urine.

Fig. 2.4 The water deprivation test. This test should only be performed on a patient with constant supervision.

Fig. 2.3 offers a systematic approach for evaluating the hypernatremic, hyperosmolar patient. Note that, due to the proximity of the osmosensors and the thirst center, there are rare patients with central lesions who can have combined defects in AVP release (partial or complete central DI) and in thirst regulation. These patients can have extreme water deprivation because their thirst mechanism does not become activated and allow them to 'drink down' to a normal serum osmolality and serum sodium. It has been demonstrated that their renal tubules have enhanced responsiveness to AVP, allowing for a high urine osmolarity even in the setting of severe AVP deficiency. This ability to maximally concentrate urine is lost as their volume deficit is partially corrected (67).

Hypervolemic hypernatremia can be managed with salt restriction, diuretics, and by correcting the free water deficit with oral water or intravenous 5% dextrose. The euvolemic patient can be managed by correcting the calculated water deficit with water or 5% dextrose. The water deficit is calculated by the equation:

$$\text{Water deficit} = 0.5^* \times \text{body weight (kg)} \, [140/\text{plasma sodium} - 1]$$
$$^*0.6 \text{ for lean males, } 0.5 \text{ for females}$$

To avoid brain edema, which can occur if the deficit is corrected too rapidly, only half of the calculated water deficit should be administered within the first 24 hours. When correcting hypovolemic hypernatremia, the best approach is to re-expand the intravascular volume with 0.9% or 0.45% saline until the patient is no longer orthostatic. Since either fluid will be hypotonic relative to the patient, brain edema can result if the sodium is corrected too quickly. Therefore, the serum sodium should not be corrected more than 12 mmol/L over the initial 24 hours. For patients with ongoing GI, renal and insensible fluid losses, a portion of those losses should be added to the calculated deficit. Concomitant hypercalcemia and hypokalemia need to be corrected as both conditions are associated with unresponsiveness of the renal tubules to AVP.

Potassium disorders

The total body potassium content is about 50 mmol/kg (40 mmol/kg for females), or roughly 3500 mmol in a 70 kg male. More than 95% of potassium is contained in the intracellular space (e.g. muscle, red blood cells, liver, bone); only 2–3% is contained in the extracellular and plasma space. Potassium will shift from the intracellular (IC) to plasma space in the presence of acidosis, whereas cellular uptake of potassium will increase in the presence of alkalosis. The presence of osmotically active particles like glucose and mannitol in the extracellular space (EC) will cause movement of water down its concentration gradient from the IC to EC space, dragging solute and potassium with it, thereby elevating serum potassium. Insulin is the body's primary defense against hyperkalemia, acting to enhance cellular uptake of potassium. Therefore diabetics with insulin deficiency, hyperglycemia, and acidosis are at particular risk for hyperkalemia. Cellular uptake of potassium is enhanced by beta 2 agonists and decreased by alpha agonists and beta 2 antagonists. Cell membrane Na/K/ATPase pumps transport sodium from the IC to EC space in exchange for potassium uptake. Digitalis overdose inhibits these pumps.

The average dietary potassium intake is 100 mmol/day, of which approximately 90% is eliminated by the kidneys and 10% via the GI tract. The major site of renal potassium regulation is in the distal tubule and collecting ducts. Aldosterone secretion stimulates Na/K/ATPase activity in distal tubule cells, resulting in sodium reabsorption and potassium secretion. In the absence of aldosterone or unresponsiveness to the hormone, serum potassium will increase. Potassium excretion is maintained by adequate urine flow rates and sodium delivery to the distal tubule.(68)

Hyperkalemia

Case report

A 69-year-old male with prostate cancer and diabetes was transferred from an outside hospital for further management of acute kidney injury, hyperkalemia, and a GI bleed which occurred while on warfarin for a mechanical heart valve. His baseline creatinine was 88.4 µmol/L. Upon admission, he had already received two units of RBCs and fresh frozen plasma and IV fluids (0.9% NS with 5 mmol/L KCl) was infusing. A urinary catheter was in place; his urine output was 50 cc over the preceding eight hours. Medications on admission included lisinopril, olmesartan, and metoprolol. Labs on admission were: WBC 8.1×10^9; Hg 79 g/L; PLT 349×10^9/L; BUN and Cr 34 mmol/L and 318 µmol/L; K 6.3 mmol/L; CO_2 16 mmol/L; glucose 18.2 mmol/L; INR 1.9; UA SG 1.010; no protein, many RBCs, no casts. A renal ultrasound showed bilateral hydroureteronephrosis with the Foley balloon within the prostate.

This patient's presentation highlights the 'perfect storm' for factors which contribute to hyperkalemia. Conceptually, hyperkalemia is straightforward (Fig. 2.5). After ruling out factitious hyperkalemia, the next step is to discern if the patient has too much potassium going in (oral or IV); not enough coming out (from the GI tract or kidneys); or if potassium is being shifted from the IC to the EC space.

Leukocytosis (WBC >100 x 10^9/L and thrombocytosis (PLT >800 x 10^9/L) can cause pseudohyperkalemia when potassium is released from cells after clotting has taken place in a serum sample (69). These patients will be asymptomatic with no typical EKG changes (peaked Ts, prolonged QRS, absent P waves). A plasma sample for potassium will clarify the diagnosis. Hemolysis at

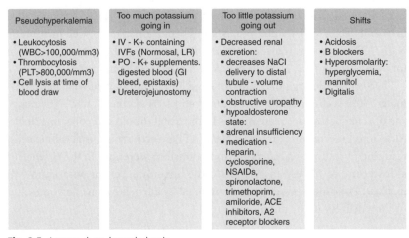

Pseudohyperkalemia	Too much potassium going in	Too little potassium going out	Shifts
• Leukocytosis (WBC>100,000/mm3) • Thrombocytosis (PLT>800,000/mm3) • Cell lysis at time of blood draw	• IV - K+ containing IVFs (Normosal, LR) • PO - K+ supplements. digested blood (GI bleed, epistaxis) • Ureterojejunostomy	• Decreased renal excretion: • decreases NaCl delivery to distal tubule - volume contraction • obstructive uropathy • hypoaldosterone state: • adrenal insufficiency • medication - heparin, cyclosporine, NSAIDs, spironolactone, trimethoprim, amiloride, ACE inhibitors, A2 receptor blockers	• Acidosis • B blockers • Hyperosmolarity: hyperglycemia, mannitol • Digitalis

Fig. 2.5 Approach to hyperkalemia.

the time of blood draw due to an overly tight tourniquet or small gauge needle may also cause pseudohyperkalemia.

Since the majority of total body potassium is contained in the IC space, intravascular hemolysis or shifts of potassium from the IC to EC space can produce clinically significant hyperkalemia. Mechanical heart valves, tumor lysis syndrome, rhabdomyolysis, thrombotic microangiopathy, and structural RBC abnormalities like hereditary spherocytosis, are all associated with intravascular hemolysis (70–4). Exogenous potassium can be delivered via K+ containing IV fluids (e.g. Normosol®) (5 mmol KCl/L), lactated ringers (4 mmol KCl/L), blood transfusions, and oral potassium supplements. Patients with upper GI bleeds or epistaxis can also absorb potassium as the blood is digested. Patients who have undergone ureteral diversions where the conduit is in contact with the jejunum can present with hyperkalemia due to absorption of urinary potassium by the jejunum (75).

Impaired renal elimination of potassium can result from ureteral or bladder neck obstruction and from abnormal secretion of aldosterone or subnormal effect of the hormone on cells in the distal tubule. A host of medications known to decrease aldosterone secretion or effect are listed in Fig. 2.5 (76–80). Additionally, chronic renal insufficiency and obstructive uropathy cause a state of hypoaldosteronism. In the setting of volume contraction, the proximal tubules avidly resorb NaCl, thereby decreasing distal sodium delivery. Decreased urine flow rate and distal sodium delivery will reduce potassium excretion. The patient presented was receiving exogenous potassium (digested blood in the GI tract and potassium containing IV fluids); had a state of effective hypoaldosteronism (ACE inhibitor, angiotensin receptor blocker, and obstructive uropathy); osmotic shift of potassium out of the cells due to hyperglycemia and presence of a beta blocker; decreased insulin levels; and was unable to excrete potassium due to a bladder neck obstruction.

Management of hyperkalemia involves a two-pronged approach: 1) shift potassium back into the intracellular space and 2) remove potassium via the kidneys and GI tract. Beta agonists (nebulizer or IV) and insulin (SQ or IV) will acutely lower serum potassium within 30–60 minutes. These medications only shift potassium and their effect will only persist for a few hours, so measures to excrete potassium also need to be employed. In a euvolemic or hypervolemic patient, furosemide and cation exchange resins (e.g. Sodium Polystyrene Sulfonate (SPS), Kayexalate®) will result in renal and GI elimination of potassium, respectively. There are rare case reports of colonic necrosis associated with exposure to cation exchange resins (81). Decreased colonic motility (from postoperative ileus or opiate administration) and concomitant sorbitol administration appear to be risk factors. In the volume-contracted patient, intravenous normal saline will increase distal sodium delivery and potassium secretion by the distal tubule. For patients with EKG abnormalities (peaked Ts, prolonged QRS, absent P waves), IV calcium gluconate or calcium chloride is needed to stabilize the cardiac membranes. Dialysis is appropriate for patients who have failed medical management; when hyperkalemia is severe; and in those situations where there is significant ongoing release of intracellular potassium (TLS, rhabdomyolysis).

Hypokalemia

Hypokalemia is one of the most common electrolyte abnormalities in hospitalized patients with incidence of up to 20% when it is defined as potassium level of <3.6 mmol/L (82). It may be even more common in malignancy and occurs in approximately 75% of cancer patients at some point during their illness (83). Although in most cases low serum potassium measurements represent true hypokalemia, spurious hypokalemia due to cellular uptake of potassium in vitro has been reported in rare patients with leukemia and markedly elevated white cell counts as well as in normal subjects when blood sample analysis is delayed in high ambient temperatures (84–5). Hypokalemia is well tolerated by healthy individuals but in patients with ischemic or scarred myocardium it may result in life-threatening arrhythmias. Severe hypokalemia of <2.5 mmol/L may lead to rhabdomyolysis and concentrations of <2.0 mmol/L can cause paralysis and respiratory arrest (86).

Hypokalemia can be caused by poor intake, excessive losses or intracellular shifts of potassium. Oral potassium intake below 1 gm (25 mEq) per day may result in hypokalemia. In cancer patients low potassium intake is usually due to anorexia, nausea, or intestinal obstruction (82–3).

Clinically significant potassium losses occur via kidneys and gastrointestinal tract as skin losses are minimal except with extreme sweating from physical exertion. Several mechanisms are responsible for renal losses in cancer patients. Thiazide and loop diuretics are the most common cause of hypokalemia due to the inhibition of sodium reabsorption in the loop of Henle and distal tubule and increased delivery to the collecting ducts where sodium is reabsorbed with resulting electrochemical gradient favoring potassium secretion (82). Hypomagnesemia is another cause of renal potassium wasting. In cancer patients, cisplatin as well as aminoglycosides, amphotericin, pamidronate, and foscarnet cause hypomagnesemia-induced hypokalemia (22). Proximal tubular dysfunction and Fanconi syndrome due to ifosfamide or light chain toxicity in multiple myeloma patients can also lead to renal potassium wasting. In rare cases, patients with acute leukemia develop severe hypokalemia and kaliuresis. The postulated mechanism for this disorder is lysozyme-induced acute tubular injury (87). Finally, penicillins when given in large intravenous doses may promote kaliuresis by increased distal delivery of sodium (82). Metabolic alkalosis is also associated with hypokalemia. It may be induced by chloride losses due to vomiting, nasogastric tube drainage, and diuretic use. Chloride depletion leads to renal potassium wasting despite low serum potassium levels. Non-chloride sensitive metabolic alkalosis and hypokalemia occur in patients with paraneoplastic syndrome of adrenocorticotropic hormone (ACTH) secretion. It is predominantly reported in small-cell tumors but is also associated with neuroendocrine neoplasms and carcinomas (renal cell tumors, colon cancers, and paragangliomas). ACTH secretion leads to glucocorticoid excess with stimulation of mineralocorticoid receptors in distal nephron resulting in enhanced potassium secretion (88). A similar effect is seen in patients on high dose steroid therapy and those receiving fludrocortisone, an oral mineralocorticoid, by its direct influence on mineralocorticoid receptors (86, 89).

The stool potassium concentration is 80–90 mmol/L but fecal losses of potassium are usually small because stool volumes are low (82). However, when diarrhea develops potassium wasting may substantial. In cancer patients causes of diarrhea include chemotherapy, radiation, infectious agents, antibiotic therapy, graft versus host disease in bone marrow transplant patients as well as villous adenoma of the colon, vasoactive peptide secreting tumors, carcinoid and Zollinger-Ellison syndrome (83). Upper gastrointestinal potassium losses due to nasogastric suction or vomiting are minimal but can lead to hypochloremic metabolic alkalosis and hypokalemia as described previously (82).

The treatment of hypokalemia is the replacement of potassium deficit and elimination of underlying cause of hypokalemia. On average, every 0.3 mmol/L decline in serum potassium concentration corresponds to a 100 mmol deficit. While hypokalemia should be corrected promptly in patients with significant deficit and those at risk for arrhythmias, overcorrection may lead to life-threatening hyperkalemia. For this reason intravenous administration should be avoided if possible. Oral potassium preparations are well absorbed but one should keep in mind that a portion of the replacement is always excreted even in the face of ongoing low serum potassium levels. These losses may be even more significant with ongoing diuretic therapy and can reach 40–100 mmol/day. In addition to supplementation, administration of potassium sparing diuretics may improve hypokalemia by inhibiting renal potassium excretion. In patients who develop hypokalemia as a result of hypomagnesemia, magnesium supplementation is essential for correction of the potassium deficit (82).

Magnesium disorders

Serum magnesium represents only 1% of total body magnesium, whereas 60% of body magnesium is contained in bone and 38% in soft tissue (90). Serum magnesium does not readily exchange with these reservoirs since most intracellular magnesium is bound to ATP and enzymes, and because it can take bone stores several weeks to compensate for losses from the extracellular space. Unlike most other elements, magnesium is not primarily resorbed in the proximal tubule but instead in the thick ascending limb of the loop of Henle (TAL LOH). The kidneys are the major organ for magnesium elimination. Since 40% of dietary magnesium is absorbed in the small intestine, disorders of the small bowel will also affect magnesium homeostasis (90).

Hypomagnesemia

Renal and GI losses are the main causes of hypomagnesemia. Decreased dietary intake, chelation in the extracellular space, and shifts to the intracellular space and bones are less common causes. Fig. 2.6 suggests an algorithm for approaching hypomagnesemia. Urinary magnesium wasting has been described with the use of ETOH and multiple anti-infective (aminoglycosides, amphotericin, pentamidine, foscarnet), diuretic (loop and thiazide) (91–2), and chemotherapeutic agents (cisplatin, carboplatin, oxaliplatin, ifosfamide,

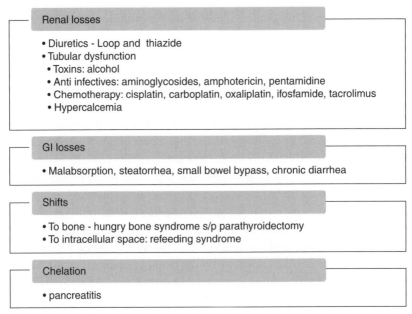

Renal losses

- Diuretics - Loop and thiazide
- Tubular dysfunction
  - Toxins: alcohol
  - Anti infectives: aminoglycosides, amphotericin, pentamidine
  - Chemotherapy: cisplatin, carboplatin, oxaliplatin, ifosfamide, tacrolimus
  - Hypercalcemia

GI losses

- Malabsorption, steatorrhea, small bowel bypass, chronic diarrhea

Shifts

- To bone - hungry bone syndrome s/p parathyroidectomy
- To intracellular space: refeeding syndrome

Chelation

- pancreatitis

Fig. 2.6 Approach to hypomagnesemia.

tacrolimus, cetuximab, panitumumab) (90, 93), as described in Chapter 5 in this book.

Some of the medications listed will also cause renal calcium and potassium wasting, leading to concomitant hypocalcemia and hypokalemia, respectively. Refractory hypokalemia and hypocalcemia can result from untreated hypomagnesemia. This is because hypomagnesemia itself potentiates kaliuresis and has a suppressive effect on PTH secretion and produces PTH resistance (94). Hypomagnesemia can be easily corrected and is short-lived when related to diuretics, once these agents have been discontinued. However, renal magnesium wasting can persist for months to years after use of cisplatin (95) and ifosfamide. The incidence of hypomagnesemia increases with successive dosing (96). Hypercalcemia causes hypomagnesemia because calcium and magnesium complete for transport in the TAL LOH (97).

The refeeding syndrome refers to the abrupt shifts of phosphorus, magnesium, and potassium into cells in chronically malnourished patients who are given a significant carbohydrate load via TPN or an oral or IV glucose infusion (34). Following parathyroidectomy for hyperparathyroidism or thyroid surgery, vigorous magnesium uptake from renewing bone can abruptly lower serum magnesium, calcium, and phosphorus. This is referred to as the hungry bone syndrome. Hypomagnesemia has been observed in the setting of pancreatitis and thought to be due to saponification (98). Lipase released in the setting of pancreatitis will cause fat necrosis and the fatty acids can bind magnesium, lowering serum magnesium levels.

The approach to treatment of hypomagnesemia varies with the severity of its clinical manifestations. When tetany or ventricular arrhythmias are present, 50 mEq of magnesium can be infused over eight hours. Serum magnesium concentration is the primary regulator of magnesium reabsorption in the TAL LOH and an acute rise in serum magnesium will result in 50% of the infused amount being excreted by the kidneys. For this reason, an infusion over 6–8 hours allows for less renal magnesium wasting. For asymptomatic hypomagnesemia, appropriate therapy is oral replacement with sustained-release preparations, which contain 5–7 mEq of magnesium per tablet. For patients who are unable to tolerate oral magnesium, infusions of 2–4 grams of magnesium (8.12 mEq/gram) over 6–8 hours is an option.

Hypermagnesemia

Because excess serum magnesium is readily excreted in the urine, renal insufficiency is the major risk factor for hypermagnesemia. Significant amounts of magnesium can be absorbed from the GI tract from ingestion of milk of magnesia, magnesium citrate, and Epsom salts. The elderly are at particular risk because they have significant reductions in GFR with only mild elevation in serum creatinine.

Treatment consists of removing any offending agents. Patients with neuromuscular involvement (hyporeflexia, muscle weakness) can be given 100–200 mg of elemental calcium over 5–10 minutes. Oliguric or anuric patients can be treated with hemodialysis.

References

1 Stewart AF (2005). Clinical practice. Hypercalcemia associated with cancer. *N Engl J Med* **352**: 373–9.

2 Vassilopoulou-Sellin R, Newman BM, Taylor SH, Guinee VF (1993). Incidence of hypercalcemia in patients with malignancy referred to a comprehensive cancer center. *Cancer* **71**: 1309–12.

3 Ralston SH, Gallacher SJ, Patel U, Campbell J, Boyle IT (1990). Cancer-associated hypercalcemia: morbidity and mortality. Clinical experience in 126 treated patients. *Ann Intern Med* **112**: 499–504.

4 Tattersall MH (1993). Hypercalcaemia: historical perspectives and present management. *Support Care Cancer* **1**: 19–25.

5 Penel N, Dewas S, Doutrelant P, Clisant S, Yazdanpanah Y, Adenis A (2008). Cancer-associated hypercalcemia treated with intravenous diphosphonates: a survival and prognostic factor analysis. *Support Care Cancer* **16**: 387–92.

6 Diercks DB, Shumaik GM, Harrigan RA, Brady WJ, Chan TC (2004). Electrocardiographic manifestations: electrolyte abnormalities. *J Emerg Med* **27**: 153–60.

7 Reikes S, Gonzales E, Martin K (2002). Abnormal Calcium and Magnesium Metabolism. In: Acid-base and Electrolyte disorders: a companion to Brenner & Rector's the kidney (ed. TD DuBose, LL Hamm), p. 453–88. Saunders, Philadelphia.

8 Lumachi F, Brunello A, Roma A, Basso U (2009). Cancer-induced hypercalcemia. *Anticancer Res* **29**: 1551–5.

9 Lumachi F, Brunello A, Roma A, Basso U (2008). Medical treatment of malignancy-associated hypercalcemia. *Curr Med Chem* **15**: 415–21.

10 Calvi LM, Bushinsky DA (2008). When is it appropriate to order an ionized calcium? *J Am Soc Nephrol* **19**: 1257–60.

11 Klontz KC, Acheson DW (2007). Dietary supplement-induced vitamin D intoxication. *N Engl J Med* **357**: 308–9.

12 LeGrand SB, Leskuski D, Zama I (2008). Narrative review: furosemide for hypercalcemia: an unproven yet common practice. *Ann Intern Med* **149**: 259–63.

13 Perazella MA, Markowitz GS (2008). Bisphosphonate nephrotoxicity. *Kidney Int* **74**: 1385–93.

14 Machado CE, Flombaum CD (1996). Safety of pamidronate in patients with renal failure and hypercalcemia. *Clin Nephrol* **45**: 175–9.

15 Lumachi F, Basso SM, Basso U (2006). Parathyroid cancer: etiology, clinical presentation and treatment. *Anticancer Res* **26**:4803–7.

16 Daugirdas J, Ross E, NIssenson A (2001). Acute hemodialysis prescription. In: Handbook of dialysis, 3 ed (ed. J Daugirdas, P Blake, T Ing), p. 102. Lippincott Williams and Wilkins, Philadelphia.

17 Abramson EC, Gajardo H, Kukreja SC (1990). Hypocalcemia in cancer. *Bone Miner* **10**: 161–9.

18 Zuradelli M, Masci G, Biancofiore G, Gullo G, Scorsetti M, Navarria P et al. (2009). High incidence of hypocalcemia and serum creatinine increase in patients with bone metastases treated with zoledronic acid. *Oncologist* **14**: 548–56.

19 Cooper MS, Gittoes NJ. Diagnosis and management of hypocalcaemia (2008). *BMJ* **336**: 1298–302.

20 Cairo MS, Bishop M (2004). Tumour lysis syndrome: new therapeutic strategies and classification. *Br J Haematol* **127**: 3–11.

21 D'Erasmo E, Celi FS, Acca M, Minisola S, Aliberti G, Mazzuoli GF (1991). Hypocalcemia and hypomagnesemia in cancer patients. *Biomed Pharmacother* **45**: 315–7.

22 Atsmon J, Dolev E (2005). Drug-induced hypomagnesaemia: scope and management. *Drug Saf* **28**: 763–88.

23 Schrag D, Chung KY, Flombaum C, Saltz L (2005). Cetuximab therapy and symptomatic hypomagnesemia. *J Natl Cancer Inst* **97**: 1221–4.

24 Tanvetyanon T, Stiff PJ (2006). Management of the adverse effects associated with intravenous bisphosphonates. *Ann Oncol* **17**: 897–907.

25 Wang-Gillam A, Miles DA, Hutchins LF (2008). Evaluation of vitamin D deficiency in breast cancer patients on bisphosphonates. *Oncologist* **13**: 821–7.

26 Shoback D (2008). Clinical practice. Hypoparathyroidism. *N Engl J Med* **359**: 391–403.

27 Izzedine H, Launay-Vacher V, Isnard-Bagnis C, Deray G (2003). Drug-induced Fanconi's syndrome. *Am J Kidney Dis* **41**: 292–309.

28 Lacy MQ, Gertz MA (1999). Acquired Fanconi's syndrome associated with monoclonal gammopathies. *Hematol Oncol Clin North Am* **13**: 1273–80.

29 Patel K, Brahmbhatt V, Ramu V (2005). Zoledronic acid-induced severe hypocalcaemia in a prostate cancer patient with extensive osteoblastic bone metastases. *Tenn Med* **98**: 83–5, 9.

30 Camp MA, Allon M (1990). Severe hypophosphatemia in hospitalized patients. *Miner Electrolyte Metab* **16**: 365–8.

31 Hoffmann M, Zemlin AE, Meyer WP, Erasmus RT (2008). Hypophosphataemia at a large academic hospital in South Africa. *J Clin Pathol* **61**: 1104–7.

32 Gaasbeek A, Meinders AE (2005). Hypophosphatemia: an update on its etiology and treatment. *Am J Med* **118**: 1094–101.

33 Amanzadeh J, Reilly RF, Jr (2006). Hypophosphatemia: an evidence-based approach to its clinical consequences and management. *Nat Clin Pract Nephrol* **2**: 136–48.

34 Marinella MA (2009). Refeeding syndrome: an important aspect of supportive oncology. *J Support Oncol* **7**: 11–16.

35 Walton RJ, Bijvoet OL (1975). Nomogram for derivation of renal threshold phosphate concentration. *Lancet* **2**: 309–10.

36 Buysschaert M, Cosyns JP, Barreto L, Jadoul M (2003). Pamidronate-induced tubu-lointerstitial nephritis with Fanconi syndrome in a patient with primary hyperparathyroidism. *Nephrol Dial Transplant* **18**: 826–9.

37 Francois H, Coppo P, Hayman JP, Fouqueray B, Mougenot B, Ronco P (2008). Partial fanconi syndrome induced by imatinib therapy: a novel cause of urinary phosphate loss. *Am J of Kidney Diseases* **51**: 298–301.

38 Glezerman I, Kewalramani T, Jhaveri K (2008). Reversible Fanconi syndrome due to lenalidomide. *Nephrol Dial Transplant Plus* **4**: 215–17.

39 Berman E, Nicolaides M, Maki RG, Fleisher M, Chanel S, Scheu K, et al. (2006). Altered bone and mineral metabolism in patients receiving imatinib mesylate. *N Engl J Med* **354**: 2006–13.

40 Hutson TE, Figlin RA, Kuhn JG, Motzer RJ (2008). Targeted therapies for metastatic renal cell carcinoma: an overview of toxicity and dosing strategies. *Oncologist* **13**: 1084–96.

41 Pollack M, Yu A (2004). Clinical disturbances of calcium, magnesium and phosphate metabolism. In: *Brenner and Rector's the kidney*. 7 ed. (ed. B Brenner), pp. 1041–76. Saunders, Philadelphia.

42 Rampello E, Fricia T, Malaguarnera M (2006). The management of tumor lysis syndrome. *Nat Clin Pract Oncol* **3**: 438–47.

43 Lane JW, Rehak NN, Hortin GL, Zaoutis T, Krause PR, Walsh TJ (2008). Pseudohyperphosphatemia associated with high-dose liposomal amphotericin B therapy. *Clin Chim Acta* **387**: 145–9.

44 Bourque CW (2008). Central mechanisms of osmosensation and systemic osmoregulation. *Nat Rev Neurosci* **9**: 519–31.

45 Berl T, Schrier R (1992). Disorders of water metabolism. In: *Renal and electrolyte disorders*. 4 ed. (ed. R Schrier), pp. 1–87. Little, Brown and Company, Boston/Toronto/London.

46 Rose B, Post T (2001). Meaning and application of urine chemistries. In: *Clinical physiology of acid-base and electrolyte disorders*. 5 ed., pp. 405–13. McGraw Hill, New York.

47 Berghmans T, Paesmans M, Body JJ (2000). A prospective study on hyponatraemia in medical cancer patients: epidemiology, aetiology and differential diagnosis. *Support Care Cancer* **8**: 192–7.

48 Glezerman IG (2009). Successful treatment of ifosfamide-induced hyponatremia with AVP receptor antagonist without interruption of hydration for prevention of hemorrhagic cystitis. *Ann Oncol* **20**: 1283–5.

49 Sorensen JB, Andersen MK, Hansen HH (1995). Syndrome of inappropriate secretion of antidiuretic hormone (SIADH) in malignant disease. *J Intern Med* **238**: 97–110.

50 Vanhees SL, Paridaens R, Vansteenkiste JF (2000). Syndrome of inappropriate antidiuretic hormone associated with chemotherapy-induced tumour lysis in small-cell lung cancer: case report and literature review. *Ann Oncol* **11**: 1061–5.

51 Raff H (1987). Glucocorticoid inhibition of neurohypophysial vasopressin secretion. *Am J Physiol* **252**: R635–44.

52 Schrier RW (2006). Body water homeostasis: clinical disorders of urinary dilution and concentration. *J Am Soc Nephrol* **17**: 1820–32.

53 Zeltser D, Rosansky S, van Rensburg H, Verbalis JG, Smith N (2007). Assessment of the efficacy and safety of intravenous conivaptan in euvolemic and hypervolemic hyponatremia. *Am J Nephrol* **27**: 447–57.

54 Raftopoulos H (2007). Diagnosis and management of hyponatremia in cancer patients. *Support Care Cancer* **15**: 1341–7.

55 Robertson GL (1984). Abnormalities of thirst regulation. *Kidney Int* **25**: 460–9.

56 Grier JF (1995). WDHA (watery diarrhea, hypokalemia, achlorhydria) syndrome: clinical features, diagnosis, and treatment. *South Med J* **88**: 22–4.

57 Rose B, Post T (2001). Hyperosmolal states—hypernatremia. Clinical physiology of acid base and electrolyte disorders. 5 ed. McGraw Hill, New York, pp. 746–93.

58 Foresti V, Casati O, Villa A, Lazzaro A, Confalonieri F (1992). Central diabetes insipidus due to acute monocytic leukemia: case report and review of the literature. *J Endocrinol Invest* **15**: 127–30.

59 Muller CI, Engelhardt M, Laubenberger J, Kunzmann R, Engelhardt R, Lubbert M (2002). Myelodysplastic syndrome in transformation to acute myeloid leukemia presenting with diabetes insipidus: due to pituitary infiltration association with abnormalities of chromosomes 3 and 7. *Eur J Haematol* **69**: 115–19.

60 Frokiaer J, Marples D, Knepper MA, Nielsen S (1996). Bilateral ureteral obstruction downregulates expression of vasopressin-sensitive AQP-2 water channel in rat kidney. *Am J Physiol* **270**: F657–68.

61 Carone FA, Epstein FH (1960). Nephrogenic diabetes insipidus caused by amyloid disease. Evidence in man of the role of the collecting ducts in concentrating urine. *Am J Med* **29**: 539–44.

62 Garofeanu CG, Weir M, Rosas-Arellano MP, Henson G, Garg AX, Clark WF (2005). Causes of reversible nephrogenic diabetes insipidus: a systematic review. *Am J Kidney Dis* **45**: 626–37.

63 Smith OP, Gale R, Hamon M, McWhinney P, Prentice HG (1994). Amphotericin B-induced nephrogenic diabetes insipidus: resolution with its liposomal counterpart. *Bone Marrow Transplant* **13**: 107–8.

64 Canada TW, Weavind LM, Augustin KM (2003). Possible liposomal amphotericin B-induced nephrogenic diabetes insipidus. *Ann Pharmacother* **37**(1): 70–3.

65 Schliefer K, Rockstroh JK, Spengler U, Sauerbruch T (1997). Nephrogenic diabetes insipidus in a patient taking cidofovir. *Lancet* **350**: 413–14.

66 Navarro JF, Quereda C, Gallego N, Antela A, Mora C, Ortuno J (1996). Nephrogenic diabetes insipidus and renal tubular acidosis secondary to foscarnet therapy. *Am J Kidney Dis* **27**: 431–4.

67 Gellai M, Edwards BR, Valtin H (1979). Urinary concentrating ability during dehydration in the absence of vasopressin. *Am J Physiol* **237**: F100–4.

68 Rose B, Post T (2001). Hyperkalemia. Clinical physiology of acid base and electrolyte disorders. 5 ed. McGraw Hill, New York, pp. 888–930.

69 Smellie WS (2007). Spurious hyperkalaemia. *BMJ* **334**: 693–5.

70 Bosch X, Poch E, Grau JM (2009). Rhabdomyolysis and acute kidney injury. *N Engl J Med* **361**: 62–72.

71 Nicolin G (2002). Emergencies and their management. *Eur J Cancer* **38**: 1365–77; discussion 78–9.

72 Alani FS, Dyer T, Hindle E, Newsome DA, Ormerod LP, Mahoney MP (1994). Pseudohyperkalaemia associated with hereditary spherocytosis in four members of a family. *Postgrad Med J* **70**: 749–51.

73 Smith HM, Farrow SJ, Ackerman JD, Stubbs JR, Sprung J (2008). Cardiac arrests associated with hyperkalemia during red blood cell transfusion: a case series. *Anesth Analg* **106**: 1062–9, table of contents.

74 Chen CH, Hong CL, Kau YC, Lee HL, Chen CK, Shyr MH (1999). Fatal hyperkalemia during rapid and massive blood transfusion in a child undergoing hip surgery—a case report. *Acta Anaesthesiol Sin* **37**: 163–6.

75 Eskandar N, Holley JL (2008). Hyperkalaemia as a complication of ureteroileostomy: a case report and literature review. *Nephrol Dial Transplant* **23**: 2081–3.

76 Pearce CJ, Gonzalez FM, Wallin JD (1993). Renal failure and hyperkalemia associated with ketorolac tromethamine. *Arch Intern Med* **153**: 1000–2.

77 Tan SY, Shapiro R, Franco R, Stockard H, Mulrow PJ (1979). Indomethacin-induced prostaglandin inhibition with hyperkalemia. A reversible cause of hyporeninemic hypoaldosteronism. *Ann Intern Med* **90**: 783–5.

78 Michelis MF (1990). Hyperkalemia in the elderly. *Am J Kidney Dis* **16**: 296–9.

79 Margassery S, Bastani B (2001). Life threatening hyperkalemia and acidosis secondary to trimethoprim-sulfamethoxazole treatment. *J Nephrol* **14**: 410–14.

80 Takami A, Asakura H, Takamatsu H, Yamazaki H, Arahata M, Hayashi T et al. (2005). Isolated hyperkalemia associated with cyclosporine administration in allogeneic stem cell transplantation for renal cell carcinoma. *Int J Hematol* **81**: 159–61.

81 Rogers FB, Li SC (2001). Acute colonic necrosis associated with sodium polystyrene sulfonate (Kayexalate) enemas in a critically ill patient: case report and review of the literature. *J Trauma* **51**: 395–7.

82 Gennari FJ (1998). Hypokalemia. *N Engl J Med* **339**: 451–8.

83 Barri YM, Knochel JP (1996). Hypercalcemia and electrolyte disturbances in malignancy. *Hematol Oncol Clin North Am* **10**: 775–90.

84 Naparstek Y, Gutman A (1984). Case report: spurious hypokalemia in myeloproliferative disorders. *Am J Med Sci* **288**: 175–7.

85 Masters PW, Lawson N, Marenah CB, Maile LJ (1996). High ambient temperature: a spurious cause of hypokalaemia. *BMJ* **312**: 1652–3.

86 Gennari FJ (2002). Disorders of potassium homeostasis. Hypokalemia and hyperkalemia. *Crit Care Clin* **18**: 273–88, vi.

87 Perazella MA, Eisen RN, Frederick WG, Brown E (1993). Renal failure and severe hypokalemia associated with acute myelomonocytic leukemia. *Am J Kidney Dis* **22**: 462–7.

88 Izzedine H, Besse B, Lazareth A, Bourry EF, Soria JC (2009). Hypokalemia, metabolic alkalosis, and hypertension in a lung cancer patient. *Kidney Int* **76**: 115–20.

89 Ben Salem C, Hmouda H, Bouraoui K (2009). Drug-induced hypokalaemia. *Curr Drug Saf* **4**: 55–61.

90 Saif MW (2008). Management of hypomagnesemia in cancer patients receiving chemotherapy. *J Support Oncol* **6**: 243–8.

91 al-Ghamdi SM, Cameron EC, Sutton RA (1994). Magnesium deficiency: pathophysiologic and clinical overview. *Am J Kidney Dis* **24**: 737–52.

92 Rose B, Post T (2001). Clinical use of diuretics. *Clinical physiology of acid base and electrolyte disorders*. 5 ed, pp. 447–77. McGraw Hill, New York.

93 Tejpar S, Piessevaux H, Claes K, Piront P, Hoenderop JG, Verslype C, et al. (2007). Magnesium wasting associated with epidermal-growth-factor receptor-targeting antibodies in colorectal cancer: a prospective study. *Lancet Oncol* **8**: 387–94.

94 Rose B, Post T (2001). *Hypokalemia. Clinical physiology of acid base and electrolyte disorders*. 5 ed. McGraw Hill, New York, p. 855.

95 von der Weid NX, Erni BM, Mamie C, Wagner HP, Bianchetti MG (1999). Cisplatin therapy in childhood: renal follow up 3 years or more after treatment. Swiss Pediatric Oncology Group. *Nephrol Dial Transplant* **14**: 1441–4.

96 Vokes EE, Mick R, Vogelzang NJ, Geiser R, Douglas F (1990). A randomised study comparing intermittent to continuous administration of magnesium aspartate hydrochloride in cisplatin-induced hypomagnesaemia. *Br J Cancer* **62**: 1015–17.

97 Quamme GA (1982). Effect of hypercalcemia on renal tubular handling of calcium and magnesium. *Can J Physiol Pharmacol* **60**: 1275–80.

98 Liamis G, Gianoutsos C, Elisaf M (2001). Acute pancreatitis-induced hypomagnesemia. *Pancreatology* **1**: 74–6.

Chapter 3

Paraneoplastic glomerulopathies

Christopher Valentine and Lee A. Hebert

Introduction

The term 'paraneoplastic glomerulopathies' refers to glomerular diseases apparently caused by cancers, via the secretion of hormones, growth factors, cytokines, or antigens. Thus, a paraneoplastic glomerulopathy is not the direct result of tumor burden, invasion, or metastases (1). The nephropathies caused by malignant or nonmalignant plasma cell dyscrasias are discussed in a separate chapter.

We begin with a case report of a patient with membranous nephropathy, which is known to be associated with malignancy. There is controversy regarding the extent of the search for malignancy.

Case report

A 56-year-old Caucasian man was evaluated for a two-month history of leg edema and nephrotic-range proteinuria. Three years earlier, he had proteinuria detected by dipstick, but was well otherwise. His edema was controlled by furosemide. There was no history of regular NSAID use. He had a 50-pack-a-year history of cigarette smoking. His weight was 98 kg, pulse 52, blood pressure 140/70 mmHg. His physical exam was otherwise unremarkable. His serum creatinine was 84 μmol/L; the proteinuria was 7.2 g/day (protein/creatinine ratio 4.4). The following tests were either normal or negative: renal ultrasound, serum protein electrophoresis, complete blood count (CBC), electrolytes, serum calcium, hepatitis B and C serologies, alanine aminotransferase (ALT), aspartate aminotransferase (AST), alkaline phosphatase, prostatic specific antigen (PSA), carcinoembryonic antigen (CEA), chest radiograph, and stool for occult blood.

His kidney biopsy contained 13 glomeruli. Under light microscopy, three were globally sclerotic and the rest were unremarkable. Of note, there was no evidence of capillary microthrombi or neutrophils, a finding reported in cancer-associated MN. A medium-sized artery showed mild arteriosclerosis with focal hyalinosis. Immunofluorescence microscopy of eight glomeruli showed IgG 4+ diffuse and granular in the glomerular basement membrane (GBM). Arterioles showed C3 1+ focally. Staining for albumin, fibrinogen, IgA, IgM, and C1q was negative. Electron microscopy revealed numerous subepithelial GBM deposits. There were no mesangial or tubular basement membrane deposits to suggest systemic lupus erythematosus. The GBM extrusion between the subepithelial deposits was moderate. The histopathologic diagnosis was membranous nephropathy (MN) stage II, probably idiopathic.

Initial therapy

A daily dosage of 10 mg enalapril was started, but as a generalized rash developed, it was changed to a daily dosage of 100 mg losartan. Two months later, the urine protein/creatinine ratio was 4.6. Five months later, it was 0.60. His blood pressure was 130/80 mmHg and serum creatinine, 84 μmol/L.

The first relapse

Six months later, i.e. one year after the kidney biopsy, his serum creatinine increased to 130 μmol/L and proteinuria to 4.3 g/day (protein/creatinine ratio 2.5). A modification of the Ponticelli protocol was begun in which oral cyclophosphamide 100 mg daily was given for one month, followed by prednisone 20 mg daily for one month. This regimen was continued for a total of six months. It was well tolerated. By the fourth month of the therapy, he was in remission. His urine protein/creatinine ratio was 0.26 and serum creatinine was 145 μmol/L.

The second relapse

About two years after completing the Ponticelli protocol, which was three years after the kidney biopsy, his proteinuria increased to 1.7 g/day (protein/creatinine ratio 1.0). Serum creatinine was stable at 145 μmol/L. Since he had already lost substantial kidney function to his MN, a decision was made to re-treat his recurrent proteinuria. He received a second course of the modified Ponticelli protocol. His proteinuria stabilized. About one year later, which was four years after the kidney biopsy, his serum creatinine began to increase. Rather than re-treat with cyclophosphamide, mycophenolate mofetil 1000 mg twice a day was begun. Because of his relapses, he was reevaluated for occult malignancy. Colonoscopy revealed a rectal adenocarcinoma.

The controversy

Was the rectal carcinoma the cause of the MN and its relapses? Should the initial search for carcinoma have been more thorough? Did the immunosuppression cause a new cancer? Should each relapse of MN be an indication to reassess for malignancy? Our analysis of the case report, based on the contents of this chapter, is discussed at the end of the chapter.

Epidemiology of malignancy-associated glomerulopathy

Table 3.1 shows the types of glomerulopathies that have been reported in association with cancer. As can be seen, MN is associated with the widest variety of cancers. In addition, MN has the strongest association with cancer (2). In retrospective analyses of paraneoplastic glomerulopathies (2–4), membranous nephropathy accounted for 44–69 % of all of the instances of paraneoplastic glomerulopathies. However, the Danish Kidney Biopsy Registry showed that membranous nephropathy accounted for only about 20% of all instances of cancer-associated primary glomerulopathy (5). Since this study is population based, it may represent a more accurate estimate of the prevalence of MN among the paraneoplastic glomerulopathies, as discussed below.

The reported incidence of cancer in patients presenting with MN varies from 5% to 22% (1). Almost all of these cancers occurred in MN patients

Table 3.1 Specific glomerulopathies and their associated malignancies

Glomerulopathy	Associated malignancies
Membranous nephropathy (MN) (6–13)	Bronchogenic carcinoma (squamous cell, small cell, adenocarcinoma)
	Adenocarcinoma of colon and rectum
	Adenocarcinoma of breast
	Undifferentiated anaplastic carcinoma
	Adenocarcinoma of stomach
	Hepatocellular carcinoma
	Squamous cell esophageal
	Carcinoid tumor
	Head and neck (palate, pharynx, hypopharynx, larynx)
	Wilm's tumor
	Renal clear cell adenocarcinoma
	Bladder (transitional cell)
	Ovarian (teratoma, adenocarcinoma)
	Cervical and endometrial
	Placental site trophoblastic tumor
	Choriocarcinoma
	Penis
	Prostate
	Skin (squamous cell, basal cell, melanoma)
	Thyroid adenocarcinoma
	Hematologic malignancies (Hodgkin's lymphoma, non Hodgkin's lymphoma, angiofollicular lymphadenopathy, angioimmunoblastic lymphadenopathy, lymphosarcoma
	Acute myeloid leukemia
	Chronic lymphocytic leukemia
	Chronic myelomonocytic leukemia
	Pheochromocytoma
	Carotid body tumor
	Spinal cord neuroma
	Neuroblastoma
	Thymoma
	Adrenal ganglioneuroma

(continued)

Table 3.1 *(continued)* Specific glomerulopathies and their associated malignancies

Glomerulopathy	Associated malignancies
Minimal Change Disease (MCD) (14–24)	Digestive tract (colon, rectal, pancreas)
	Genitourinary tract (renal clear cell, adenocarcinoma, transitional cell, Wilm's tumor, prostate)
	Hematologic malignancies (Hodgkin's lymphoma, non Hodgkin's lymphoma, angiofollicular lymphadenopathy
	Chronic lymphocytic leukemia
	Chronic myeloid leukemia
	Lung (bronchogenic carcinoma, mesothelioma)
	Mesenchymal tumors (retroperitoneal liposarcoma, malignant mesothelioma)
	Thymoma
	Ovarian
Membranoproliferative glomerulonephritis (MPGN) (25–29)	Chronic lymphocytic leukemia
	Esophagus (squamous cell)
	Gastric MALT lymphoma
	Hairy cell leukemia
	Chronic myeloid leukemia
	Hodgkin's and non Hodgkin's lymphoma
	Lymphomatoid granulomatosis
	Reticulum cell sarcoma
	Melanoma
	Wilm's tumor
	Prostate
	Non small cell lung
	Carcinoma of unknown primary site
IgA nephritis (IgA N) (30, 31)	Lung (squamous cell, small cell)
	Nasopharynx
	Hodgkin's lymphoma
	Non Hodgkin's lymphoma
	Pancreas
	Renal clear cell adenocarcinoma
	Retroperitoneal liposarcoma
	Basal cell
	Tongue (squamous cell)
	IgG lambda light chain plasmacytoma

Table 3.1 *(continued)* Specific glomerulopathies and their associated malignancies

Glomerulopathy	Associated malignancies
Focal segmental glomerulosclerosis (FSGS) (32 – 34)	Hodgkin's lymphoma
	Non Hodgkin's lymphoma
	Leukemias (CLL, AML, T cell)
	Thymoma
	Non small cell lung
Crescentic GN (CGN) (35–38)	Adenocarcinoma of lung
	Bronchogenic carcinoma
	Chronic lymphocytic leukemia
	Hodgkin's lymphoma
	Non Hodgkin's lymphoma
	Gastric adenocarcinoma
	Colon
	Larynx
	Renal cell carcinoma
	Prostate
	Penis
	Sinus histiocytosis with massive lymphadenopathy
	Thymoma
AA amyloidosis (39–42)	Hodgkin's disease
	Renal cell carcinoma
	Bladder
	Gastric
	Sarcoma of spleen
	GI stromal tumor

over the age of 50 years. Although there is general agreement that MN is significantly associated with cancer, not all centers find such high incidence rates (43). Thus, the high incidence rates of cancer-associated MN may reflect publication bias. For example, centers that observe a strong association between cancer and MN are more likely to report their results than centers that see no relationship between MN and cancer. However, studies that examine an entire population (population-based studies), rather than cohorts within a population, are less likely to suffer from publication bias. In this connection, the population-based Danish Kidney Biopsy Registry revealed a 9% incidence of cancer-associated MN (20 instances of cancer in 215 cases of MN) (5).

When MN is the cause of the paraneoplastic glomerulopathy, usually the nephrotic syndrome and the cancer are discovered simultaneously or the cancer has already manifested. It is unusual for the cancer to manifest itself later than 12 months after the onset of the MN (2–4, 44).

Minimal change disease (MCD) is a well-established paraneoplastic glomerulopathy, especially in Hodgkin's disease and lymphomas. Nevertheless, the prevalence of MCD in these conditions is low. For example, only about 0.4% of Hodgkin's disease patients have MCD (45–6).

Membranoproliferative glomerulonephritis (MPGN) has a small but significant association with hematologic malignancies, particularly those that can induce Type I or Type II cryoglobulinemia (1).

IgA nephritis (IgAN) has been reported to be paraneoplastic in 23% of patients whose onset of IgAN was at age 60 or older. The malignancy was of the mucosal immune system, especially of the head and the neck (47). In contrast to older IgAN patients, none of the IgAN patients with an onset of the disease under age 60 years had associated malignancy (47).

Henoch–Schönlein purpura, with necrotic skin lesions in the absence of cryoglobulinemia, should also prompt a search for cancer (1), particularly of the mucosal immune system of the respiratory, the gastrointestinal, and the genitourinary systems.

Crescentic glomerulonephritis (CGN) that is paraneoplastic has been reported in 7–9% of patients presented with idiopathic pauci-immune crescentic glomerulonephritis (48–9). Several of these patients were positive for antineutrophil cytoplasmic antigen (ANCA) suggesting the co-existence of idiopathic ANCA-related vasculitis or Wegener's granulomatosus. In some of these patients, the cancer was not evident at presentation (50). This suggests that patients with CGN should be routinely assessed for cancer, particularly of the lower respiratory tract (1).

AA amyloidosis can occur as a paraneoplastic syndrome in which the inflammation associated with cancer, particularly Hodgkin's disease, or renal cell carcinoma, can lead to excessive production of serum protein A with deposition in parenchymal organs, including the kidney (1). In such patients, the cancer is usually evident and chronic.

Interestingly, despite the high prevalence of breast and prostate cancer, paraneoplastic glomerulopathies are rarely seen associated with these cancers (1).

Pathogenesis of paraneoplastic glomerulopathy

Ronco (1) has suggested that to prove a causal relationship between a specific cancer and glomerulopathy, three conditions must be met: 1) clinical and histological remission of the glomerulopathy should occur after eradication or remission of the cancer; 2) if relapse of the cancer occurs, it should be followed by relapse of the glomerulopathy; and 3) there needs to be direct evidence that the tumor caused the glomerulopathy. For example, in the case of MN, elution of the immune complexes from the glomeruli should show the tumor antigens, and antibodies specific to the tumor antigen. Remarkably, no single case of paraneoplastic glomerulopathy has fulfilled all these criteria (1, 44). However, enough of these criteria linking cancer to MN have been fulfilled that most authors feel comfortable in ascribing a causal role to cancer in MN. The same cannot be said regarding the pathogenesis of most of the other paraneoplastic glomerulopathies. Thus, in the discussion that follows, generally the emphasis is on the possibility of the association of malignancy with the glomerulopathy, rather than proof of causal relationship.

Membranous nephropathy (MN)

Of the non-myeloma-related paraneoplastic glomerulopathies, MN is the best studied. With regard to the criteria for paraneoplastic causation of glomerulopathy put forth by Ronco (1), we suggest the following with respect to cancer-associated MN:

There have been numerous reports of the nephrotic syndrome of cancer-associated MN, remitting with successful tumor therapy, and relapsing with tumor recurrence (see the section on 'Treatment'). In some cases of paraneoplastic MN, tumor-specific antibodies have been eluted from the glomeruli. In other cases, tumor-related antigens have been identified in the MN glomerular deposits (1). The specific antigens include RTE (a renal brush border lipoprotein antigen that includes megalin (51)), CEA, and PSA (1). The pathogenesis of the cancer-associated MN is believed to involve glomerular deposition or in situ formation (52).

Minimal change disease (MCD)

This disorder is classically associated with Hodgkin's disease but numerous other cancers have also been implicated (Table 3.1). The MCD is thought to result from T-cell lymphokines that disrupt the glomerular filtration barrier, specifically the podocytes (53).

Membranoproliferative glomerulonephritis Type 1 (MPGN)

This paraneoplastic MPGN is usually associated with the monoclonal gammopathies of chronic lymphocytic leukemia and B-cell lymphomas (1). The monoclonal protein may be a precipitating or a nonprecipitating (in the cold) cryoglobulin, which results in the characteristic immunoglobulin containing microtubular structures in the glomerular capillaries or mesangium (1).

The cryoglobulin may be either Type I (the deposit consists of a self-aggregating monoclonal immunoglobulin) or Type II (the monoclonal protein is usually an IgM that has specificity for the Fc region of polyclonal immunoglobulins—the IgM functions as a rheumatoid factor—resulting in the formation of precipitable circulating immune complexes) (54). Included in the immune complex could also be the antigens to which the polyclonal immunoglobulin may be directed. The inflammation and proliferation caused by the glomerular deposition of the cryoglobulin is thought to be initiated by the activation of the complement system (55).

Glomerular amyloidosis

This can be AL amyloid (deposition of free monoclonal light chains from a benign or malignant clonal expansion of plasma cells (see Chapter 4) or AA amyloid (deposition of the acute phase reactant serum protein A, which is produced in excessive amounts in chronic inflammation and accumulates in the tissue). Cancer-associated AA amyloid glomerulopathy is seen in Hodgkin's disease (45, 56) and in the renal cell carcinoma-associated glomerulopathy. The secretion of IL-6 by renal cell carcinoma has proinflammatory effects that account for the fever and possibly the AA amyloidosis of renal cell carcinoma (1).

IgA nephritis (IgAN)

This is a disorder of the mucosal immune system, which constitutively secretes IgA capable of forming immune complexes (57). Tumors of the mucosal immune system, particularly of the upper respiratory tract, have a significant association with IgA nephritis, when the onset of the nephritis occurs over the age of 60 years (47). Also, at autopsy, cancers of the gastrointestinal tract have been shown to be associated with glomerular IgA deposits, possibly the result of stimulation of the mucosal immune system by the cancer (58).

Crescentic glomerulonephritis (CGN)

Most cases of pauci-immune CGN (no evidence of immunoglobulin deposition by immunofluorescent or electron microscopy) are ANCA positive. The pathogenesis of ANCA-related glomerulonephritis is unknown; however, it is widely believed that it is a T-cell-mediated disorder in which ANCA serves as an exacerbating factor (59). The mechanism of the association of pauci-immune CGN with cancer is unclear. However, it is plausible that immune activation by the cancer is responsible.

Other paraneoplastic glomerulopathies

These include fibrillary GN, immunotactoid GN, and Goodpasture's syndrome (anti-GBM disease) (1). The mechanisms by which these disorders may be associated with cancer are unclear but immune activation by the cancer is plausible.

Mechanisms of paraneoplastic nephropathy

Cancers can also cause impaired kidney function (nephropathy) by mechanisms other than that of a glomerulopathy. As shown in Fig. 3.1, cancer cells directly invade the glomeruli (60–2), or can form glomerular crescents (63). Tumors can also cause nephropathy by invasion of the renal parenchyma, occlusion of the renin vein, compression of the renal arteries, or the obstruction of ureters (1). Cancer or cancer chemotherapy associated thrombotic microangiopathy can cause a paraneoplastic glomerulopathy (64).

Assessment for malignancy in patients presenting with glomerulopathy

Table 3.2 lists clinical scenarios in which there should be a heightened awareness for the possibility of a paraneoplastic glomerulopathy.

Fig. 3.1 is an algorithm intended to optimize the search to determine if the glomerulopathy may be paraneoplastic. The assumptions underlying the algorithm are as follows:

- Proteinuria or albuminuria, usually at low levels, occurs with increased frequency in patients with malignancy (67–8). Thus, unexplained proteinuria, even if it is at a low level, is an indication for at least an age and gender appropriate search for malignancy (Table 3.3, Part 1).

- Older age is a risk factor for paraneoplastic glomerulopathy (69). Patients over 50 years with glomerulopathy should have an age and gender appropriate screening for malignancy (Table 3.3, Part 1).

- Patients with a systemic disorder such as diabetes mellitus that can explain their glomerulopathy (a secondary glomerulopathy) have a credible explanation for their glomerulopathy. Thus, except in certain instances (see Fig. 3.1), only an age and gender appropriate search for malignancy is warranted. The search described in Table 3.3, Part 1, should be sufficient.

Patients with no systemic disorder to explain their glomerulopathy are in need of an explanation for their glomerulopathy. Thus, an expanded search for malignancy (Table 3.3, Parts 1 and 2) may be appropriate, particularly for those at increased risk as highlighted in Table 3.2.

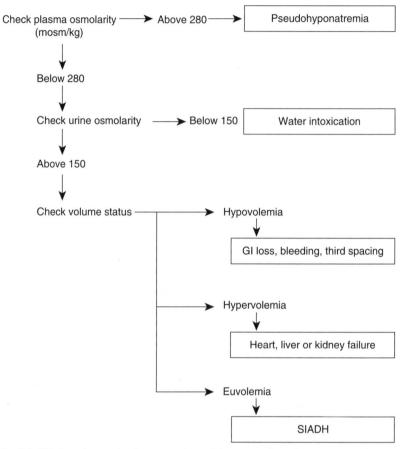

Check plasma osmolarity ⟶ Above 280 ⟶ Pseudohyponatremia
(mosm/kg)

Below 280

Check urine osmolarity ⟶ Below 150 → Water intoxication

Above 150

Check volume status ⟶ Hypovolemia

GI loss, bleeding, third spacing

⟶ Hypervolemia

Heart, liver or kidney failure

⟶ Euvolemia

SIADH

Fig. 3.1 This is a glomerulus from a patient with metastatic melanoma. Note the tumor cell emboli in the glomerular capillaries (arrows). The lesion mimics a focal proliferative glomerulonephritis; however, the nuclei of the tumor cells are much larger and more irregular than the nuclei of intrinsic glomerular cells of white blood cells (H&E, 400).

Table 3.2 Clinical and pathologic indicators that a glomerulopathy may be paraneoplastic

Indicator:
Older age (average age 73 in malignancy associated MN) (65)
> or = 20 pack years cigarette smoking (65)
Glomerular leukocytic infiltrate of > 8 cells/glomerulus. Includes polymorphonuclear and mononuclear leukocytes. (65)
Predominance of IgG_1 and IgG_2 (66)

Table 3.3 Recommended testing to search for malignancy in patients with glomerular proteinuria Part 1: Standard testing for malignancy inpatients with 1° or 2° glomerulopathy

Test	Comment
1 History	Emphasis: Personal and family history of malignancies, radiation exposure, prior chemotherapy or radiation therapy
2 Physical exam	Emphasis: Lymph nodes, skin, liver, spleen. Males: Digital rectal and testicular exam Females: Breast, pelvic, and rectal exam
3 Laboratory testing/imaging	
Complete blood count, differential count and platelets	Hematologic malignancies
Comprehensive metabolic profile	Liver disease, cancer-related hypercalcemia, hyperuricemia, hypoalbuminemia
Serum immunofixation	Monoclonal gammopathy
Urine immunofixation	Monoclonal gammopathy
Stool for occult blood	Adenocarcinoma, colon
Males: prostatic specific antigen	Prostate cancer
Females: mammogram, pap smear	Gynecologic malignancies Breast cancer
Colonoscopy	If family history of colon cancer or indicated based on age
Chest X-ray	Pulmonary renal syndrome, lymphoma

Part 2: Expanded testing for those with primary glomerulopathy or selected patients with secondary glomerulopathy (see Fig. 3.2)

Test	Comment
Colonoscopy and Esophagogastroduodenoscopy, if MN > 50 years or IgAN > 60 years	Gastrointestinal malignancies in older patients with MN or IgAN
Triple endoscopy by otolaryngologist in patient > 60 years with IgAN	Head and neck cancer in IgAN
Flow cytometry in MCD or MPGN if over age 60 years	Leukemia, lymphomas
Chest CT scan if smoking history	More sensitive than chest X-ray in screening for chest malignancy
Bone marrow examination in MPGN, if unexplained leukopenia, abnormalities of leukocyte subsets, thrombocytopenia, or anemia	Leukemia associated with MPGN

The work of Birkeland (5) and our case report emphasizes that patients with glomerulopathy may also be at an increased risk for cancer, either as the cause of the glomerulopathy, or as the result of the therapy for the glomerulopathy. In either event, it seems prudent to have a heightened awareness of cancer in patients with glomerulopathy, both at presentation and during the follow-up.

Certain therapies used to treat malignancies can themselves induce a glomerulopathy. In doing so, they could mimic the onset of a paraneoplastic glomerulopathy, suggesting that the cancer therapy was ineffective. The cancer therapeutic agents that can induce a glomerulopathy include interferon-α (70) and bevacizumab (71).

Treatment of paraneoplastic glomerulopathies

Primary management of paraneoplastic glomerulopathy

The primary approach is to treat the cancer. Cancer treatments are beyond the scope of this chapter. However, below we briefly describe examples of regression of paraneoplastic glomerulopathy by therapy.

In paraneoplastic MN, remission of nephrotic syndrome after tumor ablation has been documented in several patients (1, 44, 72).

In paraneoplastic MCD, remission has been achieved by the removal of the tumor (73–5). In those with MCD in whom cure for the malignancy was not achievable, chemotherapy of the lymphoma (76); or treatment of the MCD with prednisone (77) or cyclosporin (78) was associated with remission of the nephrotic syndrome.

In paraneoplastic MPGN associated with hematologic malignancies, remission of the nephrotic syndrome occurs if the chemotherapy is successful in controlling the hematologic disorder (1).

In paraneoplastic AA amyloidosis caused by Castleman's disease, remission has occurred with excision of the lymphoid masses (79).

Chemotherapy can remit nephrotic syndrome caused by the direct invasion of the glomeruli by leukemic cells (80–1).

Secondary management of paraneoplastic glomerulopathy

It may be appropriate to consider renoprotective therapies in patients with paraneoplastic glomerulopathies even though the malignancy underlying their nephropathy may be untreatable. The notion is that if the cancer is only slowly progressive, it would be important to protect kidney function so that the patient is not confronted with a dual problem of end-stage kidney failure and a progressive malignancy. The strongest single factor determining progression of kidney disease is the magnitude of proteinuria (82–3). The mechanism of this association is that proteinuria magnitude is the single most important mechanism of kidney disease progression. Thus, interventions that reduce proteinuria slow progression of kidney disease. In general, for every 1 gram reduction in proteinuria, GFR decline is slowed by about 1 or 2 mL/min/yr. Thus measures that result in only a modest reduction in proteinuria can have a marked effect on delaying the onset of end-stage kidney failure as shown in Fig. 3.2.

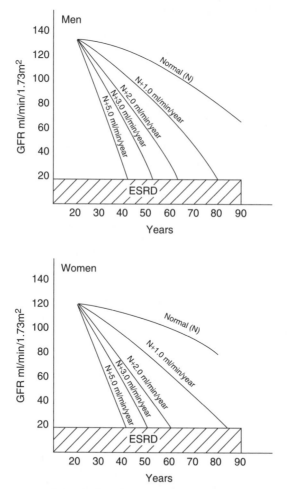

Fig. 3.2 Average rate of GFR decline due to aging (top curve) in comparison to hypothetical patients each with onset of a progressive kidney disease at age 25 years but with different rates of GFR decline superimposed on the GFR decline of aging (top panel, men; bottom panel, women). Note that small differences in the GFR decline rate can result in large differences in time to onset of ESRD [82].

A detailed discussion of renoprotective and antiproteinuric therapies is beyond the scope of this chapter. However, Table 3.4 lists the key renoprotective regimens.

In patients with MPGN induced by Type I or Type II cryoglobulins related to a hematopoietic malignancy, cryoprotein removal by plasmapheresis can be an important adjunct to chemotherapeutic agents in order to induce remission of the kidney disease.

Analysis of our case report

The analysis consists in answering the questions posed in the 'Controversy' segment of the Case Report, as follows:

Table 3.4 Key kidney protective therapies

Intervention	Goal/comment
1 Control blood pressure	The goal is a sitting systolic blood pressure in the 120s or less, if tolerated. The greater the proteinuria, the greater is the benefit of blood pressure control in slowing progression of kidney disease
2 ACE inhibitor therapy (ACEI)	Use ACEI even if the patient is normotensive. ACEI is the first choice because it is not clear whether the cardioprotective effects of angiotensin receptor blockers (ARB) are equal to ACEI. ACEI used in maximally recommended doses of ACEI, if tolerated. The goal is to reduce proteinuria to
3 Combination ACEI and ARB therapies	Adding ARB to maximum ACEI can reduce proteinuria further. However, this may also predispose to acute renal failure. Avoid ACEI and ARB combination in those with heart failure receiving a β-blocker
4 Dietary management	Avoid excessive salt intake, unless the patient has renal salt wasting. High salt intake strongly promotes proteinuria and can worsen hypertension. Appropriate salt intake is about 2 to 3 g of sodium (88 to 125 mEq of sodium) daily. To optimize the taste of salt, the salt should be added to the surface of the food just prior to eating, rather than adding the salt during preparation. Salt that is within the food (added during preparation) is less well tasted than 'surface salt'. Avoid a high protein intake. High protein intake worsens proteinuria because it causes renal vasodilatation. An appropriate intake of protein is about 0.8 to 1.0 gm/kg ideal body weight/day. Avoid 'pushing' fluids. A high-fluid intake does not protect kidney function and can worsen proteinuria. Thirst should dictate fluid intake. In general, there is no advantage to excreting more than 2 L of urine daily, unless the goal is to prevent kidney stone formation. Kidney stone formation can be a problem in patients with malignancy causing hypercalcemia.

Was the rectal carcinoma, the cause of the membranous nephropathy and its relapse?

Probably not. This conclusion is based on the assumption that the proteinuria, noted three years prior to the diagnosis of the MN, was the earliest MN manifestation. If that is the case, his rectal carcinoma would have to have been present for more than eight years, which seems unlikely.

Should the initial search for carcinoma been more thorough?

We relied on fecal testing for occult blood, the traditional testing means to screen for gastrointestinal carcinoma. This is the only screening test that has been shown to reduce colorectal cancer mortality. At presentation our patient was over 50 years of age. At that age, colonoscopy can be justified as a screening procedure for cancer.

Did the immunosuppression cause his new cancer?

Possibly. This is consistent with the insight by Birkeland (5) that patients with primary glomerulopathy have an increased incidence of cancer. These cancers were detected one to five years after the diagnosis of glomerular disease.

Should each relapse of MN be an indication to reassess for malignancy?

Maybe. This needs to be determined on a case-by-case basis.

Follow-up of our case

Since his last evaluation (2003), the patient's proteinuria is unchanged after surgery to remove his rectal carcinoma. This suggests that his rectal carcinoma is unrelated to his MN, unless he has unrecognized metastases.

References

1 Ronco PM (1999). Paraneoplastic glomerulopathies: new insights into an old entity. *Kidney Int* **56**: 355–77.

2 Eagen JW (1977). Glomerulopathies of neoplasia. *Kidney Int* **11**: 297–303.

3 Pai P, Bone JM, McDicken I, Bell GM (1996). Solid tumor and glomerulopathy. *Q J Med* **89**: 361–7.

4 Birkeland SA, Storm HH (2003). Glomerulonephritis and malignancy: A population-based analysis. *Kidney Int* **63**: 716–21.

5 Luyckx C, Van Damme B, Vanrenterghem Y, Maes B (2002). Carcinoid tumor and membranous glomerulonephritis: coincidence or malignancy-associated glomerulonephritis? *Clin Nephrol* **57**: 80–84.

6 Altiparmak MR, Pamuk ON, Pamuk GE, Ozbay G (2003). Membranous glomerulonephritis in a patient with choriocarcinoma: case report. *South Med J* **96**: 198–200.

7 Meydanli MM, Erguvan R, Altinok MT, Ataoglu O, Kafkasli A (2003). Rare case of neuroendocrine small cell carcinoma of the endometrium with paraneoplastic membranous glomerulonephritis. *Tumori* **89**: 213–17.

8 Texier F, Dharancy S, Provot F, Augusto D, Mortier PE, Mathurin P et al. (2004). Membranous glomerulonephritis complicating hepatocellular carcinoma. *Gastroenterol Clin Biol* **28**: 605–7.

9 Wadhwa NK, Gupta M, Afolabi A, Miller F (2004). Membranous glomerulonephritis in a patient with an adrenal ganglioneuroma. *Am J Kidney Dis* **44**: 363–8.

10 Sahiner S, Ayli MD, Yuksel C, Onec K, Abayli E (2004). Membranous nephropathy associated with acute myeloid leukemia. *Transplant Proc* **36**: 2618–19.

11 Batra V, Kalra OP, Mathur P, Kavita, Dev G (2007). Membranous glomerulopathy associated with placental site trophoblastic tumour: a case report. *Nephrol Dial Transplant* **22**: 1766–8.

12 Enriquez R, Sirvent AE, Marin F, Perez M, Alpera MR, Amoros F (2008). Severe renal complications in chronic myelomonocytic leukemia. *J Nephrol* **21**: 609–14.

13 Ohara G, Satoh H, Kurishima K, Ohtsuka M, Hizawa N (2009). Paraneoplastic nephrotic syndrome in patients with lung cancer. *Intern Med* **48**: 1817–20.

14 Fukuda A, Sato Y, Iwatsubo S, Komatsu H, Nishiura R, Fukudome K et al. (2009). Minimal change nephrotic syndrome complicated with recurrence of malignant thymoma: an interesting case with remission due to steroid therapy of both nephrotic syndrome and thymoma. *Nippon Jinzo Gakkai Shi* **51**: 130–7.

15 Bee PC, Gan GG, Sangkar VJ, Haris AR (2008). Nephrotic syndrome in a patient with relapsed of chronic myeloid leukemia after peripheral blood stem cell transplantation. *Med J Malaysia* **63**: 71–2.

16 Ryu DR, Yoo TH, Kim YT, Jeong HJ, Cho NH, Kang SW (2004). Minimal change disease in a patient with ovarian papillary serous carcinoma. *Gynecol Oncol* **93**: 554–6.

17 Talwar R, Dash SC, Kucheria K (2003). A case of chronic myeloid leukemia complicated with minimal change nephrotic syndrome. *Acta Haematol* **109**: 101–3.

18 Nakao K, Sugiyama H, Makino E, Matsuura H, Ohmoto A, Sugimoto T et al. (2002). Minimal change nephrotic syndrome developing during postoperative interferon-beta therapy for malignant melanoma. *Nephron* **90**: 498–500.

19 Lee HC, Cheng YF, Chuang FR, Chen JB, Hsu KT (2001). Minimal change nephrotic syndrome associated with malignant thymoma: case report and literature review. *Chang Gung Med J* **24**: 576–81.

20 Cossu A, Deiana A, Lissia A, Satta A, Cossu M, Dedola MF et al. (2004). Nephrotic syndrome and angiotropic lymphoma report of a case. *Tumori* **90**: 510–13.

21 Taniguchi K, Fujioka H, Torashima Y, Yamaguchi J, Izawa K, Kanematsu T (2004). Rectal cancer with paraneoplastic nephropathy: association of vascular endothelial growth factor. *Dig Surg* **21**: 455–7.

22 Karras A, de Montpreville V, Fakhouri F, Grunfeld JP, Lesavre P (2005). Renal and thymic pathology in thymoma-associated nephropathy: report of 21 cases and review of the literature. *Nephrol Dial Transplant* **20**: 1075–82.

23 Audard V, Larousserie F, Grimbert P, Abtahi M, Sotto JJ, Delmer A et al. (2006). Minimal change nephrotic syndrome and classical Hodgkin's lymphoma: report of 21 cases and review of the literature. *Kidney Int* **69**: 2251–60.

24 Miura N, Suzuki K, Yoshino M, Kitagawa W, Yamada H, Ohtani H et al. (2006). Acute renal failure due to IgM-lambda glomerular thrombi and MPGN-like lesions in a patient with angioimmunoblastic T-Cell lymphoma. *Am J Kidney Dis* **48**: e3–9.

25 Buob D, Copin MC (2006). Mixed cryoglobulinemia-associated membranoproliferative glomerulonephritis, disclosing gastric MALT lymphoma. *Ann Pathol* **26**: 267–70.

26 Dwyer JP, Yates KM, Sumner EL, Stone WJ, Wang Y, Koury MJ et al. (2007). Chronic myeloid leukemia-associated membranoproliferative glomerulonephritis that responded to imatinib mesylate therapy. *Clin Nephrol* **67**: 176–81.

27 Ahmed MS, Wong CF, Abraham KA (2008). Membrano-proliferative glomerulonephritis associated with metastatic prostate carcinoma—should immunosuppressive therapy be considered? *Nephrol Dial Transplant* **23**: 777.

28 Gupta K, Nada R, Das A, Kumar MS (2008). Membranoproliferative glomerulonephritis in a carcinoma with unknown primary: an autopsy study. *Indian J Pathol Microbiol* **51**: 230–3.

29 Bergmann J, Buchheidt D, Waldherr R, Maywald O, van der Woude FJ, Hehlmann R et al. (2005). IgA nephropathy and hodgkin's disease: a rare coincidence. Case report and literature review. *Am J Kidney Dis* **45**: e16–19.

30 Forslund T, Sikio A, Anttinen J (2007). IgA nephropathy in a patient with IgG lambda light-chain plasmacytoma: a rare coincidence. *Nephrol Dial Transplant* **22**: 2705–8.

31 Lin FC, Chen JY, Yang AH, Chang SC (2002). The association of non-small-cell lung cancer, focal segmental glomerulosclerosis, and platelet dysfunction. *Am J Med Sci* **324**: 161–5.

32 Gonzalez Garcia E, Olea T, Hevia C, Torre A, Azorin S, Ruiz E et al. (2007). Focal segmental glomerulosclerosis due to a relapsing non-Hodgkin's lymphoma diagnosed by positron emission tomography. *J Nephrol* **20**: 626–8.

33 Mallouk A, Pham PT, Pham PC (2006). Concurrent FSGS and Hodgkin's lymphoma: case report and literature review on the link between nephrotic glomerulopathies and hematological malignancies. *Clin Exp Nephrol* **10**: 284–9.

34 Jain S, Kakkar N, Joshi K, Varma S (2001). Crescentic glomerulonephritis associated with renal cell carcinoma. *Ren Fail* **23**: 287–90.

35 Yavuzsen T, Oztop I, Yilmaz U, Cavdar C, Sifil A, Sarioglu S et al. (2003). Gastric cancer diagnosed in a patient with crescentic glomerulonephritis. *Gastric Cancer* **6**: 267–9.

36 Parambil JG, Keogh KA, Fervenza FC, Ryu JH (2006). Microscopic polyangiitis associated with thymoma, exacerbating after thymectomy. *Am J Kidney Dis* **48**: 827–31.

37 Menendez CL, Pobes A, Corte Torres MG, Fuente E, Merino AM, Corrales B et al. (2007). A case of acquired renal cystic disease (ACDK) with oncocytosis, a dominant nodule (oncocytoma), multiple adenomas and a microscopic papillary renal cell carcinoma associated with crescentic glomerulonephritis. *Virchows Arch* **450**: 365–7.

38 Ikee R, Kobayashi S, Hemmi N, Suzuki S, Miura S (2005). Amyloidosis associated with chronic lymphocytic leukemia. *Amyloid* **12**: 131–4.

39 Jaakkola H, Tornroth T, Groop PH, Honkanen E (2001). Renal failure and nephrotic syndrome associated with gastrointestinal stromal tumour (GIST)-a rare cause of AA amyloidosis. *Nephrol Dial Transplant* **16**: 1517–18.

40 Agha I, Mahoney R, Beardslee M, Liapis H, Cowart RG, Juknevicius I (2002). Systemic amyloidosis associated with pleomorphic sarcoma of the spleen and remission of nephrotic syndrome after removal of the tumor. *Am J Kidney Dis* **40**: 411–15.

41 Ersoy A, Filiz G, Ersoy C, Kahvecioglu S, Kanat O, Vuruskan H et al. (2006). Synchronous carcinomas of stomach and bladder together with AA amyloidosis. *Nephrology (Carlton)* **11**: 120–3.

42 Alpers CE, Cotran RS (1986). Neoplasia and glomerular injury. *Kidney Int* **30**: 465–73.

43 Burstein DM, Korbet SM, Schwartz MM (1993). Membranous glomerulonephritis and malignancy. *Am J Kidney Dis* **22**: 5–10.

44 Plager J, Stutzman L (1971). Acute nephrotic syndrome as a manifestation of active Hodgkin's Disease. Report of four cases and review of the literature. *Am J Med* **50**: 56–66.

45 Kramer P, Sizoo W, Twiss EE (1981). Nephrotic syndrome in Hodgkin's disease. Report of five cases and review of the literature. *Neth J Med* **24**: 114–19.

46 Mustonen J, Pasternack A, Helin H (1984). IgA mesangial nephropathy in neoplastic diseases. *Contrib Nephrol* **40**: 283–91.

47 Whitworth JA, Morel-Maroger L, Mignon F, Richet G (1976). The significance of extracapillary proliferation. Clinicopathological review of 60 patients. *Nephron* **16**: 1–19.

48 Biava CG, Gonwa TA, Naughton JL, Hopper Jr J (1984). Crescentic glomerulonephritis associated with nonrenal malignancies. *Am J Nephrol* **4**: 208–14.

49 Edgar JDM, Rooney DP, McNamee P, McNeil TA (1993). An association between ANCA positive renal disease and malignancy. *Clin Nephrol* **40**: 22–5.

50 Ozawa T, Pluss R, Lacher J, Boedecker E, Guggenheim S, Hammond W et al. (1975). Endogenous immune complex nephropathy associated with malignancy I. Studies on the nature and immunopathogenic significance of glomerular bound antigen and antibody, isolation and characterization of tumor specific antigen and antibody and circulating immune complexes. *Q J Med* **44**: 523–41.

51 Hebert LA, Cosio FG, Birmingham DJ (1994). Circulating immune complexes. In: *Immunochemistry* (ed. C. van Oss, MHV van Regenmortel), pp. 653–80. Marcel Dekker, New York.

52 Meyers KEC, Kaplan BS (2001). Minimal-change nephrotic syndrome. In: *Immunologic renal diseases*. 2 ed. (ed. EG Neilson, WG Couser), pp. 969–85. Lippincott Williams & Wilkins, Philadelphia.

53 Agarwal A, Clements J, Sedmak DD, Imler D, Nahman Jr NS, Orsinelli DA et al. (1997). Subacute bacterial endocarditis masquerading as type III essential mixed cryoglobulinemia. *J Am Soc Nephrol* **8**: 1971–6.

54 Hebert LA, Cosio FG, Birmingham DJ (2001). Complement and complement regulatory proteins. In: *Immunologic renal diseases* 2 ed. (ed. EG Neilson, WG Couser), pp. 367–93. Lippincott Williams & Wilkins, Philadelphia.

55 Allen AC, Barratt J, Feehally J (2001). Immunoglobulin A nephropathy. In: *Immunologic renal diseases*. 2 ed. (ed. EG Neilson, WG Couser), pp. 931–47. Lippincott Williams & Wilkins, Philadelphia.

56 Beaufils H, Jouanneau C, Chomette G (1985). Kidney and cancer: results of immunofluorescence microscopy. *Nephron*, **40**: 303–308.

57 Falk RJ, Jennette JC (2001). Renal vasculitis. In: *Immunologic renal diseases*. 2 ed. (ed. EG Neilson, WG Couser), pp. 1105–25. Lippincott Williams & Wilkins, Philadelphia.

58 Aslam N, Nseir NI, Viverett JF, Bastacky SI, Johnson JP (2000). Nephrotic syndrome in chronic lymphocytic leukemia: a paraneoplastic syndrome? *Clin Nephrol* **54**: 492–7.

59 Agar JW, Gates PC, Vaughan SL, Machet D (1994). Renal biopsy in angiotropic large cell lymphoma. *Am J Kidney Dis* **24**: 92–6.

60 Sepandj F, Hirsch DJ, Jindal KK, Trillo A (1994). Metastatic lung carcinoma mimicking acute glomerulonephritis. *Am J Kidney Dis* **24**: 523–5.

61 Perl SI, Yong JC, Higgins SG (1987). Tumor crescents from intraglomerular metastases. *Clin Nephrol* **27**: 260–2.

62 Mungall S, Mathieson P (2002). Hemolytic uremic syndrome in metastatic adenocarcinoma of the prostate. *Am J Kidney Dis* **40**: 1334–6.

63 Lefaucheur C, Stengel B, Nochy D, Martel P, Hill GS, Jacquot C et al. (2006). Membranous nephropathy and cancer: Epidemiologic evidence and determinants of high-risk cancer association. *Kidney Int* **70**: 1510–17.

64 Ohtani H, Wakui H, Komatsuda A, Okuyama S, Masai R, Maki N *et al.* (2004). Distribution of glomerular IgG subclass deposits in malignancy-associated membranous nephropathy. *Nephrol Dial Transplant* **19**: 574–9.

65 Sawyer N, Wadsworth J, Wijnen M, Gabriel R (1988). Prevalence, concentration, and prognostic importance of proteinuria in patients with malignancies. *Br Med J (Clin Res Ed)* **296**: 1295–8.

66 Pascal RR (1980). Renal manifestations of extrarenal neoplasms. *Hum Pathol* **11**: 7–17.

67 Zech P, Colon S, Pointet P, Deteix P, Labeeuw M, Leitienne P (1982). The nephrotic syndrome in adults aged over 60: etiology, evolution and treatment of 76 cases. *Clin Nephrol* **17**: 232–6.

68 Dizer U, Beker CM, Yavuz I, Ortatatli M, Ozguven V, Pahsa A (2003). Minimal change disease in a patient receiving IFN-alpha therapy for chronic hepatitis C virus infection. *J Interferon Cytokine Res* **23**: 51–4.

69 Yang JC, Haworth L, Sherry RM, Hwu P, Schwartzentruber DJ, Topalian SL et al. (2003). A randomized trial of bevacizumab, an anti-vascular endothelial growth factor antibody, for metastatic renal cancer. *N Engl J Med* **349**: 427–34.

70 Barton CH, Vaziri ND, Spear GS (1980). Nephrotic syndrome associated with adenocarcinoma of the breast. *Am J Med* **68**: 308–12.

71 Gandini E, Allaria P, Castiglioni A, d'Amato I, Schiaffino E, Giangrande A (1996). Minimal change nephrotic syndrome with cecum adenocarcinoma. *Clin Nephrol* **45**: 268–70.

72 Forland M, Bannayan GA (1983). Minimal-change lesion nephrotic syndrome with renal oncocytoma. *Am J Med* **75**: 715–20.

73 Moorthy AV (1983). Minimal change glomerular disease: a paraneoplastic syndrome in two patients with bronchogenic carcinoma. *Am J Kidney Dis* **3**: 58–62.

74 Sakemi T, Uchida M, Ikeda Y, Shouno Y (1996). Acute renal failure and nephrotic syndrome in a patient with T-cell lymphoma. *Nephron* **72**: 326–7.

75 Woodrow G, Innes A, Ansell ID, Burden RP (1995). Renal cell carcinoma presenting as nephrotic syndrome. *Nephron* **69**: 166–9.

76 Orman SV, Schechter GP, Whang-Peng J, Guccion J, Chan C, Schulof RS et al. (1986). Nephrotic syndrome associated with a clonal T-cell leukemia of large granular lymphocytes with cytotoxic function. *Arch Intern Med* **146**: 1827–9.

77 Keven K, Nergizoglu G, Ates K, Erekul S, Orhan D, Erturk S et al. (2000). Remission of nephrotic syndrome after removal of localized Castleman's disease. *Am J Kidney Dis* **35**: 1207–11.

78 Omura K, Kawamura T, Utsunomiya Y, Abe A, Joh K, Sakai O (1996). Development of nephrotic syndrome in a patient with acute myeloblastic leukemia after treatment with macrophage-colony-stimulating factor. *Am J Kidney Dis* **27**: 883–7.

79 Nishikawa K, Sekiyama S, Suzuki T, Ito Y, Matsukawa W, Tamai H et al. (1991). A case of angiotropic large cell lymphoma manifesting nephrotic syndrome and treated successfully with combination chemotherapy. *Nephron* **58**: 479–82.

80 Agarwal A, Haddad N, Hebert LA (2008). Progression of kidney disease: diagnosis and management. In: *Evidence-based nephrology* (ed. D Molony, J Craig), pp. 311–22. John Wiley & Sons, Hoboken, NJ.

81 Brown C, Haddad N, Hebert LA (2009–10) Retarding progression of kidney disease. In: *Comprehensive clinical nephrology*, 4th ed. (ed. J Floege, R Johnson, J Fehally). Elsevier, Philadelphia.

82 Jefferson JA, Couser WG (2003). Therapy of membranous nephropathy associated with malignancy and secondary causes. *Semin Nephrol* **23**: 400–5.

Chapter 4

Paraproteins and the kidney

Robin G. Woolfson

Case report

A 38-year-old black Ghanaian lady was referred to our Renal Unit following emergency admission to the Medical Assessment Unit. She had presented with a 3-month history of increasing malaise, anorexia, nausea, 10 kg weight loss, low back pain with recent rib pain on coughing. Five years earlier, she had presented with arthralgia, myalgia, and facial rash and had been diagnosed with mild systemic lupus erythematosus. There had never been renal involvement and routine blood tests undertaken six months before this acute presentation had shown strongly positive ANA and polyclonal hypergammaglobulinemia but negative DNA binding, negative ENA and normal complement levels. She had been taking Hydroxychloroquine 200 mg daily for five years and Ibuprofen 400 mg twice daily. She did not smoke or drink alcohol and did not use alternative or herbal remedies.

At presentation, she was euvolemic with a normal blood pressure and visible JVP at 45°. Aside from pallor, there were no abnormal clinical findings.

Investigations

Hemoglobin 8.5 g/dL, platelets 134 10^9 /L.

Creatinine 582 μmol/L (6.61 mg/dL), urea 44 mmol/L (BUN 123 mg/dL).

Albumin 34 g/dL, corrected Ca2+ 2.5 mmol/L (normal).

CRP 33 mg/L, β_2-microglobulin 38 mg/L.

IgA 3.4 g/L [0.7–4.0], IgG 18.1 g/L [7.0–16.0], and IgM 1.1 [0.40–2.3].

Serum protein electrophoresis showed polyclonal increase in IgG with no M-band.

Free serum κ light chains 260 mg/L [3.3–19.4]; free serum λ light chains 1540 mg/L [5.7–26.3]; ratio 0.16 [0.26–1.65].

HIV negative, HBV negative, HCV negative, HHV8 negative.

Urine electrophoresis showed a M-band, identified as IgG λ on immunofixation.

Bone marrow aspirate: 50% plasma cells (λ light chain restricted) with heavy infiltrate confirmed on trephine.

Renal ultrasound normal.

Kidney biopsy showed cast nephropathy (myeloma kidney).

Management

She was oliguric on admission and for the first seven days she was dialyzed daily using a Gambro light chain filter (HCO 1100). Serum light chain measurements pre and post dialysis are outlined in Fig. 4.2. Thereafter a standard dialysis filter was used thrice weekly until sufficient renal recovery had occurred so that dialysis could be discontinued (one month following admission). Her myeloma was treated with weekly oral cyclophosphamide (1000 mg/week), fortnightly oral dexamethasone (40 mg daily for three days) and oral Thalidomide 50 mg daily. Interval high dose therapy with allograft stem cell transplant from a haplo-identical sibling is planned.

Introduction

Plasma cells are mature B lymphocytes which produce heavy and light chains and these assemble in tetramers to form different classes of immunoglobulins (IgG, IgA, IgM, IgE, IgD). Each immunoglobulin comprises two heavy chains and two light chains, either kappa (κ) or lambda (λ), based on the amino acid sequence in the constant portion of the polypeptide chain. In a plasma cell dyscrasia or malignancy, an autonomous clone produce a monoclonal paraprotein (M-band) which can be a whole immunoglobulin or a light chain or a

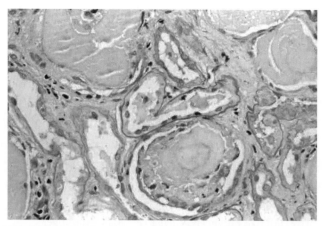

Fig. 4.1 Kidney biopsy showing cast nephropathy with classic fractured intratubular casts, tubular cell necrosis and interstitial infiltrate. Immunostaining (not shown) showed an excess of lambda over kappa light chain casts within the tubules.

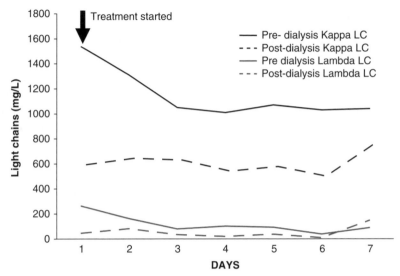

Fig. 4.2 This shows the daily levels of free serum light chains before and after the seven sessions of dialysis using the Gambro light chain filter. A marked reduction in Lambda light chain levels was observed.

heavy chain. Filtered light chains may damage glomerular mesangial cells or the epithelial cells which line the proximal or distal tubules.

Fifty-two percent of plasma cell tumors produce IgG, compared with IgA in 21%, IgM (Waldenstrom's) in 12% and light chains alone in 11%. Rarely, plasma cell tumors are non-secretory and the diagnosis is suggested by the presence of an immune-paresis due to the suppression of the normal plasma cell population. Although usually restricted to the bone marrow, extra-medullary deposits (plasmacytomas) and plasma cell leukemias can occur.

The clinical significance of an M-band is protean. In monoclonal gammopathy of unknown significance (MGUS), which comprises the largest clinical group, the M-band is not associated with any other clinical features or identifiable plasma cell dyscrasia. At the other end of the spectrum, multiple myeloma is due to a malignant plasma cell tumor with clinical presentation dependent on the tumor load present in bone marrow, plasma levels of paraprotein, and metabolic consequences. In intermediate conditions, it may be possible to identify a plasma cell dyscrasia but the clinical presentation is determined by the biochemical properties of the paraprotein and the nature and distribution of deposits within the kidney and elsewhere. *Paraprotein disease should be considered in any patient who presents with microscopic hematuria, proteinuria, nephrotic syndrome and kidney disease, either acute or chronic.*

Myeloma

All M-bands must be investigated to enable diagnosis, prognosis, and therapy. Specific diagnostic criteria differentiate myeloma from other benign and malignant disorders characterized by M-bands, which include MGUS, macroglobulinemia, B cell lymphoma, primary amyloidosis, idiopathic cold agglutinin disease, essential cryoglobulinemia, and heavy chain disease. MGUS is distinguished from myeloma by low paraprotein titers, minimal or absent urinary light chains, and less than 10% plasma cells on bone marrow biopsy. Intermediate disease is sub-classified into indolent and smouldering forms depending on the M-band level and the tumor load (Table 4.1). None of these conditions necessarily require treatment, but all patients (including those with MGUS) require careful and regular observation, so that transformation to myeloma can be diagnosed promptly.

Epidemiology

Myeloma is the second most common hematological malignancy in the USA with an estimated 20,580 cases to be diagnosed in 2009 (1). Males are more commonly affected than females (3:2) and the incidence is doubled in African-Americans and Pacific Islanders compared with Europeans and North American Caucasians, with even lower rates reported in Asians. The different racial prevalence may reflect different diets and prevalence of obesity (2). Although predominantly a disease of the elderly, significant numbers of younger individuals are affected by multiple myeloma. Of the 869 cases seen at the Mayo Clinic between 1960 and 1971, 98% of patients were 40 years of age or older; however, 35% of men and 41% of women were less than 60 years old with 75% of men and 79% of women aged below 70 years (3).

The most important risk factor for the development of multiple myeloma is a preceding MGUS which is present in 5% of the population aged over 70 years. In a 20-year database from Iceland, age-standardized incidence rates of MGUS were very low for subjects under 50 years, then increased progressively with age from 11 and 17 per 100,000 at 50–54 years, to 169 and 119 per 100,000 at 80–84 years, for men and women respectively (4). The proportion of subjects progressing to overt plasma cell malignancy can be as high as 30% over 20 years with evidence of increased relative risk of transformation with IgA paraproteins compared with IgG or IgM. Myeloma is commoner in those with a first-degree relative with the disease, a family history of any hematological malignancy and to a lesser extent, any type of cancer (5). Predisposing genetic factors have not been identified but the Cw2 HLA allele may enhance the risk of myeloma in blacks and whites but does not explain the higher incidence of this cancer among blacks.

Table 4.1 Diagnostic criteria for different plasma cell tumors

MGUS

Diagnostic criteria
1. Bone marrow plasmacytosis <10%
2. M-band: IgG <3.5 g/dL; IgA <2.0 g/dL
3. < Less than 1.0 g/24 hr of urinary light chains (Bence Jones protein)
Exclusions: constitutional symptoms, hypercalcemia and skeletal lesions

INDOLENT MYELOMA

Diagnostic criteria
1. Bone marrow plasmacytosis <10%
2. M-band: IgG <7 g/dL; IgA <5 g/dL
Additional features:
1. Up to 2 lytic skeletal lesions
2. Mild anemia, Hb >10 g/dL
3. Renal dysfunction, creatinine <2.0 mg/dL
Exclusions: constitutional symptoms, hypercalcemia

SMOLDERING MYELOMA

Diagnostic criteria
1. Bone marrow plasmacytosis < 0%
2. M-band: IgG < g/dL; IgA < g/dL
Additional features:
1. Mild anemia, Hb >10 g/dL
2. Renal dysfunction, creatinine < 2.0 mg/dL
Exclusions: constitutional symptoms, hypercalcemia, skeletal lesions

MYELOMA

The diagnosis is based on combinations of major and minor diagnostic criteria:
1. Any two major criteria
2. Major criterion 1 plus minor criterion b, c, or d
3. Major criterion 3 plus minor criterion a or c
4. Minor criteria a, b, and c, or a, b, and d
Major criteria
1. Plasmacytomas on tissue biopsy
2. Bone marrow plasmacytosis (>30% plasma cells)
3. M-band: IgG >3.5 g/dL; IgA >2.0 g/dL;
4. More than 1.0 g/24 hr of urinary light chains (Bence Jones protein)
Minor criteria
1. Bone marrow plasmacytosis (10–30% plasma cells)
2. M-band at a lower titre
3. Lytic bone lesions
4. Immune-paresis (IgM <50 mg/dL, IgA <100 mg/dL, or IgG <600 mg/dL)

Epidemiological factors influence the risk of developing MGUS or the subsequent transformation to myeloma. Biological studies support a role for aberrant class-switch recombination early in the natural history of myeloma, suggesting that factors in the environment interact with this mechanism to increase the risk of myeloma. Case-control, cohort studies and meta-analyses have identified known and suspected environmental risk factors for the development of MGUS and myeloma which include ionizing radiation, occupational exposure in the farming and petrochemical industries, engine exhaust, and hair dyes. Chronic inflammation due to allergies, autoimmune conditions, or bacterial infection also increase the risk of myeloma (6). B cell neoplasia is associated with HHV8, HIV, and HCV infection. Reports of increased incidence of myeloma following pneumococcal infection likely reflect diminished humoral immunity against encapsulated bacteria rather than causality.

Cell biology

Myeloma cells are derived from plasma cells, sharing the cell surface expression of antigens including CD38 and PCA-1. Sensitive techniques have identified molecular deletions in up to 80% of patients, with partial or complete deletions of chromosome 13q- occurring most frequently. IL-6 is both a product and a growth factor for human myeloma cells and levels correlate with greater tumor mass and adverse clinical outcome, with normal levels found in patients with smouldering disease. Hepatic synthesis of CRP is promoted by IL-6 which presumably explains its value as a surrogate prognostic indicator. Similarly, VEGF stimulates myeloma cell proliferation by both paracrine and autocrine mechanisms. Myeloma cells localize within the bone marrow via an interaction of cell-surface adhesion molecules with their respective ligands on marrow stromal cells (BMSCs) and extracellular matrix proteins. BMSCs also produce IL-6 and VEGF with secretion enhanced by binding with the myeloma cells. These autocrine loops are emerging as therapeutic targets and explain the actions of dexamethasone, thalidomide, biphosphonates, and other novel treatments. Finally, increased IL-1β production is found in 95% cases of myeloma but less than 25% of MGUS and may predict those cases which will eventually transform (7). IL-1β may be involved in the pathogenesis of osteolytic lesions and, together with IL-6, raised levels have been implicated in POEMS syndrome (8).

Prognostic factors

Several complex staging systems with prognostic significance have been developed with two remaining in common use. These systems use different parameters but are both predictive of progression-free survival and patient survival, although agreement is only 36%. Both systems rely on the prognostic importance of renal function. Salmon-Durie identifies three stages based on hemoglobin, calcium, skeletal survey, paraprotein titer, and renal function, which correlate with tumor load and prognosis. The International Staging System for multiple myeloma is based on β_2-microglobulin, albumin, CRP (which is a surrogate marker for IL-6 activity), plasma cell labelling index, absence of chromosome-13 deletion, low serum IL-6 receptor, and long duration of initial plateau phase (9). The importance of serum β_2-microglobulin levels reflects correlation with tumor mass, rate of growth, and renal function, since it is cleared by glomerular filtration. Other adverse prognostic indicators include primitive cell morphology, λ light chain production and poor performance status at diagnosis.

Renal involvement in multiple myeloma

On presentation, more than 50% of patients diagnosed with multiple myeloma will have some degree of kidney disease; and although reversible in most cases, 10% of patients will require acute dialysis. In most of these patients, the diagnosis of myeloma follows presentation with acute kidney injury. Acute kidney injury results from several different pathological processes, often in combination (see Table 4.2) but these can only be distinguished by a renal biopsy. The incidence of end-stage renal disease (ESRD) secondary to multiple myeloma is 1% (United States Renal Data System, USRDS).

Proximal tubule toxicity

In health, plasma cells normally produce more light chains than heavy chains. The molecular weight of light chains is approximately 25,000 Da and the lambda light chains dimerize and are therefore less freely filtered at the glomerulus compared with monomeric kappa chains. Filtered light chains, together with other low molecular weight proteins, are catabolized by the proximal

Table 4.2 Renal involvement in multiple myeloma

Acute tubular necrosis
Interstitial nephritis
Hypercalcemia
Cast nephropathy
Fanconi Syndrome
Nephrogenic diabetes insipidus
Fibrillary deposition disease (amyloid, fibrillary-immunotactoid, crystals)
Non-fibrillary (amorphous) deposition disease (light and heavy chain deposition diseases)
Plasma cell infiltration

renal tubule (PT). An increase in glomerular filtration of light chains, due to increased glomerular permeability or to increased light chain load (in myeloma), or a decrease in reabsorption due to PT cell injury, will lead to increased light chain levels in the urine. Filtered light chains may adversely affect glomerular mesangial cells or the epithelial cells which line the proximal and distal tubules.

Filtered light chains are endocytozed via the apical scavenger receptors cubulin and megalin, which have a particular affinity for light chains. The endosomes fuse with lysosomes to degrade the contents; however, an excessive filtered light chain load exceeds catabolic reserve and leads to the release of lysosomal contents into the cytoplasm. The activation of NFκB promotes the synthesis of inflammatory cytokines, particularly IL-6 (10), and activates signaling pathways to promote interstitial inflammation and fibrosis. Probing and inhibiting these pathways may inform future novel cytoprotective strategies (11).

Histological features include epithelial cell vacuolation, desquamation, loss of the luminal brush border, and eventually cell necrosis. Over time, local toxicity leads to irreversible chronic tubulointerstitial nephritis, which occurs independently of distal tubular cast formation. Functionally, abnormalities in glucose and water reabsorption occur early with backleak presumably contributing to the observed loss of glomerular filtration rate (GFR). Rarely, Fanconi's syndrome develops due to incompletely digested light chains, which serve as a nidus for the formation of crystals in PT endosomes which interfere with apical membrane transporters (12). Monoclonal κ light chains are usually responsible and a specific unusual amino acid sequence found in the variable segment (Vκ1) has been implicated (13).

Further evidence to support the idiosyncratic toxicity of light chains comes from perfusion experiments. Light chains from patients with renal tubular damage are more injurious to rat tubules than light chains from unaffected patients. Conversely, glomerulopathic light chains from patients with AL amyloid and light chain deposition disease (LCDD) induced morphological and inflammatory responses in cultured mesangial cells, whereas tubulopathic light chains did not (14). Variable light chain toxicity, presumably due to specific amino acid sequences and isoelectric points (pI), could reflect differing rates of endocytosis and different structural configurations of endocytozed light chains.

Distal tubule toxicity

In myeloma, depending on the tumor burden, secretory status, and PT reabsorptive capacity, an excess load of light chains is delivered to the distal tubule. Light chains with a relatively high pI (>6) have a cationic charge at the acidic urine pH found in the distal nephron and this favours binding to anionic Tamm–Horsfall mucoprotein (THP), produced by cells of the thick ascending limb of the loop of Henle, to form glutinous casts which obstruct the distal tubule and cause renal failure. Prevention and reversal of cast formation is highly desirable and understanding the protein interactions that are modified by the tubule fluid composition and volume is key.

The THP is both dissolved in tubular fluid and attached to the apical plasma membrane. Filtered light chains bind to a specific six-peptide segment of THP, which could be a target for synthetic blocking peptides. Light chains are composed of subunits with variable and constant domains. Three hypervariable segments, termed the complementarity-determining region (CDR), configure part of the antigen-binding site on the immunoglobulin molecule and CDR3 binds THP with its affinity determined by the proportion of amphipathic amino acids. When an in vivo rodent model of cast formation is used, light chains with little affinity for THP in vitro do not form casts, although this affinity can be increased by coincident dehydration and hypercalcuria (15). The CDR3 sequence variability could explain the clinical dissociation between the urinary light chain load and the nephropathy observed in the absence of other extrinsic factors.

There is also heterotypic aggregation due to ionic interactions with a central role for the carbohydrate moieties on the THP (16). Alteration of the carbohydrate moiety of Tamm–Horsfall glycoprotein with colchicine prevented intraluminal cast formation and obstruction of the rat nephron, and strategies to modify the carbohydrate components of THP or the use of oligosaccharides could decrease or prevent cast nephropathy. Aggregation rates are increased by an acidic environment, decreased extracellular fluid volume, and reduced tubule fluid flow rates, raised tubular calcium and chloride, the amount of THP and light chain load, and the presence of furosemide. Intriguingly, light chains with cast-forming potential can exert a direct effect on the loop segment to inhibit chloride reabsorption (17).

Cast nephropathy features distal tubules obstructed by multiple proteinaceous 'hard' casts which characteristically fracture during histological processing. These stain positively for κ or λ light chains. The affected tubules are surrounded by an active cellular infiltrate and, depending on the chronicity of the process, there will be a variable amount of irreversible tubular atrophy and interstitial fibrosis, which is the most important predictor of renal recovery. Acute tubular necrosis due to volume depletion, hypercalcemia, sepsis, and drug toxicity (e.g. NSAID usage) is superimposed.

Hypercalcemia causes partial nephrogenic diabetes insipidus. This is due to the reduction of both the vasopressin-mediated medullary interstitial hypertonicity which lowers the maximum urine concentration and the vaso-pressin-mediated water reabsorption in the collecting duct. Diabetes insipidus will reverse with correction of the hypercalcemia although urinary concentrating ability will remain abnormal in chronic kidney disease and patients remain at risk of volume depletion.

Presentation

Presenting features of multiple myeloma include bone pain in 68%, anemia in 62%, hypercalcemia in 30%, kidney disease in 55%, hepatomegaly in 21%, proteinuria in 88%, and skeletal abnormalities on plain X-ray in 88% (the incidence of MRI skeletal abnormalities may be higher), and M-band in 76% of patients (3). Less common renal presentations include hypercalcuria, Fanconi's syndrome, and nephrogenic diabetes insipidus. A full clinical history including drug history is essential. In the acute presentation, clinical examination should focus on circulating volume, evidence of intercurrent infection, comorbidities and general performance status, which inform the therapeutic strategy.

Myeloma kidney (cast nephropathy) must be excluded in patients with unexplained acute kidney injury, particularly in the context of ultrasound evidence of normal sized kidneys with increased echogenicity due to dense proteinaceous tubular casts and associated interstitial nephritis. This presentation usually follows a reduction in the GFR due to intercurrent sepsis, desalination, or new medication such as ACE inhibitors, AII receptor blockers, NSAIDs, and radiocontrast. Hyperosmolar radiocontrast media cause dehydration, renal vasoconstriction, and direct tubular toxicity, and thus promote cast formation. This is particularly relevant because intravenous urography is commonly used by non-nephrologists in the evaluation of the patient presenting with renal impairment. The well-recognized risk of acute kidney injury following radiocontrast administration in myeloma patients reflects direct toxicity as well as routine fluid restriction prior to the investigation and the subsequent administration of furosemide. No data show specific radiocontrast toxicity in myeloma but if such studies are unavoidable, the risk can probably be reduced by the use of non-ionic media, pre- and post-treatment with intravenous sodium bicarbonate or saline to avoid hypovolaemia and the maintenance of a diuresis.

Diagnosis

The diagnosis of myeloma is usually confirmed by serum and urine protein electrophoresis and a bone marrow biopsy (Table 4.2). Serum electrophoresis reveals an M-band in the gamma globulin region which is then characterized by specific antibodies raised against light and heavy chains (immunofixation) to confirm monoclonality. Most myelomas generate an excess of monoclonal light chains which are detected in the urine by electrophoresis and characterized by immunofixation. (Urinary light chains are the same as Bence–Jones proteins, previously identified by their capacity to precipitate and redissolve on cooling.) In patients with light chain myeloma, there may be no serum M-band and the diagnosis is dependent on urinary electrophoresis or the recently developed free serum light chain (FLC) assay.

Serum electrophoresis and immunofixation can identify FLCs at a minimum concentration of 100–150 mg/l. This is insufficient to identify the low levels of serum light chain characteristic of light chain only multiple myeloma, non-secretory, and oligo-secretory multiple myeloma, AL amyloid and light chain deposition disease. The development of the FLC assay now permits their detection to a level of 2–4 mg/l. The technique uses purified polyclonal antibodies raised against free κ and λ light chains, which have been pre-coated onto latex particles. Nephelometric or turbidometric assays are then used to quantitate the serum free light chains. This assay depends on calculation of the ratio which will be abnormal in monoclonal compared with polyclonal expansion. When used in combination with serum electrophoresis and immunofixation (which can detect whole immunoglobulins), 99% diagnostic sensitivity can be achieved, which may obviate the need for urine electrophoresis, except perhaps in AL amyloid and light-chain-deposition disease (18). In addition to diagnosis, the FLC assay is used to monitor disease course and response to treatment in plasma cell dyscrasias.

Light chain proteinuria is suggested by a negative urine stick test in the context of an elevated urine protein/creatinine ratio. Proteinuria should be characterized and quantified with a 24-hour urine collection. Urine microscopy sometimes reveals protein casts. Other essential tests are listed in Table 4.3. Hypercalcemia is usually only found in patients with renal impairment. Alkaline phosphatase is normal with osteolytic lesions characterized by the absence of osteoblastic reaction. In the absence of hypo-albuminemia, the anion gap is reduced if the paraprotein carries a positive charge. Coagulation pathway abnormalities may be due to acquired factor VIII/vWF deficiency, anti-cardiolipin activity of the paraprotein or acquired dysfibrinogenemia.

A renal biopsy is required for the precise diagnosis of patients presenting with acute kidney injury and nephrotic syndrome, and to provide information about potential for renal recovery, which usually informs the treatment of the underlying myeloma. Conventional radiology remains the 'gold standard' for staging with MRI imaging recommended in patients with normal radiography (in whom MRI may detect abnormalities in 50%) and in patients with a

Table 4.3 Routine tests (italicized tests are of prognostic value)

Blood Tests
Full blood count (*haemoglobin*, *platelet count*)
Clotting screen
Urea, *creatinine*, bicarbonate, urate
Albumin, calcium, alkaline phosphatase
CRP
β_2-*microglobulin*
Immunoglobulins and *paraprotein titre*
Serum protein electrophoresis
Serum free light chains

Other Tests
Urinalysis and microscopy
Urinary protein / creatinine ratio
Urinary immunofixation
Bone marrow biopsy
Skeletal survey
Renal ultrasound
Renal biopsy

solitary bone plasmacytoma. Bone scintigraphy should not be used for staging and other imaging techniques (e.g. PET scans) are not recommended for routine staging use (19).

Treatment

Multiple myeloma cannot be cured and although patients may meet criteria for diagnosis, the outcome for asymptomatic patients may not be improved by early treatment. When indicated, the regimen selected depends on age, comorbidity and transplantation candidacy.

Standard treatments

The aim of an initial therapy is to achieve a stable response or 'plateau' with a reduction in paraprotein level exceeding 50%. Where tested, the potency of all regimens has been improved by the addition of thalidomide and its inclusion is now standard. Regimens may include high-dose dexamethasone alone, alkylating agents (melphalan or cyclophosphamide), with or without prednisolone, or multi-drug regimens (involving combinations of vincristine, adriamycin, doxirubicin, idarubicin, and corticosteroids with or without cyclophosphamide). None of these regimens have better outcomes than melphalan/prednisolone/thalidomide, which remains the first choice for patients considered unsuitable for high-dose therapy and stem cell rescue.

Thalidomide inhibits the activities of β-FGF, VEGF, IL-6, TNF-α, and COX-2, and reduces adhesion molecule expression. The effect is to inhibit bone marrow neovascularity and binding of the myeloma cells which are essential for proliferation. Furthermore, thalidomide induces IL-12 and IFNγ which may stimulate cancer immunity. Some or all of these properties may explain the response to therapeutic thalidomide with reduced paraprotein titer, bone marrow infiltrate, and bone marrow neovascularization observed in about one-third of patients with relapsed or refractory disease in several series (20). Thalidomide is not nephrotoxic and does not require dose reduction in chronic kidney, but its important side effects include neuropathy (16%), fatigue (13%), febrile neutropenia (6%), and constipation (6%).

Lenalidomide (Revlimid) is an analogue of thalidomide with an improved safety profile. Preliminary data support its use as first-line combination therapy for myeloma with further evidence that it shows greater efficacy than dexamethasone alone in relapsed or refractory myeloma (21). Although the dose of thalidomide does not require reduction in chronic kidney disease, the dose of lenalidomide should be adjusted for patients with creatinine clearance less than 50 mL/min (22). Both drugs are under evaluation as maintenance therapy following autologous transplantation. Both thalidomide and lenalidomide are associated with a significant risk of deep venous thrombosis and prophylactic anti-coagulation should be considered.

Bortezomib (Velcade) is an inhibitor of the proteasome pathway. In the normal cell, this pathway controls the cell cycle and maintains cellular homeostasis by regulating protein expression, degrading ubiquitinated proteins, and clearing abnormal or misfolded proteins. Tumor cells are dependent on the suppression of pro-apoptotic pathways and bortezomib may work by preventing the degradation of these pro-apoptotic factors. This drug has shown improved outcome when compared with melphalan and prednisolone in the initial treatment of myeloma (23) and with high-dose melphalan when used as conditioning therapy for patients undergoing autologous bone marrow transplant (24). Patients with compromised renal function should be monitored carefully when treated with bortezomib, especially if creatinine clearance is less than 30 mL/min.

Although the role of these agents is not yet defined, the management of myeloma has been transformed and further novel agents with encouraging preliminary results are under evaluation. These include second-generation proteasome inhibitors (e.g. Carfilzomib, Salinosporamide A) with improved specificity and potency (25) and other immunomodulatory agents, such as anti-IL-6 monoclonal antibody (26).

Inhibitors of other pathways may offer complementary benefit. These include: vorinostat, a histone deacetylase inhibitor, which enhances the effects of bortezomib (27); and drugs which inhibit cellular mechanisms that normally suppress apoptosis, such as Akt (serine/threonine-specific protein kinases) and HSP-90 (28).

Differences in toxicity and dose modification in chronic kidney disease inform the choice of regime for individual patients. Initial treatment with alkylating agents should be avoided in patients potentially suitable for high-dose therapy, since they reduce the subsequent yield of peripheral blood stem cells mobilized for harvest. Following melphalan chemotherapy, the plateau phase usually lasts 18–24 months and is not prolonged by interim chemotherapy. Interferon-α therapy can prolong the plateau phase in selected patients with myeloma and is used after conventional chemotherapy or bone marrow transplantation, and may increase overall survival by up to six months. Novel agents (thalidomide, lenalidomide and bortezomib) may have a particular role in the treatment of high-risk groups with adverse cytogenetics, chromosome deletions, and high proliferative rates. Without high-dose chemotherapy, the median survival of myeloma is 2–4 years from diagnosis.

Choice of regimen in patients with chronic kidney disease

Melphalan, prednisolone, and thalidomide is the first choice for patients considered unsuitable for high-dose therapy. It is administered in low or intermediate dose regimens. The area under the dose-response curve for melphalan depends on renal function and there is an increased risk of myelosuppression in chronic kidney disease. A 50% dose reduction is advised in patients with GFR <40–50 mL/min and avoidance when the GFR <30 mL/min. This advice is probably conservative and may have led to systematic undertreatment of myeloma patients with chronic kidney disease.

Cyclophosphamide is preferred in patients presenting with neutropenia or thrombocytopenia with 25% dose reduction recommended in patients with GFR 10–50 mL/min and 50% reduction if GFR <10 mL/min. VAD (vincristine, doxirubicin, dexamethasone) or Z-Dex (idarubicin and dexamethasone) with thalidomide are the preferred initial therapies for patients to be considered for later high-dose therapy, for those patients in whom a rapid response is required, and in patients with chronic kidney disease in whom dose reduction is not required. High-dose dexamathasone alone is indicated in patients presenting with severe pancytopenia or renal failure, or those requiring extensive local radiotherapy.

Bisphosphonates and the management of acute hypercalcemia

Intravenous bisphosphonates treat hypercalcemia resistant to resalination. If the GFR <10 mL/min then 30 mg intravenous pamidronate repeated after

24 hours can be given. Alternatively, 30 mg may be given to patients with serum [Ca++] <4.0 mmol/L and 60 mg if serum [Ca++] >4.0 mmol/L. If clodronate is used, the dose should be reduced by 50% in patients with GFR 10–15 mL/min and not given if GFR <10 mL/min. Early radiotherapy is effective in patients with extensive lytic lesions and bone pain.

Eleven randomized trials involving 1113 patients receiving bisphosphonates and 1070 controls demonstrated significant prevention of pathological vertebral fractures and reduction in bone pain, particularly with clodronate and pamidronate (29). However, there was no effect of bisphosphonates on mortality, risk of nonvertebral fractures, or on the incidence of hypercalcemia; conversely, there were no significant adverse effects. The American Society of Clinical Oncology has recently issued guidelines recommending intravenous pamidronate 90 mg or zoledronic acid 4 mg administered every 3–4 weeks (30). The doses of both drugs should be reduced in renal failure, and zolendronate is not recommended in advanced chronic kidney disease. There are several case reports of collapsing focal and segmental glomerulosclerosis with nephrotic syndrome following intravenous pamidronate, and patients should be screened regularly for proteinuria. Recent data suggest that bisphosphonate-induced osteonecrosis of the jaw may be associated with polymorphisms of the cytochrome P450 CYP2C8 (31).

Role for plasma exchange

Free light chains have a high volume of distribution, with rapid plasma refilling after plasma exchange. Evidence of benefit from this intervention in the treatment of patients presenting with acute or rapidly progressive kidney injury (as opposed to hyperviscosity syndrome) remains unresolved. Improved renal recovery and 12-month survival (61% vs. 27%) was reported in patients with acute kidney injury who received additional plasma exchange compared with those receiving chemotherapy alone (32). Zucchelli et al. (33) described their experience in 29 patients with dialysis-dependent or severe kidney injury (creatinine >5 mg/dL) who were randomly allocated to receive either plasma exchange with steroids, cytotoxic drug and hemodialysis if required, or peritoneal dialysis with steroids and cytotoxic drug. Bence–Jones proteinuria was significantly reduced in the plasma exchange group who also demonstrated improved renal outcome and 12-month survival. Finally, a retrospective study reported that plasma exchange reduced the need for dialysis in 24 patients with rapidly progressive kidney injury secondary to multiple myeloma (34). These studies were compromised of small numbers and therapeutic and clinical heterogeneity.

Recent reports describe the use of high cut-off haemodialyzers to achieve much greater FLC clearance than that achieved with plasma exchange and it appears that renal function can be regained when serum levels are reduced by 50% or more in patients with biopsy-proven cast nephropathy (35–6). In the light of these encouraging findings, an open-label, multi-center randomized clinical trial has commenced to compare chemotherapy plus FLC removal with chemotherapy plus standard high flux haemodialysis. Trial chemotherapy consists of bortezomib, doxorubicin, and dexamethasone; free light chain removal is undertaken with two Gambro HCO 1100 haemodialyzers in series using an intensive treatment schedule. The primary outcome for the study is dialysis-independence at three months and the results are eagerly awaited (37).

High-dose therapy with autologous stem cell rescue

In selected patients, high-dose therapy with stem cell rescue is appropriate. After the induction of plateau phase, stem cells mobilized by treatment with cyclophosphamide and growth factors are harvested, and the patient then receives high-dose ablative therapy with melphalan. The reinfused stem cells repopulate the bone marrow.

Recent data in patients under the age of 65 years compared standard with high-dose therapy and stem cell rescue and found higher rates of response, overall survival increased by 12 months, and prolonged period of first remission with some benefit seen in every prognostic group (38). The immediate mortality rate of 5% has restricted this therapy to the newly diagnosed patients up to age 60 years with consideration of patients aged 60–70 years, if minimal comorbidity. Supplementary therapy including additional chemotherapy, total body irradiation, antibody strategies which select CD34+ cell to reduce bone marrow contamination with tumor cells, and repeated (tandem) transplants have not shown any clear survival benefit, although response rates and relapse-free survival may be improved (39). Maintenance therapy with interferon-α can prolong the plateau phase by six months, although for some patients, the side effects of fatigue, depression, and flu-like symptoms are not tolerable. For a small number of patients, autologous bone marrow transplantation offers the possibility of cure although early mortality is greater, unless sourced from a HLA-haploidentical sibling. The use of either non-myeloablative induction regimens or autologous stem cell transplantation before allogenic transplantation may improve outcomes.

Chronic kidney disease and dialysis patients have been treated with high-dose therapy with autologous stem cell transplantation. San Miguel et al. (40) reported a greater transplant-related mortality in patients with consistently abnormal renal function compared with those with normal renal function (29% vs. 3.3%), although overall survival was little different. They concluded that a creatinine exceeding 5 mg/dL (400 µmol/L) was a contraindication to a transplant. Similarly, Sirohi et al. (41) reported significant excess mortality in the first 100 days (19%) following high-dose therapy and stem cell rescue in patients with kidney disease (defined as creatinine >140 µmol/L or 1.6 mg/dL). However, overall survival was predicted by age, light chain myeloma, β_2-microglobulin levels, and performance status, but not by renal dysfunction.

More encouragingly, Badros et al. (42) have reported their experience of high-dose therapy (melphalan 140 or 200 mg/m2) and autologous stem cell therapy in 81 patients with kidney disease (creatinine >176.8 µmol/L), of whom 38 were receiving dialysis at the outset. Treatment-related mortality was 6%, mostly due to multi-organ failure, and importantly, 140 mg/m^2 melphalan was shown to be as effective as 200 mg/m^2 but associated with significantly less toxicity. Thirty-one patients (including 11 on dialysis) went on to complete the tandem therapy (treatment-related mortality 13%) although this was not shown to be beneficial. Chronic kidney disease and dialysis dependence did not affect the quality of stem cell collections, engraftment or the score at three years for event-free survival and overall survival, with the latter determined by age, sensitive disease, and albumin levels. Similarly, Raab et al. found comparable event-free and overall survival when they compared 34 dialysis-dependent patients treated with melphalan 100 mg/m^2 with matched controls with normal renal function treated with melphalan 200 mg/m^2 (43). In addition, there was no difference in transplant-related mortality, hematologic toxicity, or disease response between groups, supporting the use of lower dose melphalan regimes in this patient group.

In conclusion, the use of high-dose therapy in myeloma patients with renal failure is becoming routine although the optimum high-dose therapy regimen is not yet defined. The potential for renal recovery and the relevance of reduction of free light chain load by either high-dose or non-myeloablative therapy is emerging (44–5). The development of novel haemodialysis techniques to reduce free light chains at diagnosis appears promising and may significantly improve the outcome for the 5% of patients who are dialysis-dependent at presentation, as well as larger numbers presenting with chronic kidney disease. Patients with kidney disease should be referred to centres with active haematology and nephrology programmes where the renal diagnosis can be established by biopsy and strategies can be developed to reduce treatment-related deaths in the context of properly conducted trials.

Management of anemia

Anemia is present in two-thirds of myeloma patients in presentation and commonly complicates chemotherapy and disease progression. Erythropoiesis stimulating agents improve the hemoglobin level and reduce transfusion requirements and are indicated in all patients with renal failure, including those with myeloma (46), although no survival advantage has been demonstrated (47).

In a landmark study, Iggo et al. (48) reported the clinical outcome of 23 patients with ESRD due to multiple myeloma and found it comparable to outcome in other dialysis patients. Moreover, hemodialysis and continuous ambulatory peritoneal dialysis (CAPD) were equally effective treatments although dialysis complications, such as temporary vascular access and bacterial peritonitis, were more common than in patients with renal failure from other causes (49). Subsequent studies have shown no difference in survival when comparing the dialysis-independent myeloma patients with those requiring hemodialysis (50). In most studies, the only adverse prognostic factor identified is the poor response to chemotherapy. The biggest data set comes from USRDS with 3298 patients with ESRD due to myeloma or light chain nephropathy commencing dialysis between January 1992 and June 1997. The two-year all-cause mortality was 58% (vs. 31% for all other patients initiating dialysis, $p < 0.01$) (51). Similarly, the unadjusted median survival of 2453 patients with myeloma or light chain nephropathy from the ERA-EDTA Registry who commenced renal replacement therapy between 1986–2005 was 0.91 years compared with 4.46 years for the other 157,184 patients (52). Poorer patient survival is attributed to the increased frequency of acute presentation in worse general condition with more advanced renal failure compared with other diagnostic groups.

Specific paraprotein nephropathies

Renal disease in multiple myeloma is most commonly the result of cast nephropathy, acute tubular necrosis, or interstitial nephritis with nephropathy precipitated by desalination, hypercalcemia, or sepsis. In these situations, the paraprotein levels are high and there is a significant tumor load. However, some paraproteins have specific pathogenic properties such that kidney disease occurs in the context of low levels of paraprotein and a minimal tumor load. Diagnosis of these conditions has been facilitated by the development of the serum FLC assay although there can be overlap with myeloma, for example when cast nephropathy is found in conjunction with amyloid or light chain deposition disease. These conditions can be devastating and high-dose therapies based on the treatment of multiple myeloma have been used in an effort to eliminate the plasma cell clone responsible for paraprotein production.

In patients failing to meet the diagnostic criteria for myeloma, monoclonal immunoglobulin deposited in the glomerulus and elsewhere can lead to microscopic hematuria, proteinuria, nephrotic syndrome, and acute and chronic kidney disease. Diagnoses are classified according to the structure of deposits on electron microscopy (Table 4.4). These rare diseases are in contrast to MGUS in which the paraprotein is non-nephrotoxic and the tumor load is insignificant.

Primary (AL) amyloid

AL amyloid is due to the excess production of light chains from a single B cell clone, with very occasional cases due to deposition of heavy chains. Amyloid deposits consist of linear, nonbranching fibrils with diameter in the range 7.5–10 nm. Each fibril is composed of two twisted 3 nm filaments with an anti-parallel β-pleated sheet configuration stabilized by covalent binding. Additional stabilizing components include glycosoaminoglycans and serum amyloid-P component (SAP) (53).

Immunostaining of the bone marrow biopsy for the λ and κ isotypes demonstrates a dominant clonal population of plasma cells even when electrophoresis of serum and urine is negative (less than 10% of cases). However, the tumor mass is usually too low to meet the criteria for myeloma. Usually, the clone is λ-restricted (overall, λ:κ equals 2–3:1) and the λ-isotype is associated with greater nephrotoxicity. Clonal expansion in which the Vλ6 gene (coding for the light chain variable region) is expressed is associated with renal involvement; Vλ3 expression with 'soft-tissue' deposits; and, Vλ2 expression with cardiac involvement (54). For amyloid due to a κ-restricted clonal expansion, the Vκ1 gene is overrepresented. The formation of amyloid fibrils is influenced by certain residue amino acid sequences in the light chain variable regions and by the degree of enzymatic glycosylation. These factors presumably influence structure, stability, predisposition to aggregation, and sites of deposition, possibly by

Table 4.4 Characterization of glomerular disease in paraprotein nephropathy by electron microscopic appearance of deposits

E-M appearance of deposits		Disease
Organized	Fibrillary	AL-amyloid Fibrillary glomerulonephritis Castleman's Disease
	Microtubular	Immunotactoid glomerulonephritis Cryoglobulinemia
Non-organized	Granular	Monoclonal immunoglobulin deposition disease Cryoglobulinemia Waldenstrom's macroglobulinemia POEMS* syndrome

*POEMS: polyenuropathy, organomegaly, endocrinopathy, m-band and skin changes

affecting isolectric point (pI). Because of light chain fragmentation, only 90% of amyloid deposits contain the constant region sequence with which commercially available anti-light-chain sera react and so 10% of cases may demonstrate negative immunofluorescence despite positive Congo Red stain.

Epidemiology

The incidence of AL amyloid in the USA is nine per million per year with a median age of 64 years at diagnosis and a male predominance of 2:1. Less than 1% of the affected individuals are younger than 40 years of age. AL amyloid accounts for 10% of nephrotic syndrome in adults over 44 years of age (55).

Presentation

Most patients present with constitutional symptoms of fatigue, weight loss, and light-headedness particularly in those who are nephrotic or have significant cardiac involvement. Common clinical signs are hepatomegaly (24%), purpura (15%), macroglossia (9%), splenomegaly (5%), and lymphadenopathy (3%). All organs except the brain can be affected. Hepatomegaly may be due to infiltration or cardiac congestion. Gut involvement causes malabsorption, hemorrhage, and obstruction. Neural involvement includes sensory and motor defects, compression lesions such as carpal tunnel syndrome and autonomic neuropathy which can be extremely disabling with severe postural hypotension as well as gastrointestinal, bladder, and erectile dysfunction. Deposition in the adrenal glands can lead to their insufficiency and contribute to hypotension. Cardiac deposits cause arrhythmias, conduction abnormalities, and low voltage complexes on ECG and heart failure with early diastolic dysfunction progressing to a restrictive cardiomyopathy with markedly increased echogenic hypertrophy on echocardiography. Skin manifestations include characteristic orbital purpura, generalized bruising, infiltrative plaques, and nodules.

Chronic kidney disease is present in 45% of the patients presenting with AL amyloid (56). Fifty-five percent of AL-amyloid patients have more than 1 g proteinuria per day with nephrotic syndrome present in 40% of patients at diagnosis. Twenty percent of patients with renal involvement will require dialysis after a median interval of 13–14 months (57) with predictors of ESRD including elevated creatinine and greater proteinuria at diagnosis (58).

Bleeding complications are due to vascular infiltration with amyloid, increased fibrinolysis, reduced conversion of fibrinogen to fibrin, and circulating anti-coagulants. Clotting factor deficiencies also occur and, of these, Factor X deficiency is the most common affecting up to 9% of the AL amyloid patients, via its adsorption to amyloid fibrils.

Renal pathology

Amyloid deposits are identified on light microscopy by positive staining with Congo Red or by apple-green birefringence on polarized light, on electron microscopy by the presence of randomly orientated, parallel arrays of non-branching fibrils which are 8–10 nm wide and 30–1,000 nm long, and by immunohistochemistry with specific antisera against λ or κ light chains (Figs 4.2 and 4.4a). Early deposits are found in the mesangium close to the hilum, along the glomerular basement membrane and on either side of capillary basement membrane or the arterial media. Initially segmental, these acellular deposits gradually enlarge to produce a nonproliferative nodular and sometimes obliterative glomerulopathy. Basement membrane deposits can resemble spikes, when viewed with silver stain. An involvement of the tubular basement membrane, vasa recta, interstitium, and larger arteries and veins leads to fibrosis.

Diagnosis

Diagnosis is confirmed by finding characteristic light chain deposits on the biopsies of subcutaneous fat, rectal mucosa, skin, or bone marrow, although the increased risk of bleeding should be considered before attempting a diagnostic biopsy of deep tissues, such as the kidney. Monoclonal light chains are found in urine and/or plasma in two-thirds of patients, with increased urinary yield in patients with proteinuria exceeding 1 g/day. Using conventional assays, no serum or urine M-band can be identified in 10% of patients with AL amyloid (59). However, the development of the serum FLC assay now permits diagnosis in 92% of cases (60) and 99% of cases when combined with conventional techniques (61). The FLC level informs both severity of organ involvement and is prognostic in patients with primary systemic amyloidosis undergoing peripheral blood stem cell transplantation (62). In patients with AL amyloid, a bone marrow biopsy should be undertaken to identify clonal plasma cell expansion and to exclude underlying myeloma which confers a worse prognosis.

The finding of SAP in all amyloid deposits has provided a novel and important scintigraphic test. Radiolabeled ^{123}I-SAP can be used both to diagnose amyloid and to monitor amyloid load. The distribution of deposits permits differentiation from AA amyloid, which favours the kidney and the gut rather than the heart, liver, spleen and the tongue. However, this test is not widely available.

Therapy

Fluid retention due to nephrotic syndrome, hypotension, and cardiac failure make clinical management very difficult. Fludrocortisone is used to manage hypotensive symptoms and new oral norepinephrine-analogues (e.g. midodrine) can help. In nephrotic patients, the circulating volume is contracted and renal function is very sensitive to diuretics. Proteinuria can be diminished by AII blockade and NSAIDs but at the expense of reduced GFR. Hoyer et al. (63) have reported three out of four patients with diuretic-resistant effusions and edema who benefited from treatment with bevacizumab, a monoclonal VEGF inhibitor. Rarely, in severe nephrotic syndrome, renal embolization and dialysis are required. Both hemodialysis and peritoneal dialysis are effective treatments when ESRF supervenes with survival determined by cardiac involvement. Cardiac and renal transplantation have been undertaken in patients with a single organ failure, although disease recurs.

Chemotherapy regimens derived from the treatment of multiple myeloma are used but responses are poor, which emphazises the lesser importance of the plasma cell load compared with toxic light chain load in this condition. Historically, the assessment of treatment efficacy using M-band levels was unsatisfactory and tissue deposits regressed slowly with most patients dying before any clinical improvement became apparent (64). However, the development of the FLC assay provides a useful tool to effectively assess treatments and progress.

High-dose therapy with autologous stem cell rescue has been used successfully in AL amyloid. With a median survival of 46 months, it offers a better outcome than conventional low-dose chemotherapy (65). However, high mortality rates (reaching 40% in some series) have been reported due to intolerance of fluid shifts that occur with peripheral blood stem cell harvesting and to multi-organ failure of tissues infiltrated with amyloid deposits. In addition, the reinfusion of stem cells will inevitably also return some of the neoplastic plasma cells and in this condition only a small tumor load is required for progressive disease.

Data comparing standard-dose therapy with high-dose chemotherapy with stem cell rescue are lacking and until these are available, the identification of those patients who will benefit from more aggressive therapy is unclear. The ideal patient for high-dose therapy has single organ involvement, normal renal function, no symptomatic cardiac dysfunction, no myeloma, and is aged less than 55 years (66), effectively restricting this treatment to patients presenting with nephrotic syndrome. In patients successfully treated, proteinuria persists for some time but does eventually diminish, which presumably reflects mobilization of tissue deposits.

Prognosis

The mean survival time in AL amyloidosis is 12–18 months. Fifty percent of all deaths are secondary to cardiac involvement and, if already advanced at the time of diagnosis, the median survival is reduced to six months. The presence of cholestatic jaundice at diagnosis confers an equally grim prognosis. In contrast, when the kidney is the major organ involved, the median survival increases to 21 months (67), although if dialysis is required, then the subsequent median survival is 8.2 months (57). Concomitant myeloma confers an adverse prognosis.

The development of the free light chain assay provides a new tool for both diagnosis and the assessment of treatment which will permit future trials to compare different therapeutic strategies. This may offer greater hope in the future, particularly if coupled with the development of novel molecules (e.g. 4'-Iodo-4'-deoxydoxorubicin) which increase the mobilization and catabolism of amyloid deposits.

Monoclonal immunoglobulin deposition disease

Monoclonal immunoglobulin deposition disease (MIDD) is distinct from AL amyloid and comprises light chain deposition disease (LCDD) and heavy chain deposition disease (HCDD), which are characterized by amorphous, non-fibrillary, and Congo Red negative deposits of monoclonal light chains or heavy chains, which can occasionally occur in combination (LHCDD) (Fig. 4.3). Studies of light chain variable regions and more recently their genes derived from clonal B cell populations have identified subgroups which may affect both clinical presentation and outcome. In LCDD, 80–90% of light chains are κ, with variable regions most commonly expressing the Vκ4 precursor protein. Increased hydrophobic amino acid substitutions (leucine, isoleucine, tyrosine) in the light chain CDR may cause structural destabilization,

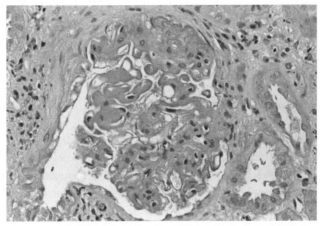

Fig. 4.3 Light chain deposition disease with nodular glomerulosclerosis and mesangial matrix accumulation.

which leads to aggregation of chains and increased interaction with matrix proteins. γ is the predominant class of heavy chain found in HCDD (associated with deletions in the constant domains, particularly CH1, and hinge regions), which accounts for the high prevalence of hypocomplementaemia due to fixation by γ1 and γ3 subclasses. Although binding to similar mesangial cell receptors, LCDD light chains exhibit different intracellular trafficking patterns and matrix metalloproteinase activation compared with AL-amyloid light chains (68). Whereas amyloid fibrils are formed in intracellular lysosomes, matrix deposits in LCDD and HCDD are extracellular and contain fibronectin, laminin, type IV collagen, and heparan sulphate proteoglycan with a possible stimulatory role for TGF-β (69). The morphological similarity of the glomerular deposits to diabetic nodular glomerulosclerosis suggests similar pathogenic pathways.

Epidemiology

MIDD is rare with a peak presentation in the sixth decade. However, significant underdiagnosis is probable since MIDD was found in 19% of the protocol biopsies performed in myeloma patients with coincident renal disease at the time of diagnosis (70).

Renal and other organ involvement

Proteinuric kidney disease with hypertension is seen almost invariably in patients with LCDD and HCDD (Table 4.5). Presentation is influenced by coexistent cast nephropathy and AL amyloid present in 19% and 7% respectively (71). Liver involvement ranges from abnormal liver function tests to hepatomegaly and rarely, fulminant hepatic failure and portal hypertension. MIDD can also cause cardiomegaly and heart failure. Thirty percent of cases have no detectable serum or urine M-band, with the serum free light chain assay offering greater diagnostic accuracy.

Pathology

Under light microscopy, the glomerulus can be normal or show evidence of mesangial expansion and proliferation, and basement membrane thickening. The most characteristic lesion found in 60% of the patients are homogeneous nodular deposits, similar to those found in diabetic nodular glomerulosclerosis, which suggests a similar pathogenic process. These nodules are PAS-positive, Congo Red-negative, and poorly argyrophilic. Tubular lesions, affecting distal tubules, loops of Henle and collecting ducts, feature PAS-positive ribbon-like material deposited in the outer part of the basement membrane. Similar basement membrane deposits are present in blood vessels.

Table 4.5 Renal presentation of 34 patients with pure MIDD on renal biopsy which comprised 12 LCDD, 5 mixed L+HCDD, 6 HCDD, and 11 LCDD with co-existent myeloma cast nephropathy (MCN) (71)

Clinical characteristic	LCDD	L+HCDD	HCDD	MIDD	LCDD+MCN
Overt multiple myeloma				39%	91%
Hypertension	83%	40%	100%	78%	64%
Proteinuria (g/day)	4.2 ± 0.8	2.9 ± 1.0	5.3 ± 2.2	4.2 ± 0.7	2.2 ± 0.7
Nephrotic (≥ 3 g/day)	50%	20%	67%	48%	18%
Microscopic hematuria	42%	60%	67%	52%	36%
Renal failure (creat ≥ 1.2mg/dL	92%	100%	100%	96%	100%

Immunostaining with light chain antisera (usually κ) shows fixation along the tubular and vascular basement membrane. This tends to be more reliable than the glomerular basement membrane staining, although the basement membrane lining the Bowman's capsule is usually positive. Staining of the glomerular nodules is variable, possibly reflecting chemical modification of the accretions. Immunostaining is negative in up to 15% of the cases although the use of heavy chain antisera identifies some cases which are positive for heavy chains and others which are positive for both light and heavy chains. In 80% of the cases, electron microscopy identifies finely granular, amorphous, electron dense deposits, which are more prominent and coarser in the tubular compared with glomerular basement membranes. The mesangial deposits are less dense and associated with mesangial matrix expansion. The apparent inconsistency of these findings and the significant prevalence of positive immunostaining in the absence of either granular deposits or electron-dense deposits could reflect the nonspecific trapping of circulating monoclonal light chains in the basement membrane.

Most other organs and tissues demonstrate positive immunostaining with deposits present in vascular and perivascular tissue. Hepatic deposits are found along the sinusoids, in the portal areas and in the centrilobular spaces with thickening of the biliary duct basement membrane and accumulation of extracellular matrix and collagen fibres. Occasionally, deposits are massive with associated dilatation and multiple ruptures of sinusoids resembling peliosis.

Prognosis

Data regarding prognosis, optimum management, and outcome in MIDD is weak, which reflects the infrequency of the diagnosis, the variability of treatment regimens, and, probably, histological imprecision with failure to specify coexistent cast and amyloid nephropathy. Reported survival is very variable and very short, if severe cardiac or hepatic involvement supervenes. In one study of 19 patients in which 18 received chemotherapy, 5-year actuarial patient survival and survival free of ESRD were 70% and 37%, respectively (72). Renal outcome is predicted by the serum creatinine at diagnosis with approximately one-third presenting in ESRD; of the remainder, two-thirds showed stability or improvement in renal function following chemotherapy (71). Consistent with this, there is evidence from serial biopsy studies that hepatic and renal deposits can regress, which emphasizes the importance of early diagnosis and treatment.

Treatment

Given the adverse prognosis from renal involvement, patients with MIDD should be managed actively, whether or not they meet diagnostic criteria for multiple myeloma. Standard myeloma chemotherapy regimens are used, including non-myeloablative therapies and high-dose therapy with stem cell rescue when appropriate (73–6). If required, patients should receive peritoneal dialysis or hemodialysis. A few patients have undergone renal transplantation, and although MIDD generally recurs in the graft, this is usually not clinically significant.

Cryoglobulins

Cryoglobulins are immunoglobulins which precipitate at 4°C and redissolve during warming. They may be a single monoclonal antibody (Type I cryoglobulinemia) which is almost always IgM or there is a polyclonal IgG fraction which is bound by monoclonal IgM (Type II) or polyclonal IgM (Type III). All three types may occur secondary to underlying lymphoproliferative disease, although there are other more important associations. In a report of 66 patients with Type II cryoglobulinaemia from the Mayo Clinic, there were 40 patients with Hepatitis C, 16 with lymphoproliferative disorders, and eight with connective tissue disease (77).

In Type I disease, the monoclonal immunoglobulin can precipitate independently, whereas in Type II and III, the IgM component has rheumatoid factor activity which binds the Fc portion of the polyclonal IgG to fix complement. Chronic circulating cryoglobulin–protein complexes increase serum viscosity, and can precipitate within small arteries and capillaries. Cryoprecipitates fix complement via the classical pathway, generating C3a, C3b, C5a, and C5b-9, which attract circulating platelets and leucocytes. This drives an inflammatory response, which leads to thrombosis and vasculitis, particularly affecting the extremities and glomerular microcirculation. See Table 4.6.

Clinical presentation

There is a female preponderance (3:1) with mean age 42–52 years at diagnosis. The presentation of Type I cryoglobulinemia commonly reflects hyperviscosity with acrocyanosis, retinal hemorrhage, severe Raynaud phenomenon, and arterial thrombosis. In contrast, patients with Types II and III cryoglobulinemia present with the symptoms of immune complex disease and vasculitis, which include rash (purpura, urticaria, vasculitis, and necrosis) in 55%, arthralgia in 21%, neuropathy in 18% and less commonly, abdominal pain (mucosal pupura and mesenteric vasculitis), pulmonary involvement (effusions, interstitial infiltrates, pulmonary hypertension, and intra-alveolar hemorrhage), and renal disease in 26% (77). Variable renal involvement includes proteinuria and microscopic hematuria, nephrotic syndrome, chronic kidney disease, and rapidly progressive (acute) kidney injury. Resistant and unexplained hypertension is a frequent concomitant symptom.

The commonest association with Types II and III cryoglobulinemia is underlying HCV infection, which is observed in 70–90% of these cases. The mechanism remains obscure, but involves the production of a IgMκ rheumatoid factor from an expanded B cell clone, possibly stimulated by a HCV–IgG complex. After ten years of HCV infection, approximately 50% of patients have evidence of a cryoglobulin, although it is pathological in only a minority. The B cell clone

Table 4.6 Cryoglobulin classification

Type	Classes of immunoglobulin	Clinical diagnosis
I	Monoclonal IgG or IgM	Multiple myeloma MGUS Waldenstrom's Macroglobulinaemia (IgM) Lymphoproliferative diseases including CLL, Lymphoma
II	Monoclonal IgM +Polyclonal IgG	Chronic hepatitis C infection Lymphoproliferative diseases including CLL, Lymphoma Idiopathic
III	Polyclonal IgG + IgM	Lymphoproliferative diseases Chronic infection (viral, bacterial, parasitic) Autoimmune disease (SLE, RA)

can become autonomous and 10–40% of patients meet diagnostic criteria for lymphoma or chronic lymphocytic leukemia within 10 years of diagnosis (78).

Investigations

Cryoglobulins should be suspected in the presence of reduced complement and a positive rheumatoid factor. Activation of the classical pathway results in low levels of C4 and CH50 with low or normal levels of C3. Patients should be screened for HCV, HBV, and other chronic infections (including HIV, CMV, EBV, endocarditis, chronically infected shunts, syphilis, leprosy, Lyme disease, Q fever, brucellosis, coccidiomycosis, schistosomiasis, malaria, toxoplasmosis) as appropriate.

Renal pathology

Types II and III cryoglobulinemia are usually associated with Type I membranopro-liferative glomerulonephritis. Immune deposits in mesangium and subendothelial space are associated with the mesangial proliferation, glomerular basement membrane thickening, and reduplication. Silver stain reveals double contoured GBM ('tram-lining') with granular deposits of IgM, IgG, C3, C1q, and C4 present in the capillary wall on immunostaining. Intracapillary PAS-positive cryoglobulin deposits can sometimes be seen, often associated with a macrophage infiltrate. Cellular crescents on renal biopsy correlate with a rapidly progressive clinical course and as with all glomerular diseases, the degree of tubulo-interstitial damage predicts renal prognosis. Electron microscopy shows dense deposits in the subendothelial and mesangial spaces with an organized tubular structure (Fig. 4.4(b)).

Type I membranoproliferative glomerulonephritis can also occur in the absence of serologically and histologically demonstrable cryoglobulin. In some cases, this may be due to the failure to identify a low titer of cryoglobulin.

Management

Conventional protocols are used when underlying myeloma, CLL, and lymphoma have been diagnosed. In patients with severe vasculitis, particularly if there is renal involvement, then steroids and cytotoxic therapy (cyclophosphamide and azathioprine) are commonly used. Plasma exchange, preferably using a centrifugal plasma separator, is a helpful adjunctive therapy. Given the role of platelets, aspirin and dipyridamole have been used with reports of reduced proteinuria and improved renal outcome.

Pegylated interferon-α may suppress HCV-related cryoglobulinemia although benefit takes weeks rather than days to accrue and is therefore not the treatment of choice in acute severe disease. There are also encouraging reports that HCV-driven lymphoma can regress with interferon-α (79).

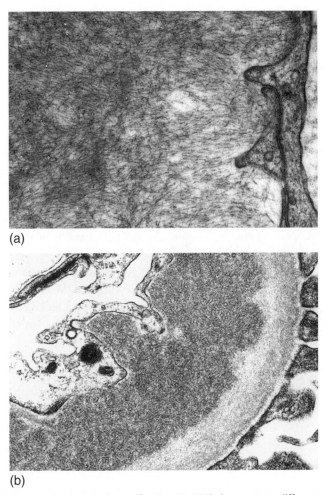

(a)

(b)

Fig. 4.4 Electron micrographs (magnification 55 000) demonstrate different arrangements of fibrils. (A) AL amyloid fibrils: randomly oriented, nonbranching fibrils, 8–15 nm wide; (B) Cryoglobulin: dense deposits with organized tubular structure.

Antiviral therapy may also be effective (80) and there are encouraging reports that rituximab, an anti-CD20 chimeric monoclonal antibody, may be effective for cryoglobulinemic glomerulonephritis and other disease manifestations although viral titers may rise (81).

Prognosis

The overall prognosis in cryoglobulinemia depends on concomitant disease, such as the presence of primary lymphoproliferative disease or viral hepatitis.

Morbidity due to cryoglobulinemic vasculitis can be significant, with arterial thrombosis, painful skin ulceration, and renal disease. Renal involvement is associated with worse survival (50% after 10 years) which reflects the severity of systemic involvement, infection, and cardiovascular disease rather than the renal outcome itself.

Waldenstrom's macroglobulinemia

Waldenstrom's macroglobulinemia is a low-grade lymphoplasmacytic lymphoma characterized by a circulating monoclonal IgM which causes a hyperviscosity syndrome. Presenting symptoms include constitutional symptoms, headaches, visual disturbance, and a history of abnormal bleeding due to coagulation abnormalities, thrombocytopenia, and anemia. Clinical signs include lymphadenopathy, hepatosplenomegaly, and peripheral neuropathy due to IgM deposition.

Significant renal involvement is rare but proteinuria, nephrotic syndrome, and renal impairment can occur. Within the kidney, IgM aggregates in the glomerular capillaries or is deposited within the basement membrane as PAS-positive Congo Red-negative deposits. Urinary light chains (usually κ) are present in 40% of patients and can cause cast nephropathy or an acquired Fanconi's syndrome with glycosuria, acidosis, generalized aminoaciduria, and hypophosphatemia (12). The kidneys can be infiltrated with tumor cells and cases of AL amyloid (Congo Red-positive) have been described. Waldenstrom's macroglobulinemia can present as Type I cryoglobulinemia causing glomerular disease.

POEMS syndrome

Originally described by Crow in 1956 and then Fukase in 1968, POEMS syndrome (Polyneuropathy, Organomegaly, Endocrinopathy, M-protein and Skin changes) is a rare multisystem disease with diagnosis requiring three or more of these five features. The pathogenesis remains obscure but is the consequence of an underlying plasma cell dyscrasia associated with elevated levels of IL-6, IL-1β, TNF-α, and VEGF (82). VEGF may promote increased vascular permeability leading to oedema, extravasation of plasma cell derived material, cytokines and complement, and vascular proliferation. These factors may drive neuropathy, lymphadenopathy, serositis, arteriopathy, and renal involvement.

Epidemiology and presentation

The median age at presentation is 51 years with 63% patients being male. Given the complexity of system involvement and the rarity of the condition, the diagnosis is frequently made late.

A sensorimotor polyneuropathy is always present and tends to be peripheral, symmetrical, and progressive with EMG showing components of both axonal degeneration and demyelinization, without cranial nerve or autonomic involvement. Organomegaly is present in 50% of patients and affects liver, spleen, and lymph nodes leading to lymphoedema. Although the histology of hepatomegaly is nonspecific, enlarged spleen and lymph nodes are present in 15% of patients and show evidence of Castleman disease. Endocrinopathy is present in 67% of the patients and include hypogonadism (55%), pituitary–adrenal axis insufficiency (18%), hypothyroidism (14%), diabetes mellitus or glucose intolerance, impotence and gynecomastia (due to elevated oestrogen levels), and hypoparathyroidism, although involvement may be restricted to blunted responses to dynamic testing.

Although Nakanishi et al. (83) identified a monoclonal plasma cell dyscrasia in only 42/52 cases, subsequent studies have almost invariably demonstrated a monoclonal λ light chain which is usually IgA or IgG (84–5). Use of plasma and urine immunofixation as well as the more sensitive FLC assay may define the presence of an M-band as an essential diagnostic feature. Some patients fit diagnostic criteria for plasmacytoma, Castleman's Disease or Waldenstrom's macroglobulinemia, but the tumor load is usually low and does not correlate with the clinical presentation. Skin changes are described in 68% of patients and most commonly feature hyper-pigmentation, skin thickening, acrocyanosis, hypertrichosis, and leuconychia, and cutaneous glomeruloid hemangioma, although unusual, are diagnostic. Pulmonary manifestations are prognostically important and include pulmonary hypertension, pleural effusions, restrictive lung disease, respiratory muscle weakness, and reduced alveolar-capillary gas transfer factor. Bone lesions (sclerotic, lytic, or both) were reported in 97% of cases and other features include thrombocytosis, weight loss, fatigue, diarrhoea, polycythemia, clubbing, thrombotic events, ascites, and congestive heart failure (85).

Nakamoto et al. (86) have reported the spectrum of renal involvement in 52 patients with the POEMS syndrome. Seventy-five percent of patients had less than 1 g proteinuria per day and none were nephrotic. Microscopic hematuria was reported in less than one-third of cases. Hypertension occurred in less than 25% of patients and 50% had plasma creatinine greater than 1.5 mg/dL. Asymmetrical renal atrophy was present in two cases. Most patients had an IgA-λ (46%) or IgG-λ (35%) paraprotein with no monoclonal protein identified in the remainder.

Renal pathology

The most common glomerular lesion is membranoproliferative glomerulonephritis, usually with negative immunostaining for heavy and light chains, immunoglobulins, complement, and fibrin. However, in biopsies with positive immunostaining, electron dense deposits may be present. Glomeruli are enlarged by mesangiolysis, micro-aneurysms, nodular lesions, and swollen endothelial-mesangial cells. Interstitial fibrosis and tubular atrophy may be present with subcapsular atrophy associated with a noninflammatory thrombotic microangiopathic process with intimal proliferation and severe luminal narrowing (85).

Treatment

In the case of isolated plasmacytomas, surgical excision may be curative. Radiation therapy of solitary osteosclerotic lesions is first-line therapy for patients with an isolated plasmacytoma.

Treatment should be aggressive with the emerging evidence of benefit from high-dose therapy with autologous stem cell rescue, when appropriate. Dispenzieri et al. (87) have reported treatment of 30 patients with high-dose chemotherapy followed by autologous hematopoietic stem cell transplantation. There was a 3% treatment-related mortality and 50% of patients achieved engraftment with clinical improvements and reduction in plasma VEGF levels. In patients with bony deposits, more than 50% of the patients responded to radiation; 22–50% of the patients responded to prednisolone and combined melphalan–prednisolone, respectively.

Bevacizumab (Avastin) is a monoclonal antibody which binds and inhibits VEGF to reduce plasma levels. There are reports of clinical improvement following treatment but no long-term data are available. In addition, there are worrying reports of adverse outcomes, possibly due to profound endothelial dysfunction in the context of reduced circulating VEGF levels, and, of course, this treatment strategy does not reduce clonal plasma cells.

Thalidomide is cytotoxic against plasma cells and reduces production of proinflammatory and proangiogenic cytokines with some reports to support its use in POEMS. Better results may be achieved with lenalidomide (Revlemid) which is a derivative of thalidomide that is a much more potent inhibitor of TNF-α and associated with fewer adverse side effects. There are also encouraging reports following the use of bortezomib (Velcade) which causes neoplastic cell apoptosis by proteasome inhibition. Neither intravenous immunoglobulin nor plasmapheresis have shown therapeutic benefit.

Prognosis

The median survival of 99 patients reported in 2003 was 165 months and only clubbing and extravascular volume overload at presentation correlated with an adverse outcome. Patients died from cachexia, infections, cardio-respiratory failure and progressive inanition rather than from plasma cell expansion (85). A recent retrospective review of 137 patients emphasized the importance of respiratory involvement with muscle weakness and cough being associated with reduced survival (87 vs. 139 months, p <0.05) (88).

Castleman's disease

Castleman's disease is a rare lymphoproliferative disorder which may be unicentric (commonly in the mediastinum) or multicentric. Histology may show hyaline-vascular variant, plasma cell variant, or mixed variant, with each type associated with increased IL-6 production which is either endogenous or secondary to infection with human herpesvirus 8 (vIL-6). HHV-8 infection is present in almost all HIV-associated disease and 50% of HIV negative cases.

Presenting symptoms include malaise, weight loss, anemia, and elevated markers of systemic inflammation (CRP, SA-A), particularly with the plasma cell variant. Rarely, patients present with proteinuria and nephrotic syndrome and a variety of glomerular lesions have been described. These include membranoproliferative glomerulonephritis, crescentic glomerulonephritis, anti-glomerular basement membrane disease, membranous glomerulonephritis, fibrillary glomerulonephritis, AA amyloid, and interstitial nephritis.

Unicentric disease (usually hyaline-vascular variant) may be cured by surgical excision and this has been associated with renal remission including regression of AA amyloid (89). The treatment of multicentric disease may include antiviral therapy (including both antiretroviral and anti-HHV-8), single-agent chemotherapy, combination chemotherapy, interferon α, rituximab (anti-CD20 antibodies) to achieve B cell depletion, monoclonal anti-IL6 receptor antibodies (e.g. tocilizumab), and thalidomide (90).

Fibrillary and immunotactoid glomerulonephritis

These rare histological entities are characterized by extracellular deposits of nonbranching isodense fibrils or microtubules with an electron-lucent core within the mesangium and the glomerular capillary walls on electron microscopy. Thicker than amyloid fibrils, deposits lack the β-pleated sheet structure and are Congo Red-Negative. In addition to their characteristically wider and microtubular structure, immunotactoid deposits demonstrate a parallel array compared with the random distribution of fibrillary deposits. The importance of trying to differentiate between these two entities is emphasized by two studies (91–2) in which immunotactoid disease was associated with monoclonal paraproteinemia, lymphoproliferative disease (plasma cell dyscrasia, CLL, and non Hodgkin's lymphoma), adenocarcinoma, and hypocomplementemia.

In contrast, fibrillary glomerulonephritis was associated with connective tissue disease (including mixed connective tissue disease, primary Sjögren's, and anti-phospholipid syndrome), HCV, and leucocytoclastic vasculitis.

Renal pathology

Immunotactoid deposits

PAS-positive deposits are associated with mesangial expansion, hypercellularity, and capillary wall thickening and lead to diagnosis of membranous, mesangiocapillary, or mesangioproliferative glomerulonephritis, occasionally with crescents. Vascular and tubulo-interstitial involvement are common. Immunostaining is usually positive for the coarse deposits of IgG and C3 along capillary basement membrane and in the mesangium. Electron microscopy is required to demonstrate the microtubules deposited in the subepithelial space and mesangium with diameters that usually exceed 30 nm arranged in parallel arrays (Fig. 4.4(d)). Of renal biopsies with immunotactoid deposits 50% to 95% are histochemically positive for light chains, although circulating M-bands are less frequently detected on immunofixation. Intracytoplasmic IgG deposits, of the same type as those found in the kidney, may be demonstrated in lymphocytes from blood or bone marrow, especially in patients with underlying CLL or B cell lymphoma (91). Alveolar capillary membrane and dermal deposits have also been reported in patients with pulmonary-renal and skin involvement respectively.

Fibrillary deposits

These deposits occur in association with membranous, mesangiocapillary or mesangioproliferative glomerulonephritis with positive immunostaining for IgG. Vascular and tubulo-interstitial involvement is common. Electron microscopy demonstrates narrow fibrils deposited in the subepithelial space and mesangium with diameters less than 30 nm but arranged randomly (Fig. 4.4(c)). Deposits tend to be polyclonal, with no evidence of plasma cell dyscrasia or underlying lymphoproliferative disorder, and intriguingly, frequently involve IgG$_4$. This particular subclass may have structural properties, which predispose to fibril formation. This polyclonal activation favors an autoimmune pathogenesis.

Clinical presentation

Fibrillary glomerulonephritis is extremely rare (<1% of native kidney biopsies) with immunotactoid disease tenfold rarer. Patients present with hypertension, microscopic hematuria, proteinuria, nephrotic syndrome, and CKD. Rapidly progressive disease with crescentic glomerulonephritis is

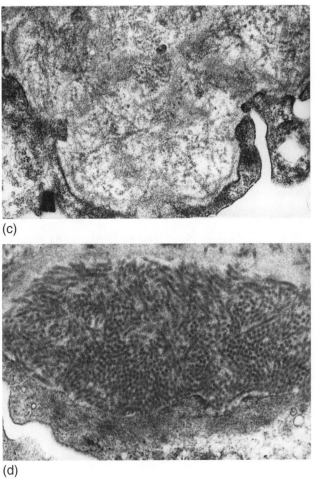

Fig. 4.4 (*continued*) (C) Fibrillary glomerulonephritis: randomly oriented, amyloid-like fibrils, less than 30 nm wide; (D) Immunotactoid glomerulonephritis: thick-walled microtubules arranged in parallel arrays, diameter usually exceeds 30 nm.

reported to be more common in fibrillary disease and, overall, 50% of patients will progress to ESRF within four years (93). Extra-renal presentation with pulmonary alveolar hemorrhage and cutaneous leucocytoclastic vasculitis is reported.

Treatment

The overall response to steroid and cytotoxic therapy is not encouraging, with slightly better renal survival in patients with immunotactoid as opposed to fibrillary glomerulonephritis. However, disease recurrence following renal transplantation is more common amongst patients with a monoclonal gammopathy (94). The prognosis of these extremely rare diseases will hopefully improve as treatment of the underlying plasma cell dyscrasia becomes more effective.

References

1 American Cancer Society: http://www.cancer.org/docroot/CRI/CRI_2_1x. asp?rnav=criov&dt=30.

2 Calle EE, Rodriguez C, Walker-Thurmond K, Thun MJ (2003). Overweight, obesity, and mortality from cancer in a prospectively studied cohort of U.S. adults. *N Engl J Med* **348**: 1625–38.

3 Kyle RA (1975). Multiple myeloma: review of 869 cases. *Mayo Clin Proc* **50**: 29–40.

4 Ogmundsdottir HM, Haraldsdottir V, M Johannesson G, et al. (2002). Monoclonal gammopathy in Iceland: a population-based registry and follow-up. *Br J Haematol* **118**: 166–73.

5 Brown LM, Linet MS, Greenberg RS, et al. (1999). Multiple myeloma and family history of cancer among blacks and whites in the U.S. *Cancer* **85**: 2385–90.

6 Bourguet CC, Logue EE (1993). Antigenic stimulation and multiple myeloma. A prospective study. *Cancer* **72**: 2148–54.

7 Lacy MQ, Donovan KA, Heimbach JK, Ahmann GJ, Lust JA (1999). Comparison of interleukin-1 beta expression by in situ hybridization in monoclonal gam-mopathy of undetermined significance and multiple myeloma. *Blood* **93**: 300–5.

8 Gherardi RK, Belec L, Fromont G, et al. (1994). Elevated levels of interleukin-1 beta (IL-1 beta) and IL-6 in serum and increased production of IL-1 beta mRNA in lymph nodes of patients with polyneuropathy, organomegaly, endocrinopathy, M protein, and skin changes (POEMS) syndrome. *Blood* **83**: 2587–93.

9 Greipp PR, San Miguel J, Durie BG, et al. (2005). International staging system for multiple myeloma. *J Clin Oncol* **23**: 3412–20.

10 Sengul S, Zwizinski C, Simon EE, et al. (2002). Endocytosis of light chains induces cytokines through activation of NF-kappaB in human proximal tubule cells. *Kidney Int* **62**: 1977–88.

11 Li M, Maderdrut JL, Lertora JJ, et al. (2008). Renoprotection by pituitary adenylate cyclase-activating polypeptide in multiple myeloma and other kidney diseases. *Regul Pept* **145**: 24–32.

12 Lacy MQ and Gertz MA (1999). Acquired Fanconi's syndrome associated with mono-clonal gammopathies. *Hematol Oncol Clin North Am* **13**: 1273–80.

13 Decourt C, Bridoux F, Touchard G, Cogne M (2003). A monoclonal V kappa l light chain responsible for incomplete proximal tubulopathy. *Am J Kidney Dis* **41**: 497–504.

14 Russell WJ, Cardelli J, Harris E, Baier RJ, Herrera GA (2001). Monoclonal light chain—mesangial cell interactions: early signaling events and subsequent pathologic effects. *Lab Invest* **81**: 689–703.

15 Ying WZ and Sanders PW (2001). Mapping the binding domain of immunoglobulin light chains for Tamm-Horsfall protein. *Am J Pathol* **158**: 1859–66.

16 Huang ZQ and Sanders PW (1995). Biochemical interaction between Tamm-Horsfall glycoprotein and Ig light chains in the pathogenesis of cast nephropathy. *Lab Invest* **73**: 810–17.

17 Sanders PW, Booker BB, Bishop JB, Cheung HC (1990). Mechanisms of intranephronal proteinaceous cast formation by low molecular weight proteins. *J Clin Invest* **85**: 570–6.

18 Dispenzieri A, Kyle R, Merlini G, et al. (2009). International Myeloma Working Group guidelines for serum-free light chain analysis in multiple myeloma and related disorders. *Leukemia* **23**: 215–24.

19 Dimopoulos M, Terpos E, Comenzo RL, et al. (2009) International myeloma working group consensus statement and guidelines regarding the current role of imaging techniques in the diagnosis and monitoring of multiple Myeloma. *Leukemia.* **23**: 1545–56.

20 Kumar S, Gertz MA, Dispenzieri A, et al. (2003). Response rate, durability of response, and survival after thalidomide therapy for relapsed multiple myeloma. *Mayo Clin Proc* **78**: 34–9.

21 Weber DM, Chen C, Niesvizky R, et al. (2007). Lenalidomide plus dexamethasone for relapsed multiple myeloma in North America. *N Engl J Med* **357**: 2133–42.

22 Chen N, Lau H, Kong L, Kumar G, Zeldis JB, Knight R, Laskin OL (2007). Pharmacokinetics of lenalidomide in subjects with various degrees of renal impairment and in subjects on hemodialysis. *J Clin Pharmacol* **47**: 1466–75.

23 San Miguel JF, Schlag R, Khuageva NK, et al. (2008). Bortezomib plus melphalan and prednisone for initial treatment of multiple myeloma. *N Engl J Med* **359**: 906–17.

24 Roussel M, Moreau P, Huynh A, et al. (2010). Bortezomib and high dose melphalan as conditioning regimen before autologous stem cell transplantation in patients with de novo multiple myeloma: a phase II study of the Intergroupe Francophone du Myelome (IFM). *Blood,* **115**: 32–7.

25 Shah JJ, Orlowski RZ (2009). Proteasome inhibitors in the treatment of multiple myeloma. *Leukemia* **23**: 1964–79.

26 Fulciniti M, Hideshima T, Vermot-Desroches C, et al. (2009). A high-affinity fully human anti-IL-6 mAb, 1339, for the treatment of multiple myeloma. *Clin Cancer Res* **15**: 7144–52.

27 Badros A, Burger AM, Philip S, et al. (2009). Phase I study of vorinostat in combination with bortezomib for relapsed and refractory multiple myeloma. *Clin Cancer Res* **15**: 5250–7.

28 Mitsiades CS, Hideshima T, Chauhan D, et al. (2009). Emerging treatments for multiple myeloma: beyond immunomodulatory drugs and bortezomib. *Semin Hematol* **46**: 166–75.

29 Djulbegovic B, Wheatley K, Ross J, et al. (2002). Bisphosphonates in multiple myeloma. *Cochrane Database Syst Rev* **3**: CD003188.

30 American Society of Clinical Oncology (2007). Clinical practice guideline update on the role of bisphosphonates in multiple myeloma. http://www.guideline.gov/summary/summary.aspx?doc_id=10857&nbr=005670

31 Sarasquete ME, García-Sanz R, Marín L, et al. (2008) Bisphosphonate-related osteonecrosis of the jaw is associated with polymorphisms of the cytochrome P450 CYP2C8 in multiple myeloma: a genome-wide single nucleotide polymorphism analysis. *Blood* **112**: 2709–12.

32 Pozzi C, Pasquali S, Donini U, Casanova S, Banfi G, Tiraboschi G, Furci L, Porri MT, Ravelli M, Lupo A. et al. (1987). Prognostic factors and effectiveness of treatment in acute renal failure due to multiple myeloma: a review of 50 cases. Report of the Italien Renal Immunopathology Group. *Clin Nephrol* **28**: 1–9.

33 Zucchelli P, Pasquali S, Cagnoli L, Ferrari G (1988). Controlled plasma exchange trial in acute renal failure due to multiple myeloma. *Kidney Int* **33**: 1175–80.

34 Moist L, Nesrallah G, Kortas C, Espirtu E, Ostbye T, Clark WF (1999). Plasma exchange in rapidly progressive renal failure due to multiple myeloma. A retro-spective case series. *Am J Nephrol* **19**: 45–50.

35 Leung N, Gertz MA, Zeldenrust SR, et al. (2008). Improvement of cast nephropathy with plasma exchange depends on the diagnosis and on reduction of serum free light chains. *Kidney Int* **73**: 1282–8.

36 Hutchison CA, Cockwell P, Reid S, et al. (2007). Efficient removal of immunoglobulin free light chains by hemodialysis for multiple myeloma: in vitro and in vivo studies. *J Am Soc Nephrol* **18**: 886–95.

37 Hutchison CA, Cook M, Heyne N, Weisel K, Billingham L, Bradwell A, Cockwell P. (2008). European trial of free light chain removal by extended haemodialysis in cast nephropathy (EuLITE): a randomised control trial. *Trials* **9**: 55.

38 Child JA, Morgan GJ, Davies FE, et al. (2003). High-dose chemotherapy with hematopoietic stem-cell rescue for multiple myeloma. *N Engl J Med* **348**: 1875–83.

39 Cavo M, Tosi P, Zamagni E, et al. (2007). Prospective, randomized study of single compared with double autologous stem-cell transplantation for multiple myeloma: Bologna 96 clinical study. *J Clin Oncol* **25**: 2434–41.

40 San Miguel JF, Lahuerta JJ, Garcia-Sanz R, et al. (2000). Are myeloma patients with renal failure candidates for autologous stem cell transplantation? *Hematol J* **1**: 28–36.

41 Sirohi B, Powles R, Mehta J. et al. (2001). The implication of compromised renal function at presentation in myeloma: similar outcome in patients who receive high-dose therapy: a single-center study of 251 previously untreated patients. *Med Oncol* **18**: 39–50.

42 Badros A, Barlogie B, Siegel E. et al. (2001). Results of autologous stem cell transplant in multiple myeloma patients with renal failure. *Br J Haematol* **114**: 822–9.

43 Raab MS, Breitkreutz I, Hundemer M., et al. (2006). The outcome of autologous stem cell transplantation in patients with plasma cell disorders and dialysis-dependent renal failure. *Haematologica* **91**: 1555–8.

44 Parikh GC, Amjad AI, Saliba RM, et al. (2009). Autologous hematopoietic stem cell transplantation may reverse renal failure in patients with multiple myeloma. *Biol Blood Marrow Transplant* **15**: 812–16.

45 Matsue K, Fujiwara H, Iwama KI, et al. (2010) Reversal of dialysis-dependent renal failure in patients with advanced multiple myeloma: single institutional experiences over 8 years. *Ann Hematol*, **89**: 291–7.

46 U.K Myeloma Forum (2001). Diagnosis and management of multiple myeloma. *Br J Haematol* **115**: 522–40.

47 Wilson J, Yao GL, Raftery J, et al. (2007). A systematic review and economic evaluation of epoetin alpha, epoetin beta and darbepoetin alpha in anaemia associated with cancer, especially that attributable to cancer treatment. *Health Technol Assess* **11**: 1–202, iii–iv.

48 Iggo N, Palmer AB, Severn A, et al. (1989). Chronic dialysis in patients with multiple myeloma and renal failure: a worthwhile treatment. *Q J Med* **73**: 903–10.

49 Korzets A, Tam F, Russell G, Feehally J, Walls J (1990). The role of continuous ambulatory peritoneal dialysis in end-stage renal failure due to multiple myeloma. *Am J Kidney Dis* **16**: 216–23.

50 Sharland A, Snowdon L, Joshua DE, Gibson J, Tiller DJ (1997). Hemodialysis: an appropriate therapy in myeloma-induced renal failure. *Am J Kidney Dis* **30**: 786–92.

51 Abbott KC and Agodoa LY (2001). Multiple myeloma and light chain-associated nephropathy at end-stage renal disease in the United States: patient characteristics and survival. *Clin Nephrol* **56**: 207–10.

52 Tsakiris DJ, Stel VS, Finne P, et al. (2010). Incidence and outcome of patients starting renal replacement therapy for end-stage renal disease due to multiple myeloma or light-chain deposit disease: an ERA-EDTA Registry study. *Nephrol Dial Transplant*, **25**: 1200–6.

53 Merlini G and Bellotti V (2003). Molecular mechanisms of amyloidosis. *N Engl J Med* **349**: 583–96.

54 Abraham RS, Geyer SM, Price-Troska TL, et al. (2003). Immunoglobulin light chain variable (V) region genes influence clinical presentation and outcome in light chain-associated amyloidosis (AL). *Blood* **101**: 3801–7.

55 Haas M, Meehan SM, Karrison TG, Spargo B.H. (1997). Changing etiologies of unexplained adult nephrotic syndrome: a comparison of renal biopsy findings from 1976–1979 and 1995–1997. *Am J Kidney Dis* **30**: 621–31.

56 Kyle RA and Gertz MA (1995). Primary systemic amyloidosis: clinical and laboratory features in 474 cases. *Semin Hematol* **32**: 45.

57 Gertz MA, Kyle RA, O'Fallon WM (1992). Dialysis support of patients with primary systemic amyloidosis. A study of 211 patients. *Arch Intern Med* **152**: 2245–50.

58 Sezer O, Eucker J, Jakob C, Possinger K (2000). Diagnosis and treatment of AL amyloidosis. *Clin Nephrol* **53**: 417–23.

59 Gertz NA, Lacy MQ, Dispensieri A (2002). Immunoglobulin light chain amyloidosis and the kidney. *Kidney Int* **61**: 1–9.

60 Lachmann HJ, Gallimore R, Gillmore JD, Carr-Smith HD (2003). Outcome in systemic AL amyloidosis in relation to changes in concentration of circulating immunoglobulin light chains following chemotherapy. *Br J Haematol* **122**: 78–84.

61 Gertz MA, Comenzo R, Falk RH, et al. (2005) Definition of organ involvement and treatment response in immunoglobulin light chain amyloidosis (AL): a consensus opinion from the 10th International Symposium on Amyloid and Amyloidosis. *Am J Haematol* **79**: 319–28.

62 Dispenzieri A, Lacy MQ, Katzmann JA, et al. (2006). Absolute values of immunoglobulin free light chains are prognostic in patients with primary systemic amyloidosis undergoing peripheral blood stem cell transplantation. *Blood* **107**: 3378–83.

63 Hoyer RJ, Leung N, Witzig TE, Lacy MQ (2007). Treatment of diuretic refractory pleural effusions with bevacizumab in four patients with primary systemic amyloidosis. *Am J Hematol* **82**: 409–13.

64 Kyle RA, Gertz MA, Greipp PR, et al. (1999). Long-term survival (10 years or more) in 30 patients with primary amyloidosis. *Blood* **93**: 1062–9.

65 Gertz MA, Lacy MQ, Dispenzieri A. (2000). Myeloablative chemotherapy with stem cell rescue for the treatment of primary systemic amyloidosis: a status report. *Bone Marrow Transplant* **25**: 465–70.

66 Comenzo RL and Gertz MA (2002). Autologous stem cell transplantation for primary systemic amyloidosis. *Blood* **99**: 4276–82.

67 Falk RH, Comenzo RL, Skinner M (1997). The systemic amyloidoses. *N Engl J Med* **337**: 898–909.

68 Teng J, Russell WJ, Gu X, et al. (2004). Different types of glomerulopathic light chains interact with mesangial cells using a common receptor but exhibit different intracellular trafficking patterns. *Lab Invest* **84**: 440–51.

69 Zhu L, Herrera GA, Murphy-Ullrich JE, et al. (1995). Pathogenesis of glomerulosclerosis in light chain deposition disease. Role for transforming growth factor-beta. *Am J Pathol* **147**: 375–85.

70 Montseny JJ, Kleinknecht D, Meyrier A, et al. (1998). Long-term outcome according to renal histological lesions in 118 patients with monoclonal gammopathies. *Nephrol Dial Transplant* **13**: 1438–45.

71 Lin J, Markowitz GS, Valeri AM, et al. (2001). Renal monoclonal immunoglobulin deposition disease: the disease spectrum. *J Am Soc Nephrol* **12**: 1482–92.

72 Heilman RL, Velosa JA, Holley KE, Offord KP, Kyle RA (1992). Long-term follow-up and response to chemotherapy in patients with light-chain deposition disease. *Am J Kidney Dis* **20**: 34–41.

73 Royer B, Arnulf B, Martinez F, et al. (2004). High dose chemotherapy in light chain or light and heavy chain deposition disease. *Kidney Int* **65**: 642–8.

74 Firkin F, Hill PA, Dwyer K, Gock H (2004). Reversal of dialysis-dependent renal failure in light-chain deposition disease by autologous peripheral blood stem cell transplantation. *Am J Kidney Dis* **44**: 551–5.

75 Lorenz EC, Gertz MA, Fervenza FC, et al. (2008). Long-term outcome of autologous stem cell transplantation in light chain deposition disease. *Nephrol Dial Transplant* **23**: 2052–7.

76 Kastritis E, Migkou M, Gavriatopoulou M, et al. (2009). Treatment of light chain deposition disease with bortezomib and dexamethasone. *Haematologica* **94**: 300–2.

77 Bryce AH, Kyle RA, Dispenzieri A, Gertz MA (2006). Natural history and therapy of 66 patients with mixed cryoglobulinemia. *Am J Hematol* **81**: 511–18.

78 Saadoun D, Sellam J, Ghillani-Dalbin P, et al. (2006). Increased risks of lymphoma and death among patients with non-hepatitis C virus-related mixed cryoglobulinemia. *Arch Intern Med* **166**: 2101–8.

79 Hermine O, Lefrere F, Bronowicki JP, et al. (2002). Regression of splenic lymphoma with villous lymphocytes after treatment of hepatitis C virus infection. *N Engl J Med* **347**: 89–94.

80 Enomoto M, Nakanishi T, Ishii M, Tamori A, Kawada N (2008). Entecavir to treat hepatitis B-associated cryoglobulinemic vasculitis. *Ann Intern Med* **149**: 912–13.

81 Quartuccio L, Soardo G, Romano G, Zaja F, Scott CA, De Marchi G, et al. (2006). Rituximab treatment for glomerulonephritis in HCV-associated mixed cryoglobulinaemia: efficacy and safety in the absence of steroids. *Rheumatology* **45**: 842–6.

82 Watanabe O, Arimura K, Kitajima I, Osame M, Maruyama I (1996). Greatly raised vascular endothelial growth factor (VEGF) in POEMS syndrome. *Lancet* **347**: 702.

83 Nakanishi T, Sobue I, Toyokura Y, et al. (1984). The Crow-Fukase syndrome: A study of 102 cases in Japan. *Neurology* **34**: 712–20.

84 Soubrier MJ, Dubost JJ, Sauvezie BJ (1994). POEMS syndrome: a study of 25 cases and a review of the literature. *Am J Med* **97**: 543–53.

85 Dispenzieri A, Kyle RA, Lacy MQ, et al. (2003). POEMS syndrome: definitions and long-term outcome. *Blood* **101**: 2496–506.

86 Nakamoto Y, Imai H, Yasuda T, Wakui H, Miura AB (1999). A spectrum of clinicopathological features of nephropathy associated with POEMS syndrome. *Nephrol Dial Transplant* **14**: 2370–8.

87 Dispenzieri A, Lacy MQ, Hayman SR, et al. (2008). Peripheral blood stem cell transplant for POEMS syndrome is associated with high rates of engraftment syndrome. *Eur J Haematol* **80**: 397–406.

88 Allam JS, Kennedy CC, Aksamit TR, Dispenzieri A (2008). Pulmonary manifestations in patients with POEMS syndrome: a retrospective review of 137 patients. *Chest* **133**: 969–74.

89 Lachmann HJ, Gilbertson JA, Gillmore JD, Hawkins PN, Pepys MB (2002). Unicentric Castleman's disease complicated by systemic AA amyloidosis: a curable disease. *QJM* **95**: 211–18.

90 Dispenzieri A, Gertz MA (2005). Treatment of Castleman's disease. *Curr Treat Options Oncol* **6**: 255–66.

91 Bridoux F, Hugue V, Coldefy O, et al. (2002). Fibrillary glomerulonephritis and immuno-tactoid (microtubular) glomerulopathy are associated with distinct immunologic features. *Kidney Int* **62**: 1764.

92 Rosenstock JL, Markowitz GS, Valeri AM, et al. (2003). Fibrillary and immunotactoid glomerulonephritis: Distinct entities with different clinical and pathologic features. *Kidney Int* **63**: 1450–61

93 Pronovost PH, Brady HR, Gunning ME, Espinoza O, Rennke HG (1996). Clinical features, predictors of disease progression and results of renal transplantation in fibrillary /immunotactoid glomerulopathy. *Nephrol Dial Transplant* **11**: 837–42.

94 Czarnecki PG, Lager DJ, Leung N, et al. (2009). Long-term outcome of kidney transplantation in patients with fibrillary glomerulonephritis or monoclonal gammopathy with fibrillary deposits. *Kidney Int* **75**: 420–7.

Chapter 5

Nephrotoxicity of chemotherapy agents and chemotherapy administration in patients with renal disease

Carlos D. Flombaum

Case report

A woman with a history of breast cancer was hospitalized with acute pulmonary edema following a blood transfusion (Fig. 5.1). She had been treated for one year with mitomycin C (MMC) (total cumulative dose 86 mg/m^2). During the latter part of the treatment she developed worsening anemia, thrombocytopenia, and other changes compatible with a microangiopathic hemolytic anemia (rising lactic acid dehydrogenase (LDH) levels and schistocytes in the peripheral blood smear). During the two months preceding the present hospitalization, she had also developed worsening hypertension, dyspnea, and a progressive rise in blood urea nitrogen (BUN) and creatinine levels. During the three months after her first episode of pulmonary edema, she again was hospitalized for pulmonary edema which occurred in association with recalcitrant hypertension. Her hematological abnormalities improved, but she later died following a hemorrhagic stroke.

Nephrotoxicity of chemotherapy agents

The kidneys normally receive 20% of the cardiac output. Drugs are filtered and/or secreted and then progressively concentrated in the urine. Therefore, these organs are especially vulnerable to the toxic effects of many drugs, including chemotherapy agents (1–3).

Nephrotoxicity is often a dose-limiting adverse effect of chemotherapy. Chemotherapy agents can affect the microvasculature, the glomerulus, or the tubules. Depending on the site of the nephron more adversely affected, the clinical manifestations may vary from a hemolytic process resembling the hemolytic uremic syndrome (HUS) or a tubular-interstitial injury causing asymptomatic decreases in the glomerular filtration rate (GFR), overt renal failure requiring dialysis, or a variety of electrolyte disorders.

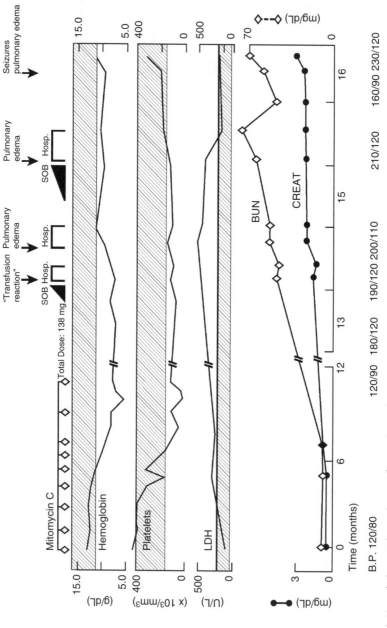

Fig. 5.1 Hemolytic-uremic syndrome after prolonged mitomycin C chemotherapy. SOB, shortness of breath; Hosp, hospitalization.

Because the kidneys are one of the major routes of elimination of many drugs, nephrotoxicity is a serious complication in patients undergoing chemotherapy. The dose of renally eliminated drugs has to be adjusted in order to prevent systemic toxicity, and the administration of other potentially nephrotoxic drugs, such as chemotherapy agents or antibiotics, may have to be interrupted, making management of the patient more difficult.

This section will review the nephrotoxic effects of different chemotherapy agents and some preventive measures to avoid their nephrotoxicity. The metabolism of those chemotherapy agents that are predominantly renally excreted and the recommended dose modifications in patients with renal insufficiency will be reviewed in the second part of this chapter. The most common methods utilized to estimate GFR are the creatinine clearance (CrCl) or the clearance of radiolabeled compounds. The creatinine clearance can be determined from a 24-hour urine collection or based on formulas which use the plasma creatinine concentration (like the Cockcroft–Gault equation). More recently, clinical laboratories are using the Modification of Diet in Renal Disease (MDRD) equation to report GFR (4), but it needs to be stressed that up to now, the vast majority of pharmacokinetic studies in oncology did not use this formula and were performed by measuring CrCl or estimating it by the Cockcroft–Gault equation. For practical purposes and because they are close to each other in absolute value, creatinine clearance and GFR are used interchangeably throughout this chapter.

Agents causing thrombotic microangiopathy and hemolytic-uremic syndrome

Mitomycin C

Case report

A patient with a history of rectal carcinoma was evaluated because of chronic renal disease and worsening hypertension. Six years earlier, he had been treated with MMC for approximately ten months. During the five months following the MMC chemotherapy, he developed mild anemia and thrombocytopenia together with elevated LDH levels and undetectable haptoglobin in blood. His BUN and creatinine, which were 4.6 mmol/L (13 mg/dL) and 97 μmol/L (1.1 mg/dL) respectively prior to starting chemotherapy, had risen to 14 mmol/L (38 mg/dL) and 195 μmol/L (2.2 mg/dL). Six years later, at the time of the consultation, BUN and creatinine levels were 15 mmol/L (41 mg/dL) and 24.8 μmol/L (2.8 mg/dL), he still had mild anemia, but the thrombocytopenia had resolved. His blood pressure was 220/120 mmHg. His hypertension was easily controlled with antihypertensive medications. His renal disease was attributed to chronic MMC nephrotoxicity.

Mitomycin C is an alkylating antibiotic used in the treatment of breast, gastrointestinal, pancreatic, and lung cancers. MMC nephrotoxicity typically manifests with the development of the HUS, which is usually detected six to twenty months after the initiation of chemotherapy. A characteristic triad of microangiopathic hemolytic anemia (MAHA), thrombocytopenia, and renal failure is present. Worsening Coombs-negative hemolytic anemia and thrombocytopenia are the earliest detectable hematological abnormalities (5–8). The typical features of MAHA are present, and they include the presence of schistocytes in the peripheral smear, decreased serum haptoglobin, and rising LDH levels in conjunction with normal coagulation tests. The MAHA usually precedes the development of renal failure by weeks and in some cases may have resolved by the time azotemia develops. Some patients may present with a more indolent course with isolated renal impairment without overt MAHA (9). The renal insufficiency shows a pattern of subacute progression with BUN and creatinine levels increasing slowly and progressively within weeks after the initial detection of azotemia. Some patients require dialysis, but in others, renal function stabilizes and in some cases there may be a slow improvement with time. Microhematuria with red blood cell casts, together with mild proteinuria are present in most cases. Other manifestations commonly seen include the development of severe hypertension and episodes of noncardiogenic pulmonary edema often precipitated by blood transfusions (5–6). Severe hypertension usually precedes the onset of other severe complications such as pulmonary edema, hypertensive encephalopathy, or seizures. The renal biopsy findings are those of a thrombotic microangiopathy as seen in most cases of HUS (5–6). These changes typically include occlusive thrombi in small arteries and arterioles, glomerular mesangiolysis, and a widening of the subendothelial space due to detachment of the endothelial cells from the glomerular basement membrane with accumulation of electron-lucent material.

The nephrotoxicity of MMC is dose-dependent and appears usually after cumulative doses of more than 40–60 mg/m^2 given over a period of several months (8). Based on this observation, MMC is presently given for only two or three doses and the incidence of nephrotoxicity and HUS have decreased markedly. Direct endothelial injury appears to be responsible for the renal damage as evidenced by the appearance of the classic microangiopathic changes when MMC is infused directly into the rat renal artery (10).

High-dose corticosteroids, plasmapheresis, and antiplatelet drugs have been tried as therapy, with variable success (11). Some patients may also have a spontaneous improvement in the MAHA and thrombocytopenia with conservative treatment alone, and therefore, it is difficult to make conclusions of the effectiveness of the above interventions.

Gemcitabine

Case report

A patient with lung cancer was initially treated with taxol and trastuzumab for ten months. Because of the progression of the disease, she received nine additional months of treatment with gemcitabine (Fig. 5.2). Five months after starting chemotherapy with this drug, she developed worsening hypertension, which had been preceded by leg edema necessitating the use of a diuretic. High LDH, low haptoglobin, and anemia occurred, then rising BUN and creatinine at 9 months after the start of gemcitabine. Transient and mild thrombocytopenias were also noted. A urinalysis revealed microscopic hematuria with red cell casts and 3+ proteinuria. After discontinuation of chemotherapy with gemcitabine, her renal function improved over the ensuing six months although it did not return to baseline.

Gemcitabine is a new chemotherapy drug used against pancreatic, pulmonary, urothelial, and ovarian carcinomas. The main toxicities of gemcitabine

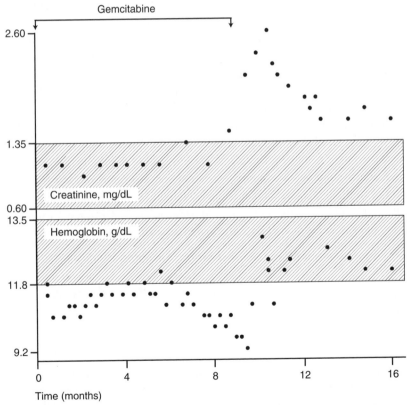

Fig. 5.2 Hemolytic-uremic syndrome after Gemcitabine chemotherapy. Shaded area represents normal range.

include mild myelosuppression, reversible elevation in liver function tests, and transient flu-like symptoms. Although it is generally well tolerated, it has potential for nephrotoxicity and can also lead to the development of the HUS (12–15). Mild proteinuria and microscopic hematuria have been described in clinical trials in up to 50% of patients, and elevations in BUN and creatinine levels in 17% and 8% of cases, respectively (16). In a small number of patients, the full-blown HUS can appear. Clinically, these patients present with worsening anemia and thrombocytopenia, elevated LDH levels with low haptoglobin, renal insufficiency, and worsening hypertension. Dyspnea, peripheral edema, and in some cases, neurological manifestations may also be present. In contrast to mitomycin C, the time interval between the initiation of gemcitabine chemotherapy and the onset of the HUS is variable, with no clear-cut relationship to total duration of therapy and/or cumulative dose. In one report, the median duration between the initiation of chemotherapy and the onset of HUS was eight months (with a range of two to 34 months) (12). Renal biopsy specimens show the characteristic features of thrombotic microangiopathy. Previous chemotherapy with MMC may accelerate the development of HUS. The diagnosis is often delayed because the anemia and thrombocytopenia are attributed to bone marrow suppression from chemotherapy. In some cases, the onset of renal dysfunction can appear after the drug is discontinued. Although some patients rapidly progress to end-stage renal disease requiring dialysis, in many cases renal function stabilizes after discontinuation of the drug and may even spontaneously improve in association with a resolution of the hemolytic anemia and thrombocytopenia (12). As with MMC, a variety of treatments have been tried with variable success. It is difficult to draw conclusions about their effectiveness when a spontaneous improvement can also occur (17). We do not routinely recommend plasmapheresis and consider supportive treatment (control of hypertension and fluid overload) and immediate discontinuation of MMC or gemcitabine as the main therapeutic interventions.

Angiogenesis Inhibitors (see section on 'Targeted therapies')

Agents with predominant tubulointerstitial damage
Cisplatin

Case report

An elderly patient with laryngeal cancer was treated with radiation to the neck and cisplatin-based chemotherapy (the 'larynx preservation protocol'). The serum creatinine level rose immediately after cisplatin administration, peaked on the 5th day and decreased thereafter (Fig. 5.3). While receiving 3–5 L of intravenous (IV) fluids daily, her urine volume was

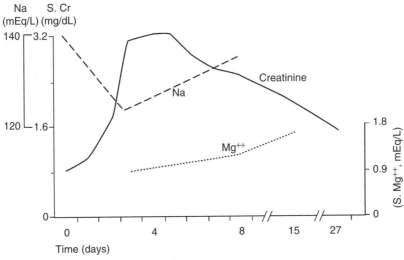

Fig. 5.3 Acute renal failure after high-dose cisplatin (CDDP).

between 2–4 L/day, but hyponatremia developed, associated with a weight gain of 3 kg and high urinary sodium levels. Approximately one month after cisplatin administration, mild renal insufficiency persisted and carboplatin was given instead of cisplatin, because of concern about further nephrotoxicity.

Cisplatin is a chemotherapy agent effective in the treatment of genitourinary malignancies, head and neck cancers, and osteosarcoma among others. Ototoxicity, nephrotoxicity, neuropathy, and a variety of ill-defined vascular changes are the main side effects. Cisplatin nephrotoxicity is its major dose-limiting side effect that constrains therapy with this drug. Cisplatin becomes rapidly bound to proteins and renal excretion is minimal but becomes very concentrated in renal tissue by undetermined mechanisms.

The manifestations of cisplatin nephrotoxicity include: acute declines in renal function, which may range from transient and subclinical decreases in GFR to overt acute renal failure; a progressive decline in glomerular filtration after repeated doses of therapy; salt-wasting nephropathy; and magnesium-wasting nephropathy (18–19).

When cisplatin chemotherapy was introduced, renal damage was the dose-limiting toxicity that prevented the repeated administration of the drug. More recently, however, the incidence and severity of nephrotoxicity has been markedly reduced by regimens of vigorous hydration with saline and mannitol infusion and patients can thus be treated with repeated courses (20–21).

The most commonly observed change in renal function has been a subclinical fall in GFR occurring after the first or the second course of chemotherapy (22).

These changes are mild and transient in many patients (23–24) and elevations in serum creatinine above 133 μmol/L (1.5 mg/dL) are rare (24). In one study of 95 patients, only four ever developed a serum creatinine level above 133 μmol/L (1.5 mg/dL) (24). Azotemia was transient in each case and three of these patients received further cisplatin chemotherapy without worsening in renal function (24). The development of cisplatin nephrotoxicity also appears to depend on the cumulative effect of the drug. Following repeated cycles, creatinine clearance decreases to 60–80% of baseline (22), but progressive renal failure is rare. In one study of 54 patients followed for more than three months, only one developed late onset azotemia (24). Although long-term follow-up studies indicate that renal function either remains stable or improves over time (22–6), some patients may have a significant reduction in creatinine clearance despite normal serum creatinine levels (27–28).

Cisplatin-induced acute renal failure (ARF) rarely occurs with single doses of less than 50 mg/m^2, but its incidence increases progressively with higher doses. Although renal damage resulting in subtle degrees of renal dysfunction is a well-recognized complication of conventional-dose cisplatin therapy (50–100 mg/m^2), overt ARF requiring dialysis is uncommon. In cisplatin-induced ARF, serum creatinine typically rises soon after administration of the drug, peaks in 3–10 days and returns to normal within 2–4 weeks, although recovery may be delayed for several months in some cases. Cisplatin nephrotoxicity has usually been associated with IV administration, but it can also occur after intraperitoneal and regional intra-arterial delivery. Renal failure is nonoliguric and BUN levels are usually disproportionately low because of the large amounts of fluids administered concomitantly. Hypomagnesemia and hypokalemia often occur as a consequence of the associated tubular defect and a solute diuresis resulting from vigorous saline administration. Progression to chronic renal failure is uncommon and dialysis is rarely required. Although underlying renal insufficiency has been considered grounds for exclusion from treatment with cisplatin, a report describes 4 children with pre-existing renal insufficiency (baseline GFR of 17–45 mL/min/m^2) who received a mean of 3.5 courses of cisplatin-based chemotherapy without an additional loss of renal function (23). In addition, cisplatin has been given to patients who suffered previous episodes of cisplatin-induced acute renal failure (24, 29–30), or with already diminished renal function by virtue of age (31), single kidney (32), or who have had a renal transplant (32), without apparent risk of increased nephrotoxicity.

Prevention or reduction of nephrotoxicity requires that the patient be adequately hydrated prior to the administration of the drug. The provision of a high chloride concentration in the intravenous fluids minimizes the formation of toxic, highly reactive platinum compounds, and infusion of saline solution to maintain a urine volume of above 150 mL/h is now routine. The concurrent use of hypertonic (3%) saline has allowed the administration of up to 200 mg/m^2 of cisplatin without any significant decline in creatinine clearance. Amifostine, an organic thiophosphate, may be useful in the prevention of cisplatin nephrotoxicity but it is not used routinely.

Cisplatin use may be followed by a salt-losing tendency (33). In one report, seven of 70 patients treated with cisplatin in the preceding 2–4 months, developed a salt-losing nephropathy characterized by hyponatremia, volume depletion, orthostatic hypotension, and inappropriately high urine salt losses (33). The incidence of this complication is probably higher than what has been reported. It is not unusual for patients to need to be hospitalized shortly after receiving cisplatin chemotherapy because of failure to thrive and worsening renal failure associated with prerenal azotemia from hypovolemia, related, in turn, to this salt-losing tendency. The urinary salt and volume losses are exacerbated by poor food intake related to chemotherapy-induced anorexia, and difficulties in swallowing because of drug or radiation-induced stomatitis and mucositis, especially in patients with a history of head and neck cancer. Because of this salt-losing tendency and the anorexia-induced weight loss associated with this type of chemotherapy, patients become sensitive to antihypertensive medications. Because of this reason, this author recommends discontinuing, at least temporarily, all angiotensin-converting enzyme inhibitors or angiotensin receptor blockers as an additional measure to prevent ARF due to cisplatin.

Of note, hyponatremia can also be seen in some patients during the first few days immediately following cisplatin administration. The development of hyponatremia in these cases is best explained by the syndrome of inappropriate antidiuretic hormone secretion (SIADH) brought about by high ADH levels induced by the emetogenic chemotherapy and the high volume of fluids given to prevent cisplatin nephrotoxicity.

Renal-magnesium wasting occurs in almost all patients treated with cisplatin, and 50% manifest clinically significant hypomagnesemia (19, 34). When hypomagnesemia is severe, hypocalcemia as well as hypokalemia are usually present. The hypocalcemia results from decreased parathyroid hormone secretion as well as resistance of the bones to its action. The hypokalemia is secondary to increased urinary loses. Both associated metabolic abnormalities resolve after correction of the magnesium deficits.

A variety of vascular phenomena have also been described in patients receiving combination chemotherapy with cisplatin (26, 35–39). The Raynaud's phenomenon can occur in up to 50% of patients with testicular cancer treated with cisplatin-based chemotherapy (35–36), but bleomycin, which is used simultaneously with cisplatin, is now thought to be largely responsible for this complication. Increased plasma renin and aldosterone levels associated with chronic hypomagnesemia (37), and an increased incidence of hypertension have also been reported as events possibly related to the long-term toxicity of cisplatin (26, 39).

Carboplatin

While nephrotoxicity is the main side effect with cisplatin, myelosuppression and neuropathy are the main toxic effects of carboplatin. Acute renal failure is rare after carboplatin (40–42). Although decreases in GFR of up to 20% can be seen after repeated courses of carboplatin (43), this drug is significantly less nephrotoxic than cisplatin, when given in the usual doses (400–600 mg/m^2). This significantly reduced potential for nephrotoxicity may be explained by the fact that carboplatin is significantly less protein bound than cisplatin. Hypomagnesemia occurs less often than with cisplatin and salt wasting is only rarely seen (44). Transient acute renal failure has been described in patients receiving very high doses (1600–2400 mg/m^2) followed by autologous bone marrow transplant (45–48).

Oxaliplatin

Oxaliplatin is a new cisplatin analogue with a different spectrum of activity, effective in the treatment of colorectal cancer. Unlike carboplatin, oxaliplatin produces only mild to moderate myelosuppression, has no nephrotoxicity (49) and its administration appears to be safe in patients with pre-existing mild renal impairment (50).(See also oxaliplatin section in the second part of this chapter 'Administration of chemotherapy in patients with renal failure').

High-dose methotrexate

Case report

This elderly man was treated for a primary brain lymphoma with high-dose methotrexate, procarbazine, and vincristine. For his first course of chemotherapy, methotrexate was given intravenously at a dose of 3.5 g/m^2. Leucovorin, 25 mg every six hours orally, was administered for three days to counteract the potential systemic toxicity of methotrexate (the so-called leucovorin rescue). Except for a mild increase in serum creatinine from 80 to 124 µmol/L (0.9 to 1.4 mg/dL), this first cycle of chemotherapy was tolerated well (Fig. 5.4). Two weeks later, he received a second course of high-dose methotrexate which was complicated by nonoliguric acute renal insufficiency (serum creatinine rose from 106 to 256 µmol/L [1.2 to 2.9 mg/dL]). As a consequence of the acute renal dysfunction, blood methotrexate levels rose above what are considered toxic concentrations and remained elevated for seven days. Leucovorin was given at higher doses than previously (40 mg every four hours) and continued for eight days. With the increased dose of leucovorin there was no evidence of systemic toxicity. Because of the concern for excessive systemic toxicity due to the loss of

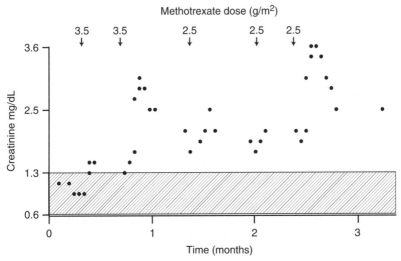

Fig. 5.4 Acute renal insufficiency secondary to high-dose methotrexate chemotherapy. Shaded area represents normal range.

renal function (creatinine clearance had decreased from 131 to 53 mL/min), the patient was treated with two additional courses of high-dose methotrexate, but at lower doses (2.5 g/m^2) in conjunction with leucovorin given at higher doses than usual, and continued until the plasma methotrexate level fell below 0.1 μmol/L. With the reduction in methotrexate dose and supplemental leucovorin rescue, no undue gastrointestinal or hematological toxicity developed. Unfortunately, a more severe degree of nonoliguric acute renal failure occurred with the 5th and last course of high-dose methotrexate when the serum creatinine rose from 150 to 318 μmol/L (1.7 to 3.6 mg/dL). Blood methotrexate levels remained in the toxic range for ten days, but with continued leucovorin therapy at a daily dose of 240 mg given for 11 days, the patient suffered only mild and short lived neutropenia. Renal function returned to baseline six weeks later.

Methotrexate is a cytotoxic agent that blocks folinic acid (leucovorin) synthesis by inhibiting the enzymes dihydrofolate reductase and thymidylate synthetase. Gastrointestinal ulcerations, mucositis, and bone marrow suppression are its prime extra-renal toxicities. Methotrexate and its 7-hydroxy metabolite are eliminated predominantly by the kidneys, through glomerular filtration and tubular secretion. After intravenous administration, 70–100% of the drug appears in the urine in the first 24 hours. Both the parent drug and its metabolite are highly insoluble, especially in acid and concentrated urine. Thus, when large doses are administered and subsequently excreted and concentrated in the urine, acute renal failure (ARF) can occur due to intratubular precipitation of the drug and possibly a direct tubulotoxic effect (51–54). Methotrexate-induced ARF is usually mild and nonoliguric and dialysis is rarely required for azotemia. Renal impairment is totally reversed in 70–100% of patients with conservative medical management. Recovery usually occurs after an average of 12 ± 7 days (55). Methotrexate given in the usual low doses is not nephrotoxic unless there is underlying renal dysfunction. ARF is seen mostly in patients receiving high doses ($1–12$ g/m^2), usually given as therapy for osteosarcoma, certain non-Hodgkin lymphomas, or central nervous system lymphomas. Treatment with cisplatin enhances methotrexate nephrotoxicity (56).

With proper hydration (to ensure an adequate urine volume) and bicarbonate administration (to alkalinize the urine), high-dose methotrexate is usually well tolerated. However, life-threatening myelosuppression and gastrointestinal toxicity can occur as a result of delayed methotrexate elimination if ARF develops. The duration and intensity of these acute toxicities, in general, depend on the level and duration of the elevated methotrexate levels. Even prolonged low plasma concentrations but higher than 0.05 to 0.1 µmol/L may be toxic. Therefore, it is crucial to monitor methotrexate plasma concentrations if serum creatinine increases by 50% or more. Systemic toxicity is observed when plasma concentrations are higher than 5 to 20 µmol/L 24 hours after drug administration, 0.5 to 2 µmol/L at 48 hours, and 0.05 to 0.1 µmol/L at 72 hours. In addition to impaired renal function, enhanced systemic toxicity due to delayed methotrexate clearance can also be seen in patients with ascites or pleural effusions; when nonsteroidal anti-inflammatory drugs are used together with methotrexate; or prior treatment with cisplatin (57).

To avoid untoward methotrexate toxicities, administration of leucovorin is critical. Leucovorin does not prevent or treat the renal toxicity, but is used to prevent the systemic toxicity due to methotrexate retention. This compound is converted in vivo to metabolites which can bypass the block to dihydrofolate reductase caused by methotrexate. Administration of leucovorin supplies the product of the inhibited enzyme and 'rescues' normal cells. Leucovorin by itself is retained in renal failure. The excess leucovorin not only bypasses the metabolic block but also prevents the further entry of methotrexate into, and favors its efflux from, the cell. Drug concentration and duration of exposure are the main determinants of cytotoxicity, and the longer the interval between methotrexate administration and initiation of leucovorin rescue, the higher the danger of systemic toxicity. Therefore, leucovorin should be started soon (within the first 24 to 36 hours) after methotrexate administration and continued until the serum methotrexate levels decrease below 0.05–0.1 µmol/L. Small doses of leucovorin are unable to prevent toxicity in patients with elevated drug levels, even when leucovorin is continued beyond 48 hours. In such cases leucovorin in increased doses is required and the dose must be increased in proportion to the plasma concentration of methotrexate. Nomograms and different treatment protocols have been proposed to treat patients with elevated methotrexate concentrations (54, 58–60). According to one review, methotrexate levels above 0.5 µmol/L at 48 hours after methotrexate administration require continued leucovorin rescue (60). These authors recommend giving leucovorin at a dose of 15 mg/m^2 every six hours for a methotrexate level of 0.5 µmol/L, 100 mg/m^2 every six hours for methotrexate levels of 1 µmol/L, 200 mg/m^2 every six hours for a level of 2 µmol/L, and to further increase the dose in proportion to the methotrexate level up to a maximum of 500 mg/m^2 (60) (see Table 5.1). Subsequent leucovorin dose adjustments should be based on repeated methotrexate levels taken at 24-hour intervals until the methotrexate level is less than 0.05 µmol/L. Because the bioavailability of oral leucovorin is limited above doses of 40 mg, it is recommended that it should be administered IV when given at higher doses (60).

To minimize systemic toxicity, removal of methotrexate by regular peritoneal dialysis or hemodialysis is ineffective because the drug is extensively protein-bound. Charcoal hemoperfusion removes methotrexate more effectively, but methotrexate blood levels rebound after discontinuation of the procedure and the hemoperfusion cartridges have to be repeatedly changed because of rapid saturation (61–62). Daily, high-flux hemodialysis (63–64), intensive peritoneal dialysis (64) as well as carboxypeptidase (an enzyme which inactivates methotrexate) (65–67) have also been used to treat these patients. Carboxypeptidase is given intravenously at a dose of 50 U/Kg and is available in the USA from the National Cancer Institute (NCI) on a compassionate basis. When using carboxypeptidase, methotrexate levels have to be measured by high-performance liquid chromatography, rather than by immunoassay, because methotrexate metabolites interfere with the latter. In a recent study of patients at high risk for methotrexate toxicity because of ARF, high-dose leucovorin alone was a safe and effective therapy (for the methotrexate blood levels observed in these patients) (55).

Table 5.1 Recommendations for leucovorin rescue in patients with delayed methotrexate clearance. Methotrexate levels above 0.5 µmol/L at 48 hours after the start of methotrexate infusion require continued leucovorin rescue

Methotrexate level	Leucovorin dose
0.5µmol/L	15 mg/m^2 every 6h x 8 doses
1.0µmol/L	100 mg/m^2 every 6h x 8 doses
2.0µmol/L	200 mg/m^2 every 6h x 8 doses

Adapted from 60. Chu ET. and Allegra C. Antifolates In: Chabner B, Longo DL, editors. *Cancer chemotherapy and biotherapy: Principles and practice*. 2nd ed. Philadelphia: Lippincott-Raven; 1996. pp. 109–148.

Pemetrexed

Pemetrexed is also an antifolate agent structurally related to methotrexate being used in patients with malignant mesothelioma and non small cell lung cancer. Mild, transient renal dysfunction can occur in up to 20% of patients (68), and occasional cases of ARF have been reported (69, 70), although cisplatin was given together with this drug in some cases (71). Pemetrexed is also eliminated mainly by the kidneys, and a decreased GFR results in increased drug exposure and hematological toxicity (72). Like methotrexate, pemetrexed is retained in pleural effusions and in ascites, and recirculation of the drug from these sites may lead to delayed clearance and prolonged drug exposure (71).

Ifosfamide

Case report

A middle-aged man with metastatic, high-grade synovial sarcoma was evaluated because of worsening renal insufficiency. For the previous 18 months, he had been treated with 19 cycles of high-dose ifosfamide therapy (Fig. 5.5). His renal function remained stable until the end of the first year of chemotherapy when serum creatinine levels begun to increase. Despite the rising BUN and creatinine levels, he exhibited persistent hypouricemia, hypokalemia, and hypophosphatemia as well as hyperchloremic, non-gap metabolic acidosis. Numerous urinalyses revealed microscopic hematuria, mild proteinuria, persistent glucosuria (despite normal blood glucose levels), and urine pH values of 6–7 (despite the presence of metabolic acidosis). His renal function continued to deteriorate and he had to be placed on hemodialysis approximately 15 months after discontinuation of chemotherapy with ifosfamide.

Ifosfamide is an alkylating drug, a structural analog of cyclophosphamide. Its main side effects include myelosuppression, neurotoxicity, and nephrotoxicity. Although both agents can produce hemorrhagic cystitis, only ifosfamide has a potential for significant nephrotoxicity (73–78). Proximal tubular impairment is the most common and prominent feature of toxicity, which frequently presents as the Fanconi's syndrome manifesting as hyperchloremic metabolic acidosis, hypophosphatemia, hypokalemia, renal glucosuria, and aminoaciduria (73–74, 79–80). Transient enzymuria, nonselective nephrotic proteinuria, and, rarely, nephrogenic diabetes insipidus may also be present. Hypophosphatemia and hypokalemia (which may be severe) are related to excessive urinary losses of phosphorous and potassium. Chronic hypophosphatemia may lead to rickets and growth failure in children (73). This tubulopathy can either be transient or long-lasting with cumulative doses. Ifosfamide nephrotoxicity may also manifest as ARF (73, 77). In one report, 10% of patients experienced an acute rise in serum creatinine (78). Ifosfamide nephrotoxicity

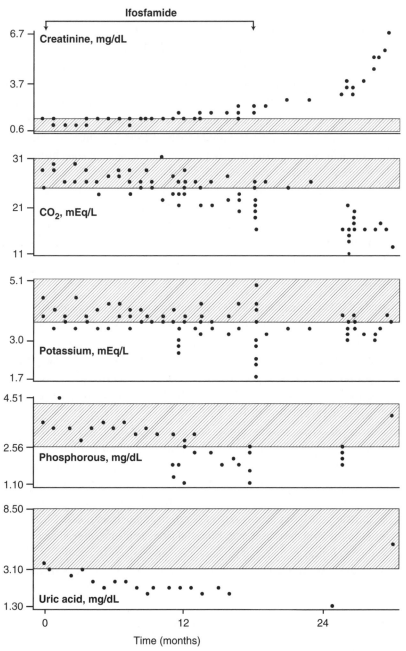

Fig. 5.5 Chronic renal failure secondary to prolonged chemotherapy with ifosfamide.

is dose-dependent; in the study of Van Dyk et al. (75), 13% of patients receiving 20 mg/kg had a rise in BUN levels, while 66% of those who received 150 mg/kg had a rise in their BUN levels (75). The onset of azotemia varied between 1–5 days and transient cylindruria with granular casts was common. Examination of renal tissue in those patients who died showed evidence of acute tubular necrosis. Progression to chronic renal failure has also been reported. In one study, progressive and irreversible renal failure developed in two patients after cumulative ifosfamide doses of 26 and 28 g/m^2 (81). Biopsies in both patients showed extensive tubular interstitial damage and chronic vascular changes. Chronic ifosfamide nephrotoxicity may have a late onset (76); in one study, six of 37 children developed decreased renal function and elevated creatinine levels which were first noted 19–36 months after completion of ifosfamide chemotherapy (76). Affected children were older and had received high cumulative doses of ifosfamide. Previous or concomitant treatment with cisplatin potentiates ifosfamide nephrotoxicity (82).

Nitrosoureas

Methyl-CCNU (semustine), BCNU (carmustine) and CCNU (lomustine) are lipid-soluble alkylating agents used in the treatment of malignant brain tumors, melanomas, and other malignancies. All these three drugs can produce dose-related nephrotoxicity which can progress to advanced renal failure, especially with cumulative doses of greater than 1200–1500 mg/m^2 given over long periods of time (83, 84, 85, 86). In one study of 161 patients treated with either semustine or carmustine in doses of 200 mg/m^2 every eight weeks, 17 of 18 patients who received six courses and all nine patients who received more than ten courses developed renal disease, including four patients who progressed to end-stage renal failure (85). In another report, the incidence of nephrotoxicity appeared to be significantly lower and only 26% of patients receiving more than 1400 mg/m^2 of semustine developed abnormalities of renal function (86). Nephrotoxicity develops insidiously without overt abnormalities in the urinalysis and with minimal or absent proteinuria. In patients developing clinical evidence of toxicity, increases in serum creatinine may be delayed until months after the completion of chemotherapy. Pathological findings in affected patients include extensive glomerular and interstitial fibrosis and tubular atrophy.

Streptozocin is another nitrosourea used to treat pancreatic islet-cell tumors and malignant carcinoid. The most frequent manifestations of streptozocin nephrotoxicity are abnormalities of proximal tubular dysfunction and proteinuria (87, 88). Hypophosphatemia and proteinuria may be early manifestations of this nephrotoxicity (87, 88). ARF can also occur, and in one case, it was related to extensive intraureteral uric acid deposits despite normal serum uric acid levels (89).

Pentostatin

Pentostatin (2'-deoxycoformycin) is a purine antimetabolite that inhibits adenosine deaminase. It is used in the treatment of hairy cell leukemia and some low-grade lymphomas. The dose-limiting adverse effects of this drug are myelosuppression, neurotoxicity (lethargy, seizures), and nephrotoxicity. Pentostatin-related nephrotoxicity is a dose-related adverse effect and overt ARF is rarely seen with doses of less than 4 mg/m^2 (90–91). In patients with normal renal function, mild and reversible creatinine elevations occur in less than 5% of patients (90–91). Patients with impaired renal function and poor performance status may have severe renal and systemic toxicity (90–91). The risk of nephrotoxicity is reduced by adequate hydration before and after drug administration. Another uncommon manifestation of nephrotoxicity is the appearance of a thrombotic microangiopathy with a typical triad of microangiopathic hemolytic anemia, thrombocytopenia and renal failure (92).

5-Azacitidine

Metabolic abnormalities compatible with proximal tubular dysfunction can occur in a significant number of patients receiving this drug. In one study, renal glucosuria, metabolic acidosis, and hypophosphatemia were observed in 28%, 73%, and 66% of treatment courses, respectively (93). Polyuria, salt wasting, and orthostatic hypotension were also frequent. Transient elevations in serum creatinine occurred in 20% of patients (94).

High-dose melphalan

High-dose melphalan (140–200 mg/m^2 given IV) is being used routinely as cytoreductive therapy preceding autologous hematopoietic transplantation in patients with multiple myeloma or primary systemic amyloidosis. One study of patients with amyloidosis reported ARF caused by this drug (95), although it is difficult to ascertain the pathogenetic role of other contributing factors frequent in this patient population, such as the use of diuretics for fluid retention, hypotension, liver disease, and/or congestive heart failure.

Targeted therapies

Angiogenesis inhibitors (See also Chapter 6.)

The growth of tumors and metastasis is in part influenced by vascular endothelial growth factor (VEGF). Presently, two types of compounds are being used as VEGF antagonists: monoclonal antibodies targeting circulating

VEGF (bevacizumab and VEGF-trap) and tyrosine kinase inhibitors (TKIs) that block the activity of the VEGF receptor (96–97).

Of patients receiving bevacizumab, hypertension and proteinuria of varying degrees have been described in up to 36% and 63%, respectively (98). Patients who develop proteinuria tend to develop hypertension, and both increase with the duration of therapy and are dose-dependent, with higher doses associated with a greater degree of proteinuria. Reducing the dose and/or increasing the interval between drug administrations may allow continuation of therapy in patients with worsening proteinuria. Concomitant use of pamidronate increases the incidence of proteinuria. Hypertension and proteinuria resolve with discontinuation of bevacizumab. In the vast majority of patients, proteinuria is usually asymptomatic, nephrotic proteinuria may occur, but nephrotic syndrome is rare and renal function remains stable. On occasion, a more severe complication is the development of renal thrombotic microangiopathy (99).

Hypertension, proteinuria, and rarely even thrombotic microangiopathy, can also be seen in patients receiving VEGF-Trap (100–101).

Hypertension is also a common complication of therapy with sunitinib, sorafenib, and other oral anti-VEGF TKIs (102–103). Sunitinib is usually administered once daily in a 4-weeks-on, 2-weeks-off schedule and blood pressure levels tend to rise as the cycle progresses, peaking by week 4 and decreasing in the subsequent two weeks, but remaining elevated (104). Proteinuria is less frequent than with bevacizumab, but acute kidney injury and a picture resembling HUS have been also described with sunitinib and sorafenib (105–106). It appears, therefore, that hypertension and proteinuria of varying degrees, depending on the agent used, are toxic effects of all therapies that target the VEGF pathway and should be routinely monitored in patients (107).

A marked increase in the occurrence of hypertension, proteinuria, renal dysfunction, and thrombotic microangiopathy was observed when two inhibitors of the VEGF pathway (sunitinib or sorafenib and bevacizumab) were used in combination, suggesting synergistic toxic effects (108–110). Some of this increased toxicity may be related to the fact that many of these patients had had a previous nephrectomy, as treatment for renal cell cancer.

Early detection and treatment of hypertension in patients receiving angiogenesis inhibitors are critical, not only to ameliorate proteinuria, but also to avoid more severe complications, such as reversible posterior leukoencephalopathy or hypertensive encephalopathy (97, 111–112). No definitive recommendations exist as to the antihypertensive agents of choice for this patient population (113). In theory, drugs that inhibit the renin-angiotensin axis have the potential advantage of not only treating the hypertension but also of decreasing proteinuria. Sorafenib is partially metabolized by cytochrome P450, which is inhibited by certain calcium-channel blockers (i.e. verapamil and diltiazem), and in this situation, other agents may need to be chosen.

Epithelial growth factor receptor antibodies

Cetuximab, matuzumab, and panitumumab are antibodies directed against the epithelial growth factor receptor (EGFR). They are being used in patients with colorectal and head and neck cancer, and non small cell lung carcinoma. Progressive decreases in serum magnesium concentrations are seen in up to 97% of patients (114–115). The hypomagnesemia is due to renal magnesium wasting. The incidence and severity increases with total treatment duration and can be severe, necessitating intermittent (and at times, daily) intravenous magnesium replacement (115). Hypocalcemia can also be seen but is due to magnesium depletion and improves once the hypomagnesemia is corrected. Hypomagnesemia resolves once treatment is discontinued.

Abl Tyrosine Kinase inhibitors

Imatinib, nilotinib, and dasatinib are oral TKIs being used in patients with chronic myeloid leukemia and gastrointestinal stromal tumors. Nephrotoxicity is very rare, but fluid retention may occur. Peripheral edema is the most common manifestation, but ascites, pleural, and pericardial effusions, and anasarca can be occasionally seen (116–117).

Biphosphonates

This group of drugs are potent inhibitors of osteoclast-mediated bone reabsorption and are extensively used in the treatment of hypercalcemia of malignancy and in the treatment and prevention of bone metastases, especially in patients with multiple myeloma and breast cancer. Rapid intravenous administration of large doses has produced nephrotoxicity in animals, and there are occasional reports of acute renal failure in humans. Pamidronate is extensively used and is well tolerated, and it is unusual to see nephrotoxicity from this agent. In a retrospective review, an elevation in serum creatinine was observed in 8% of patients after etidronate but only in 2% of those receiving pamidronate (118). A recent report describes the development of acute tubular necrosis following treatment with zoledronate in six patients, five of whom had multiple myeloma as the underlying diagnosis (119). In most of the patients, this agent had been administered for three to four months before the serum creatinine levels rose, and 5 of the 6 patients had evidence of renal dysfunction prior to starting treatment with zoledronate (119–120). It appears that the nephrotoxicity of zoledronate is dose-dependent and infusion time dependent (it is usually given over 5–15 min, in contrast to pamidronate which is infused over 2–4 hours). Therefore, it is recommended that serum creatinine be monitored prior to each dose of the drug (119). Another described complication is the development of collapsing focal and segmental glomerulosclerosis after long-term therapy with pamidronate (120). In this report, 7 patients developed renal failure and nephrotic syndrome 15–48 months after initiation of monthly therapy with pamidronate (120). Although 5 of these patients were receiving what are considered high doses (180–360 mg monthly), two were not. Renal biopsy studies showed collapsing focal and segmental glomerulosclerosis and extensive tubular injury. There is an additional report of renal failure and nephrotic syndrome associated with minimal change disease in a patient who received pamidronate in regular doses over a one-year period (121). We have also seen several patients who developed worsening renal function and proteinuria after long-term pamidronate given at regular doses (60–90 mg once a month).

Interferons

Although an uncommon occurrence, there are case reports of nephrotic syndrome appearing during therapy with interferons (IFN) (122–126). Some of these patients also presented with renal failure (123, 126) and kidney biopsy showed focal segmental glomerular sclerosis (122, 124) or interstitial nephritis (126). Proteinuria and renal function often improved after discontinuation of INF therapy. In some of the cases reported, it is difficult to ascribe the renal dysfunction exclusively to the use of INF as these patients are seriously ill with other conditions. A review of 23 patients receiving INF for chronic hepatitis C infection reported exacerbation of proteinuria and/or hematuria during therapy with this drug (127). Nephrotoxicity associated with INF has also been described in reviews of cancer patients being treated with this drug (128). Subclinical nephrotoxicity may be more common: evidence of tubular damage, shown as an increase in urinary enzymes, was found in a study of 58 patients receiving INF for myeloproliferative disorders (129). Mild increases in serum creatinine were seen in 5–10% and proteinuria in 20% of the patients (129). There are also occasional reports of thrombotic microangiopathy as a complication of interferon therapy (130).

Agents causing urinary tract obstruction

Both cyclophosphamide and ifosfamide can cause severe urologic toxicity manifesting as hemorrhagic cystitis, which may range from mild cystitis to severe bleeding, necessitating cystectomy. Acute cystitis has a variable onset occurring within days to months of drug exposure and usually resolves within two to three weeks of discontinuing the drug. This toxicity is due to the excretion in the urine of toxic metabolites such as acrolein. The irritation of the bladder mucosa is exacerbated by the prolonged exposure of the bladder to these toxic metabolites and their concentration in the urine. Consequently, the incidence and severity of this complication can be lessened by intensive hydration in order to produce a vigorous diuresis, and frequent bladder emptying. In addition, the parenteral administration of MESNA (2-mercaptoethane sulfonate) is the most effective measure for preventing hemorrhagic cystitis and is now routine during chemotherapy with ifosfamide or high-dose cyclophosphamide. This compound conjugates with the toxic metabolites and prevents cystitis. The risk of hemorrhagic cystitis is proportional to the dose of intravenous cyclophosphamide or ifosfamide, but may also occur suddenly after prolonged therapy with oral cyclophosphamide. Acute renal failure can be seen during the phase of acute hemorrhagic cystitis due to ureteral obstruction from the associated bladder wall edema, blood clots, and also bladder outlet obstruction.

Chronic complications of this uroepithelial toxicity include bladder wall fibrosis and late development of bladder cancer (131). This is proportional to the dose, being greater when the total cumulative dose is above 30 g. Bladder contraction, outlet obstruction, and ureteral obstruction, due to scarring, may develop late in the course of therapy or long after chemotherapy has been discontinued.

Administration of chemotherapy in patients with renal failure

The kidneys are one of the major elimination routes of many chemotherapy drugs and their metabolites. Therefore, many drugs require dose adjustment when administered in patients with underlying renal dysfunction. The use of antineoplastic agents in patients with renal failure is hampered by the narrow therapeutic index of these drugs and the fact that measurement of serum drug levels is not performed routinely. In addition, because most clinical trials exclude patients with any significant degree of renal failure, there is often a paucity of experience on the use of chemotherapy in this group. For those drugs that are renally eliminated, dose adjustments are typically based upon the predicted behavior of a particular drug (using an estimation of the GFR by formulas based on serum creatinine levels, measured creatinine clearance, or, less often, GFR measured by a radioisotopic method); titrating the dose based on clinical signs of drug toxicity (i.e. myelosuppression); and limited information from either case reports or prospective studies in a small number of patients. The method of calculating dose adjustments in patients with renal failure, extrapolating from pharmacokinetic studies, may not always conform to what is observed in clinical practice. For example, the parent drug may not be renally eliminated, as opposed to a metabolite which can either be toxic by itself or inhibit metabolism of the parent drug. Finally, chronic renal failure and the 'uremic environment' can alter the hepatic metabolism of many drugs leading to unexpected toxic effects (132–135).

The recommendations provided in this section are based on published guidelines of chemotherapy drug prescribing in renal failure (136–139, 141–143) and, with special emphasis, on the information gathered from the review of articles describing the experience with the use of individual drugs in patients with impaired renal function and on dialysis. In the absence of prospectively validated studies, any recommendations for changes in dose can be considered only as guidelines and subsequent dose administration should be based on observation of any untoward clinical effects and the tolerance of a particular patient. For many drugs, the prudent course of action is to initiate therapy with a low dose and escalate the dose as tolerated, especially in older individuals.

Alkylating agents

Nitrogen mustards

Mechlorethamine (nitrogen mustard) This drug is rapidly metabolized and has minimal urinary excretion. No dose adjustment is indicated in patients with decreased renal function.

Cyclophosphamide Cyclophosphamide dosing varies from 60 to 120 mg/m^2 per day orally to 400 to 2000 mg/m^2 per day IV every three to four weeks. High-dose regimens (4–6 g/m^2) have also been used in combination with bone marrow transplant. Cyclophosphamide is a drug which is predominantly eliminated by hepatic metabolism. Although only 6–20% of the drug is excreted unchanged in the urine, both cytotoxic and detoxified metabolites are renally excreted (144–145). The need for dose reduction for cyclophosphamide in patients with renal impairment is controversial. Although some authors have described increased and prolonged plasma levels of cyclophosphamide and/or its metabolites in patients with renal failure (145–148), others found no correlation between GFR and cyclophosphamide clearance or clearance of alkylating metabolites (144, 149). Similarly, there appears to be no correlation between the severity of renal insufficiency and the depth or duration of myelosuppression when patients with renal disease are given cyclophosphamide, even at doses of up to 60 mg/kg (144, 150). Furthermore, high-dose cyclophosphamide has been used for peripheral blood stem cell mobilization (151, 152) and in one study, advanced renal insufficiency did not compromise the quality of peripheral blood stem collection, as long as cyclophosphamide was given with granulocyte-macrophage colony stimulating factor (151). High-dose cyclophosphamide has also been given to patients on dialysis as a cytoreductive agent prior to bone marrow transplant without enhanced toxicity (152–154). Hemodialysis effectively removes cyclophosphamide and its alkylating metabolites (148, 153, 155–156). For patients with renal insufficiency receiving cyclophosphamide as treatment for autoimmune diseases (IV in monthly doses of 0.5 to 1.0 gm/m^2) Haubitz et al. recommend a dose reduction of 20 to 30% (148).

Ifosfamide Ifosfamide is the chemotherapy drug of choice in patients with soft-tissue sarcomas. It is also used in hematological malignancies, uroepithelial cancers, breast, and ovarian tumors. It is often given every three to four weeks in the following doses: 1–1.2 g/m^2 per day for five days, 2–3 g/m^2 per day for three days, or 5 g/m^2 as a single dose. MESNA (60% of the ifosfamide dose) must also be given to prevent hemorrhagic cystitis. Like cyclophosphamide, ifosfamide is metabolized by the liver and converted into active metabolites. Urinary excretion of ifosfamide and its metabolites has been reported to vary between 6–50% of the dose given, depending on the method and measurement utilized, and the age of the patient (157). Although no published studies reporting ifosfamide pharmacokinetics in patients with renal failure are available, increased nephrotoxicity and myelosuppression have been reported in patients with decreased renal function such as nephrectomized patients, patients with elevated serum creatinine, and after previous or concomitant treatment with cisplatin (presumably related to subclinical decreases in GFR). Neurotoxicity, manifesting as changes in mental status, tremors, and seizures, has also been reported during treatment with ifosfamide and is thought to be related to retention of chloroacetaldehyde, a neurotoxic renally excreted metabolite. Neurotoxicity is also increased in patients with compromised renal function. Dose adjustments appear to be indicated in patients with decreased GFR, but published guidelines include withholding the drug if the serum creatinine is above 265 umol/ L(3 mg/dL) and reducing the dose by 25–50% if the serum creatinine is between 133 to 265 umol/L (1.5 to 3 mg/dL); reducing the dose by 20%, 25%, and 30% for creatinine clearance of 60, 45, and 30 mL/min respectively (138); or a dose reduction of 25% for patients with creatinine clearance less than 10 mL/min only (140).

There is also a report of an anephric child on hemodialysis who received ifosfamide (158). In this study, the doses of ifosfamide varied between 1–1.6 g/m^2, administered over 30 min at intervals of 24–72 hours between doses and repeated up to four times in one course of treatment. Each ifosfamide course of treatment was given every three weeks for a total of four separate courses.

The first course consisted of a single dose of 1.6 g/m^2; the second course of two doses of 1.6 and 1.0 g/m^2 72 hours apart; the third course of three doses of 1.0 g/m^2 48 hours apart; and the last course of four doses of 1.0 g/m^2 24 hours apart. Hemodialysis was performed 7–24 hours after each dose of ifosfamide. The degree of myelosuppression seen with each course appeared to correlate with the total number of doses given. Although dose-related myelosuppression did occur, the patient tolerated the treatments without experiencing excessive hematologic toxicity. CNS toxicity, manifesting as tremors, sedation, and, on one occasion, seizures (which occurred after the patient had received four daily doses of 1 g/m^2) were also observed. In this case, hemodialysis was shown to remove ifosfamide and its metabolites and also to reverse ifosfamide-related neurotoxicity (158).

Our own experience consists of an adult patient with metastatic synovial sarcoma, who was on chronic hemodialysis. Ifosfamide was administered initially in a dose of 1 g/m^2 per day, for two consecutive days per course. Each course of treatment was given every 3–4 weeks and the daily ifosfamide dose was gradually increased to 2 g/m^2 per day over the next three months. Hemodialysis was performed 16–18 hours after each dose and the patient was able to tolerate chemotherapy with ifosfamide for one year without developing excessive myelosuppression or neurotoxicity.

In order to prevent hemorrhagic cystitis, vigorous hydration is routinely administered together with ifosfamide or high-dose cyclophosphamide. It is important to keep in mind that this maneuver is contraindicated in patients on dialysis because of the danger of fluid overload, and moreover it may not be necessary because of the decreased urinary elimination of the parent drug or toxic metabolites in these patients.

Melphalan Melphalan is an effective chemotherapeutic agent for the treatment of multiple myeloma and amyloidosis. It is used in doses of 6–9 mg/m^2/day or 0.25 mg/kg/day orally for 4 days, every 4–6 weeks. High-dose melphalan (140–200 mg/m^2 intravenously) followed by bone marrow reconstitution with bone marrow transplant or peripheral blood stem cells has been administered as treatment for multiple myeloma or amyloidosis. Pharmacokinetic studies have shown interindividual variation with a mean urinary excretion of unchanged melphalan of 18–34% of the dose. Plasma elimination and renal clearance may be decreased in the presence of renal dysfunction (159), and patients with renal insufficiency have a higher frequency of myelosuppression and infection after receiving conventional doses of melphalan compared to individuals with normal renal function (160–161). Therefore, dose reductions of 25% and 50% have been recommended for patients with creatinine clearance between 10 and 50 mL/min and less than 10 mL/min respectively (140).

High-dose melphalan has also been given to patients with advanced renal failure and those on dialysis (151). Although the patients with renal failure had a longer duration of mucositis, fever, and hospitalization compared to normals, dose reduction was not recommended (151).

Chlorambucil Chlorambucil is extensively metabolized by the liver and urinary elimination is minimal. Therefore, dose reduction appears not to be indicated in patients with decreased renal function (138), although another review recommends giving 75% or 50% of the regular dose for patients with CrCl of 10–50 mL/min and less than 10 mL/min respectively (140).

Ethylenimines and methylmelamines

Altretamine (Hexamethylmelamine) Altretamine is extensively metabolized by the liver. Less than 1% of the unchanged drug is eliminated in the urine, but up to 50–60% of a daily dose is renally excreted as metabolites of undefined activity (138). There is no information on the use of this drug in patients with renal failure.

Thiotepa Thiotepa is extensively metabolized by the liver. Renal elimination accounts for less than 2% of the parent drug and approximately 25–30% of alkylating metabolites. There is no information on the use of this drug in renal failure.

Alkyl sulfonates

Busulfan Busulfan is metabolized to several compounds which are partially eliminated in the urine. According to one review, the dose does not have to be changed in patients with decreased GFR (140).

Nitrosoureas

Carmustine (BCNU), lomustine (CCNU), and semustine (methyl-CCNU) These drugs are compounds that can cross the blood–brain barrier and are used to treat brain tumors. They all have significant renal excretion with up to 50–60% of the parent drugs and metabolites being eliminated in the urine. Recommended dose reductions vary from between 25% and 50% of the dose in patients with a creatinine clearance of 10 to 50 mL/min (138, 139, 140) to withholding these drugs altogether in patients with GFR <30 mL/min (138). Because of the danger of delayed myelosuppression and cumulative nephrotoxicity, these agents should not be given more often than every six weeks.

Streptozocin Streptozocin is another nitrosurea used in patients with pancreatic islet-cell tumors and malignant carcinoid. Only 10–20% of a streptozocin dose is renally excreted. One review recommends a 25% dose reduction for a creatinine clearance of 10–50 mL/min and a 50% reduction for a creatinine clearance <10 mL/min (140), but another recommends that patients with significant renal impairment should be treated with other drugs if possible (138).

Triazenes

Dacarbazine (DTIC) This drug is used in the treatment of metastatic melanoma and also as a secondary line of therapy for patients with Hodgkin's disease. Forty percent of the dose appears unchanged in the urine and dose reductions of 20%, 25%, and 30% are recommended for patients with creatinine clearance of 60, 45, and 30 mL/min, respectively (138).

Temozolomide (TMZ) This drug is being used in the treatment of brain tumors and melanoma. Renal clearance of the parent drug and its metabolites does not play a significant role in the elimination of temozolomide (162), and population pharmacokinetics indicate that in patients with creatinine clearance over the range of 36–100 mL/min, renal function has no clinically significant impact on the clearance of the drug (163). There is no reported experience in patients with severely impaired renal function.

Antimetabolites

Folic acid analogs

Methotrexate (Amethopterin) Because methotrexate is eliminated predominantly by the kidney, its use has been considered relatively contraindicated in patients with renal failure. There are several reports describing enhanced systemic toxicity in patients with varying degrees of renal insufficiency who were treated with methotrexate for cancer or rheumatological conditions (164–167). Even low doses (5–15 mg given only once or at weekly intervals) produced prolonged neutropenia, severe gastrointestinal toxicity, and even death (164–167). However, in these cases, methotrexate levels were not monitored and the patients did not receive leucovorin rescue routinely or, when it was done, it was initiated several days after methotrexate administration. Conversely, it appears that with close monitoring of methotrexate levels and earlier administration of leucovorin, in doses adjusted to the measured methotrexate levels (see the section 'High-dose methotrexate'), chemotherapy with this drug is possible in patients with renal failure. There are at least five reports documenting the use of methotrexate in patients on dialysis (63–64, 168–170). In the study by Thomson et al. (168), a patient with laryngeal carcinoma received three-weekly methotrexate doses of 12 mg/m^2 followed by leucovorin (30 mg every six hours) starting 24 hours after methotrexate administration and continued until the methotrexate concentration was less than 0.1 μmol/L. Yokogi et al. (169) successfully treated a hemodialysis patient with ureteral carcinoma with a methotrexate dose of 20 mg. Tokunaga et al. (170) also treated a hemodialysis patient with advanced ureteral carcinoma with the M-VAC protocol (which includes methotrexate, cisplatin, Vinblastin, and Doxorubicin). After 4 consecutive cycles of chemotherapy, the tumor was resected and the patient entered a complete remission. Although, as expected methotrexate elimination was slow, the timely administration of leucovorin in adequate doses prevented significant toxicity in these cases. It also appears that even higher methotrexate doses can be safely given to patients on dialysis, as long as the drug is removed by intensive, high-flux hemodialysis, and high leucovorin doses are utilized as well. Wall et al. (63) reported effective clearance of methotrexate using daily HD with high-flux dialyzers and were able to treat two hemodialysis patients with osteosarcoma with methotrexate doses of 2.2–9.5 g/m^2. Chemotherapy in these patients was followed one hour later by daily 6-hour dialysis treatments until the methotrexate concentration was less than 0.3 μmol/L (63). In another report, a patient on peritoneal dialysis received six cycles of high-dose methotrexate while receiving either daily, high-flux hemodialysis, or intensive peritoneal dialysis (64).

Pemetrexed Pemetrexed is used to treat malignant pleural mesothelioma. It is given intravenously at a dose of 500 mg/m^2 every three weeks. Like methotrexate, it is also fully eliminated by renal excretion, and decreased renal function leads to accumulation of the drug and increased systemic toxicity. According to one study (72), pemetrexed is not recommended in patients with GFR <45 mL/min, and patients with GFR of 45 to 79 mL/min (measured by radio-isotope serum clearance) can tolerate the usual dose if given together with oral folic acid and parenteral vitamin B12 supplementation.

Pyrimidine analogs

5-Fluorouracil (5-FU) 5-FU is used in the treatment of solid tumors (breast, colorectal, and head and neck cancers). The usual dose varies widely, as it can be given as IV push for five days, every four weeks, or by continuous infusion. Although less than 10% of unchanged drug undergoes renal excretion, 5-FU undergoes extensive metabolism in the liver and other tissues, and its main metabolite α-fluoro-β-alanine (FBAL) is largely eliminated in the urine. 5-FU is not retained in patients with renal failure, but FBAL is and it may increase toxicity in these patients (171–2). In the latter study, plasma clearance of 5-FU measured one hour after hemodialysis was completed, was faster than when measured later on and it was postulated that the uremic environment inhibited 5-FU metabolism (172). While in one report patients with mild renal impairment tolerated weekly doses of 1000 to 2600 mg/m^2 (173), another group described increased toxicity in patients with CrCl of 30–50 mL/min, but the regimen of 5-FU administration was different (425 mg/m^2 as an IV bolus, daily for five days) (174). 5-FU in varying doses and regimens, at times in combination with oxaliplatin or irinotecan, has been given to patients on dialysis and appears to be tolerated with acceptable toxicity (172, 175–7), although in some patients excessive gastrointestinal toxicity occurred (171, 178). For patients on hemodialysis, one review recommends giving 50% of the dose recommended for individuals with normal renal function, but no adjustment for patients with renal failure who are not yet on dialysis (140). It may be prudent to administer a reduced dose in the beginning and escalate the dose as tolerated (174).

Capecitabine Capecitabine is an orally administered fluoropyrimidine designed to generate 5-FU preferentially within tumoral tissues (179). Capecitabine is used for breast and colorectal cancer. It is usually administered orally at a dose of 1–1.25 g/m^2 twice daily given in 3-week cycles consisting of two weeks of treatment followed by one week of rest. Although renal impairment has no effect on the pharmacokinetics of capecitabine or 5-FU, reduced renal function leads to retention of active metabolites, with a risk of increased systemic toxicity (174, 179). The manufacturer recommends that patients with creatinine clearance of 30–50 mL/min should be treated with 75% of the recommended standard starting dose. Patients with CrCl above 50 mL/min should be given the regular dose and the drug should be avoided in patients with severe renal impairment (CrCl < 30 mL/min) (179).

Cytarabine (Cytosine arabinoside, ARA-C) Cytarabine is an antimetabolite used primarily for the treatment of leukemias and lymphomas and is one of the most active agents in the treatment of acute non-lymphocytic leukemia. Adult dosages range between 0.1–0.2 g/m^2/day—by continuous infusion over 24 hours for 5–7 days (low-dose regimen) or 2–3 g/m^2 every 12 hours for two to three days (high-dose regimen). Cytarabine is rapidly and extensively converted to uridine-arabinoside (Ara-U). Approximately 10% to 30% of cytarabine and 80% of its inactive metabolite are eliminated by urinary excretion (139). The primary toxicity is myelosuppression, but CNS toxicity manifesting as cerebral or cerebellar dysfunction has also been observed after high doses (above 1 g/m^2). The incidence of this type of neurotoxicity is markedly increased in patients with renal insufficiency (180). This increased neurotoxicity may be related to retention of Ara-U, which in itself delays cytarabine catabolism. Although dose reduction may not be required with low-dose regimens, chemotherapy with high-dose cytarabine should be used with caution in patients with reduced GFR and dosed relative to renal dysfunction to reduce the potential for neurotoxicity. Smith et al. recommend reducing the dose in adults to 1 g/m^2 for patients with serum creatinine of 133–168 μmol/L (1.5–1.9 mg/dL), or with an increase in serum creatinine during treatment of 44–106 μmol/L (0.5–1.2 mg/dL), and reducing the dose further to 0.1 g/m^2 per day for serum creatinine levels of ≥ 177 μmol/L (2 mg/dL) or increase in serum creatinine levels greater than 106 μmol/L (1.2 mg/dL) (180). There are no guidelines for patients on dialysis, but there are two reports of patients on hemodialysis who received this drug by continuous infusion at a dose of 0.1 g/m^2 per day for seven days (153, 181). The treatment was tolerated well and one study showed that both cytarabine and Ara-U are removed by hemodialysis (181).

5-Azacitidine Azacitidine is primarily renally excreted and has not been studied in patients with renal impairment.

Gemcitabine Gemcitabine is usually administered at a dose of 1000 mg/m^2 weekly for three weeks with a week of rest per cycle. Only 10% of a dose appears in the urine as unchanged drug and the rest is metabolized to difluorodeoxyuridine (dFdU), an inactive compound which is eliminated entirely into the urine. Accumulation of this inactive metabolite occurs in patients with compromised renal function and this is an issue in patients with uroepithelial malignancies who often have pre-existing renal disease. In four studies of patients with varying degrees of renal impairment, chemotherapy with gemcitabine was well tolerated with an acceptable toxicity profile, although some patients needed a dose reduction or increased intervals between chemotherapy sessions (182–185). Conversely, Venook et al. reported significant toxicity in patients with serum creatinine levels of 141–442 umol/L (1.6–5.0 mg/dL) receiving gemcitabine, even at reduced doses of 650–850 mg/m^2 (186). There is also a report of a patient with end-stage renal disease who received two cycles of gemcitabine at a standard dose of 1000 mg/m^2 on days 1 and 10 followed by a regular hemodialysis treatment 24 hours after each chemotherapy administration (187). The pharmacokinetics of gemcitabine were normal but there was a significant retention of dFdU, which was effectively removed by dialysis. Both cycles of chemotherapy were tolerated well without unexpected side effects and the authors recommended no adjustment in the gemcitabine dose, as long as hemodialysis is performed 6–12 hours after drug administration. Two other studies reported similar pharmacokinetics (i.e. retention of dFdU and clearance with dialysis) in three patients on hemodialysis (188–189).

Purine analogs and related inhibitors

6-Thioguanine, azathioprine and 6-mercaptopurine Thioguanine is eliminated via hepatic metabolism to inactive metabolites. Dose adjustment is not necessary in patients with renal impairment (138). Azathioprine is rapidly metabolized to 6-mercaptopurine, which in turn is converted to inactive metabolites. Renal dysfunction does not alter the pharmacokinetics of either drug (190–191), and renal failure does not influence the degree of myelosuppression in patients receiving azathioprine (192). Nevertheless, the manufacturer advises reduction of the dose of 6-mecaptopurine in patients with impaired renal function while another review recommends reduction of the dose of azathioprine by 25% and 50% for creatinine clearance of 10–50 mL/min and less than 10 mL/min respectively (140). Dose reduction is imperative if allopurinol is given together with azathioprine or 6-mecaptopurine.

Pentostatin Pentostatin is usually given IV every two weeks at a dose of 4 mg/m^2.This drug undergoes significant renal clearance and also has a potential for nephrotoxicity. Therefore, its administration has not been recommended for patients with renal dysfunction. Nonetheless, a study on the pharmacokinetic parameters of pentostatin in 13 patients with varying degrees of renal function showed that, with appropriate dose reduction, pentostatin administration appears to be safe in patients with mild to moderate renal insufficiency (creatinine clearance above 20 mL/min) (193). Seven of these patients had impairment in renal function and the pentostatin dose was reduced to 3 mg/m^2 for creatinine clearance between 41 and 60 mL/min and 2 mg/m^2 for creatinine clearance between 21 and 40 mL/min (193). There was a good correlation between the creatinine clearance and pentostatin plasma clearance. The area under the plasma concentration–time curve (AUC) values in the patients with abnormal renal function, who received the drug at lower doses, were similar to those of patients with normal renal function, and the toxicities were similar as well (193).

Fludarabine and cladribine Fludarabine is used for the treatment of chronic lymphocytic leukemia and other low-grade lymphoproliferative malignancies. The main toxicities include myelosuppression and infections related to immunosuppression. The usual dose is 15–30 mg/m^2 per day for 5 days every 28 days. When given intravenously, this drug is rapidly dephosphorylated to an active metabolite (F-ara-A) which is primarily eliminated in the urine (approximately 60% within the first 24 hours) (194). The total body clearance of F-ara-A is directly correlated with creatinine clearance, and the dose of fludarabine should be reduced in patients with decreased renal function (194). In one study of patients with varying degrees of renal function, dose adjustments based on creatinine clearance provided equivalent F-ara-A exposure and allowed treatment without undue toxicity in those with renal insufficiency (195). In this report, patients received a five-day course of treatment with daily fludarabine doses of 25 mg/m^2, if the creatinine clearance was more than 70 mL/min, 20 mg/m^2 for a clearance of 70–30 mL/min, and 15 mg/m^2 for a clearance less than 30 mL/min (195). Fludarabine has also been given to two patients on hemodialysis in association with stem cell transplantation at a dose of 6 mg/m^2 for 4 days and hemodialysis performed daily (196–197).

Renal clearance accounts for approximately 50% of the total systemic clearance of cladribine and 20–35% of an IV administered dose is excreted unchanged in the urine during the first 24 hours (198). There is no information about dose adjustments for patients with renal impairment, although because of the significant renal elimination, caution should be used if giving this drug to this group of patients.

Natural products

Epipodophyllotoxins

Etoposide (VP–16) Forty percent of an administered dose of etoposide is excreted in the urine unchanged, and approximately 40% is eliminated by hepatic metabolism with inactive metabolites also excreted in the urine. Etoposide is highly protein bound, and pharmacokinetic studies have shown substantial inter- and intrapatient variability.

Patients with impaired renal function have decreased drug clearance rates and renal impairment has been shown to be predictive of toxicity (199, 200, 201, 202). No dose reduction is recommended for patients with a creatinine clearance above 50 mL/min, but the dose should be reduced by 25% in patients with a creatinine clearance of 10–50 mL/min, and by 50% for clearance <10 mL/min (140). Nonetheless, etoposide has been given to patients on dialysis without evidence of increased toxicity (203–213). The doses administered in these studies varied between 50 mg/m^2 daily for two days to 100 mg/m^2 daily for four days. Myelosuppression occurred in some patients but they had also received other drugs such as carboplatin or cyclophosphamide, which could have contributed to this toxicity. Etoposide is not removed by dialysis and the pharmacokinetics of this drug are not affected by the interval between chemotherapy and hemodialysis. Despite the significant renal elimination shown in other studies, when measured in three hemodialysis patients, the pharmacokinetic parameters were similar to those in patients with normal renal function (203, 213).

Vinca alkaloids

Vinblastine, vincristine, vindesine, and vinorelbine Hepatic metabolism and biliary excretion constitute the main routes of elimination of the Vinca alkaloids and dose-adjustments are not indicated in patients with renal dysfunction.

Taxanes

Paclitaxel This drug is extensively metabolized by the liver and secreted in bile. Renal clearance contributes minimally to drug elimination and less than 10% appears unchanged in the urine (214). It has been administered to patients with impaired renal function (215–217) and to patients on dialysis (218–220) without increased systemic toxicity. The pharmacokinetics of this drug were comparable to that in patients with normal renal function when studied in an anephric patient receiving hemodialysis (219). Dose reduction is not recommended in patients with reduced renal function.

Docetaxel The metabolism and elimination of this agent is similar to those of paclitaxel and urinary excretion is minimal. No dose reduction is recommended in patient with impaired renal function or on dialysis (221–223).

Camptothecins

Topotecan Topotecan is used in patients with small-cell lung cancer and ovarian cancer. When given IV, the usual dose is 1.5 mg/m^2 per day for five days every three weeks. Renal elimination accounts for 30–70% of total drug disposition. Significant correlations exist between GFR and the plasma clearance of both topotecan and its main metabolite, and life-threatening myelosuppression has been described in patients with renal impairment, as a consequence of increased systemic exposure (224–225). Since a significant amount of the drug is eliminated by the kidneys, patients with renal impairment are at an increased risk of toxicity, including myelosuppression and other systemic effects (224–227). No dose adjustments are recommended for patients with creatinine clearance higher than 60 mL/min. For patients with extensive prior chemotherapy or radiation therapy, who are at an increased risk for myelosuppression, the dose of topotecan should be reduced to 1 mg/m^2 per day for a creatinine clearance of 40–59 mL/min and to 0.5 mg/m^2 per day for creatinine clearance of 20–39 mL/min (224–225) (see Table 5.2). For patients without previous extensive chemotherapy or radiation, no dose adjustments are recommended if the creatinine clearance is higher than 40 mL/min, but it should be reduced to 0.75 mg/m^2 per day for a creatinine clearance of 20–39 mL/min (224–225). There is no published information for patients with more advanced degrees of renal insufficiency (creatinine clearance less than 20 mL/min) except for one case report where a patient on hemodialysis received two courses of topotecan (1 mg/m^2 per day for two days) with tolerable hematological toxicity (228). Of note, topotecan was found to be dialyzable but plasma levels rebounded after discontinuation of dialysis. There are two more reports of topotecan administration in two children with ESRD (one on hemodialysis and one on peritoneal dialysis) and both tolerated five daily infusions of 0.75 mg/m^2 (229–230).

Irinotecan Irinotecan is another topoisomerase inhibitor. When given intravenously, about 15–30% of the drug and its metabolites appear in the urine, and biliary excretion and fecal elimination account for the rest of drug elimination (231–233). One prospective study of nine patients with CrCl of

Table 5.2 Recommendations of dose adjustments of topotecan in patients with impaired renal function

Creatinine clearance	Minimal prior therapy	Extensive prior therapy
>60 mL/min	1.5 mg/m^2/day	1.5 mg/m^2/day
40–59 mL/min	1.5 mg/m^2/day	1.0 mg/m^2/day
20–39 mL/min	0.75 mg/m^2/day	0.5 mg/m^2/day
<20 mL/min	Not Established	Not Established

Adapted from O'Reilly S, Armstrong DK, Grochow LB. Life-threatening myelosuppression in patients with occult renal impairment receiving topotecan. *Gynecol Oncol* 1997 Dec; **67**(3):329–30. With permission from Elsevier.

20–60 mL/min (serum creatinine 141–309 umol/L (1.6–3.5 mg/dL) reported no alteration in pharmacokinetics or excessive myelosuppression (234). In a larger, retrospective study, of 187 patients with CrCl of 35 mL/min or above, the clearance of irinotecan was not correlated with renal function, but 31 patients with the lowest CrCl (35–66 mL/min) had increased hematological toxicity (235). Of note, is the finding that the active irinotecan metabolite SN-38 was found to be retained in a patient on dialysis (236) and the authors attributed this delayed clearance to inhibition of its metabolism by uremic toxins. In patients on hemodialysis, irinotecan given at weekly doses of 50–80 mg/m^2 is well tolerated (176–177, 236–239). Higher doses are associated with severe diarrhea and myelosuppression, although in one study, a hemodialysis patient tolerated six courses of irinotecan given at a dose of 100 mg/m^2 on days 1, 8, and 15 of a 28-day cycle (238).

Antibiotics

Anthracyclines The anthracycline antibiotics, daunorubicin, doxorubicin, epirubicin, and idarubicin, are rapidly and extensively metabolized and less than 20% of the drug is eliminated in the urine. Therefore, dosage reduction has not been recommended in patients with reduced renal function (138, 140). In a study of patients with urothelial cancer and impaired renal function (CrCl of 30–60 mL/min./1.73 m^2), doxorubicin at a dose of 50 mg/m^2 and gemcitabine 2000 mg/m^2, given every other week, was tolerated without unusual toxicity (240). There is, nevertheless, a pharmacokinetic study of doxorubicin in five hemodialysis patients which showed decreased clearance of this drug and its main active metabolite (241).The authors postulated that the delayed doxorubicin clearance and accumulation of its metabolite may have resulted from impaired hepatic metabolism related to the renal failure, as has been described for other drugs (132–135). Based on this observation, the authors recommended close monitoring of hemodialysis patients receiving this drug. Because of this uncertainty, it may be prudent to start therapy at a reduced dose and escalate as tolerated.

Bleomycin Up to 70% of an intravenous dose of bleomycin is eliminated in the urine within the first 24 hours (242–243). The metabolism of bleomycin has not been systematically studied in patients with renal impairment, but there are several reports of decreased bleomycin elimination in patients with renal insufficiency (243–245). Moreover, renal dysfunction can predispose patients to the development of bleomycin pulmonary toxicity, which is the major dose-limiting toxicity of this drug (246–248). Therefore, the dose should be reduced in patients with impaired renal function. A dose reduction of 25–50% has been recommended for patients with creatinine clearance between 10–60 mL/min (138, 140, 248). For more advanced degrees of renal dysfunction (creatinine clearance less than 10–30 mL/min) some authors recommend withholding the drug altogether (138, 248). Because of the potential for cumulative pulmonary toxicity in patients with advanced renal failure, bleomycin should be given with caution and serial measurements of pulmonary function should be performed prior to each drug administration. When this agent is given with nephrotoxic drugs, the renal function should be checked prior to each administration of bleomycin.

Mitomycin C (MMC) Mitomycin C is usually given in doses of 10–20 mg/m^2 once every 6–8 weeks and is primarily metabolized by the liver. It is rapidly cleared from plasma, and less than 20% of a dose is excreted in the urine within a few hours after drug administration (138). Guidelines for patients with underlying renal insufficiency vary from reducing the dose by 50% when serum creatinine is ≤212 µmol/L (2.4 mg/dL) and avoiding this agent altogether for higher serum creatinine levels (249) to reducing the dose by 25% only for creatinine clearance less than 10 mL/min (140). In any case, close monitoring for signs and symptoms of HUS should be carried out. MMC can be removed by dialysis if given during the hemodialysis procedure (250–251). There is one report of a patient on hemodialysis who received two courses of MMC at a dose of 10 mg/m^2 (250).

Biological response modifiers

Interferons

These antiviral and antineoplastic agents have been used in the treatment of Kaposi's sarcoma, renal cell carcinoma, melanoma, and a variety of hematological malignancies. The clearance of these agents from plasma is dependent on adequate kidney function. In nephrectomized animals the pharmacokinetics of interferon is altered and patients with advanced renal failure and on dialysis have an impaired metabolism with decreased clearance, increased plasma concentrations, and higher AUCs (252). In patients with normal renal function, the doses used may vary from 3 to 10 million units daily or thrice weekly, to 20 million units per dose. In dialysis patients, the most commonly used regimen is 3 million units subcutaneously, three times a week (253–255). Although this dose has been tolerated relatively well, there are several reports describing severe neurologic side effects such as changes in mental status, seizures, and the syndrome of posterior leukoencephalopathy, especially in patients on dialysis (256–258).

Miscellaneous agents

Platinum coordination complexes

Cisplatin In patients with normal renal function (creatinine clearance above 60 mL/min), cisplatin is administered in doses of 50–100 mg/m^2, either as a single infusion or given in divided doses over 3–5 days and repeated every 3–4 weeks. Cisplatin rapidly binds to plasma and tissue proteins and no drug remains free in the circulation at 24 hours. This explains the fact that only 20–25% of the drug is excreted in the urine during the first 24 hours after administration and that hemodialysis is ineffective in removing cisplatin, unless performed concomitant with or immediately after drug administration. Impaired renal function has been considered to be a contraindication for cisplatin-based chemotherapy and oncologists usually use carboplatin in patients with creatinine clearance less than 60 mL/min, although for some tumors (i.e. testicular and, possibly, uroepithelial cancers) this drug is not as effective as cisplatin. Moreover, there is anecdotal evidence that even in these patients cisplatin may be safe. For patients on chronic dialysis in whom nephrotoxicity is not an issue, cisplatin administration appears to be safe. There are many case reports of patients on dialysis who received cisplatin-based chemotherapy (169–170, 204, 211, 259–271). Although most patients received doses ranging between 13 and 70 mg/m^2, some received up to 100 mg/m^2 given every 3–4 weeks (204, 211, 260, 265). Treatment was tolerated well and when hematological toxicity occurred, it could be attributed to concomitant myelosuppressive chemotherapy.

Cisplatin-based chemotherapy in the renal-transplant recipient The incidence of cancer in patients who have undergone renal transplantation is higher than that of the general population (see also Chapter 13). Although skin cancer and lymphomas are by far the most common neoplasia in this patient population, other malignancies also occur. If cisplatin-based chemotherapy is needed, several concerns arise: is the patient at increased risk for nephrotoxicity; should carboplatin be used instead, considering that it is less nephrotoxic than cisplatin; is it safe to use cyclosporin together with cisplatin in view of its own potential nephrotoxicity and the influence of cyclosporin in the metabolism of other drugs; should other immunosuppressive therapy be temporarily discontinued or reduced, as chemotherapy by itself may have immunosuppressive effects? Although the experience with cisplatin-based chemotherapy in renal transplant recipients is limited, there are at least 13 cases reported in the literature (32, 272–273). Seven patients received cisplatin-based chemotherapy for metastatic testicular cancer, four had advanced bladder cancer, one patient suffered from metastatic ovarian cancer, and one had leukemia. The number of cisplatin-containing courses of chemotherapy in an individual patient varied from one to eight and most of the patients received regular doses of cisplatin. Most of the patients with testicular cancer underwent complete remission resulting in long survivals. In the patients with bladder cancer, chemotherapy induced an initial remission, but the duration of the response was short-lived. With vigorous hydration and other preventive measures, no patient developed overt renal failure during or shortly after administration of chemotherapy, although one patient suffered mild and transient rises in serum creatinine.

Carboplatin In contrast to cisplatin, carboplatin binds only slowly to proteins and 70–90% is excreted in the urine in the first 24 hours. Renal clearance of carboplatin is closely correlated with GFR and pre-treatment renal function markedly affects the severity of myelosuppression, which is its main toxicity (274–275). Because of minimal nephrotoxicity, carboplatin can be used in patients with renal failure, but the dose has to be adjusted in proportion to the GFR. In patients with normal renal function, a common dose is 300–400 mg/m^2 given intravenously every four weeks. Higher doses (up to 1600 mg/m^2) have been used in combination with other agents as part of high-dose chemotherapy regimens followed by bone marrow or peripheral stem cell transplants. An alternative dosing scheme is based on the Calvert formula (275), which considers GFR or creatinine clearance and the desired target AUC: carboplatin total dose (mg) = target AUC × (GFR + 25). The target AUC is typically 4–7 mg/m^2 min, depending on the patient's prior and concurrent therapy (other myelosuppressive drugs and/or radiation). Pharmacokinetic studies done in patients on dialysis revealed significant retention of carboplatin, with a high proportion of the drug remaining free in plasma as the biologically active ultrafilterable fraction, but unbound carboplatin is extensively removed from the circulation by hemodialysis, without rebound in drug levels (204, 207, 210, 276–277). Thus, carboplatin can be given to patients on dialysis, but at reduced doses (usually 100–200 mg/m^2) and with hemodialysis carried out 4–24 hours later in order to remove free unbound drug to limit systemic exposure to carboplatin and avoid toxic side effects (204, 210, 212, 276–277).

Oxaliplatin Following the administration of oxaliplatin, its binding to plasma proteins and red cells is rapid and extensive. The reactive oxaliplatin derivatives are present as a fraction of the unbound platinum in plasma ultrafiltrate. As with carboplatin, the major route of oxaliplatin elimination is renal excretion, with 50% of the platinum administered recovered in the urine within the first five days after drug administration (278–279).In one study of oxaliplatin kinetics, renal clearance of ultrafilterable platinum was significantly correlated with GFR and was decreased in patients with renal impairment (278). As a result, the AUC of the platinum in the plasma increases as renal function decreases. Thus, renal impairment results in a greater systemic exposure to platinum (278). However, this study failed to show any relationship between moderate renal impairment (creatinine clearance 27–57 mL/min) and the acute toxicity associated with oxaliplatin when given at a dose of 130 mg/m^2 (278). In patients with normal renal function the usual dosing of this drug is 80–100 mg/m^2 every two weeks or 100–135 mg/m^2 every three weeks, given intravenously. A recent study describes the use of this drug in 37 patients with impaired renal function (280). Oxaliplatin was given intravenously in doses of up to 130 mg/m^2 every three weeks. Although patients with abnormal GFR had a decreased clearance of plasma ultrafilterable platinum, chemotherapy was well tolerated in all patients with a creatinine clearance of ≥20 mL/min and no dose-limiting toxicities were observed, even when oxaliplatin was given at a dose of 130 mg/m^2. One patient with a creatinine clearance of 13 mL/min received two cycles of oxaliplatin at a dose of 60 mg/m^2. The authors also studied the possible cumulative nephrotoxicity of this drug. Although serum creatinine levels rose in two patients, the deteriorating renal function was ascribed to progression of disease and urinary tract obstruction. Therefore dose adjustment appears to be not necessary with CrCl of 20mL/min or above. In another study, oxaliplatin 85 mg/m^2 and gemcitabine 1200 mg/m^2 were given twice a month to 25 patients with CrCl of less than 60 mL/min (11 with CrCl less than 30 mL/min) and treatment was tolerated well (184). At present, there are no published guidelines on how to adjust the dose of this drug in patients on dialysis but oxaliplatin has been given either just before or in conjunction with hemodialysis in doses of 32 to 85 mg/m^2 (281–283). Oxaliplatin has also been given via a hepatic artery catheter in a dialysis patient with hepatic metastasis from colon cancer, and tolerated for a period of four months (284).

Targeted therapies (see also Chapter 6)

Monoclonal antibodies

There are two reports of bevacizumab administration in two patients on hemodialysis (5 mg/Kg every two weeks) and the treatment was well tolerated (177, 285). Treatment with cetuximab at a weekly dose of 250 mg/m^2 has also been given to patients on hemodialysis (in one case together with bevacizumab and in another with irinotecan) without undue toxicity (177, 239, 286).

Tyrosine Kinase inhibitors (TKIs)

Sunitinib and sorafenib are oral TKIs used in patients with renal cell cancer.

Sunitinib and its main metabolite are mainly eliminated via the fecal route, with less than 20% of the drug cleared by the kidneys. Sunitinib has been given at full recommended dose to patients with severe renal function impairment and also to patients on dialysis, and was tolerated well (287–291). According to one study, the pharmacokinetics of sunitinib in patients on dialysis is in the range of patients with normal renal function (288).

Sorafenib is primarily metabolized in the liver and has been given to patients with renal dysfunction and on dialysis (292–294). A pharmacokinetic study in patients with varying degrees of renal dysfunction and on dialysis revealed no differences between groups (292). The authors of this study recommended starting therapy with the usual dose of 400 mg twice daily for individuals with a CrCl of 40 mL/min or above, and reducing it to 200 mg twice daily and 200mg daily for patients with CrCl between 20 to 39 mL/min and on dialysis, respectively. Because there were no patients with CrCl of less than 20mL/min but not yet on dialysis, no recommendation was given for this group. Dose escalation in patients tolerating treatment well was also suggested. In another report, two patients on hemodialysis tolerated a dose of 200 mg twice daily, which was increased to the standard dose of 400 mg twice daily in one of the two patients.

Imatinib and dasatinib are Bcr-Abl TKIs used in patients with gastrointestinal tumors and chronic myelogenous leukemia. Imatinib, given in doses of 200 to 800 mg/day, has been studied prospectively in patients with renal impairment (CrCl 20–60 mL/min) (295). Although imatinib is mainly eliminated by hepatic metabolism, with less than 10% of renal excretion, there was an unexpected decrease in drug clearance and increased drug exposure, which the authors attributed to decreased hepatic metabolism due to renal failure. Serious adverse events were more common in patients with renal impairment but treatment was generally well tolerated and the authors recommend no dose modification if the CrCl is 20 mL/min or higher. Imatinib, at a dose of 400 mg/day, has been given to patients with chronic kidney disease and to hemodialysis patients (even up to a year in one patient) and was well tolerated (296–297).

Dasatinib is also primarily metabolized by the liver and has been given to a 64-year-old patient with a GFR of 30 mL/min (SCr 194.5 umol/L, 2.2 mg/dL) at a dose of 70 mg twice daily for six months (298).

Erlotinib and gefitinib are used in patients with lung cancer. Erlotinib is metabolized by the liver and urinary excretion is less than 10%. It has been studied prospectively in patients with renal dysfunction (SCr 141 to 433 umol/L,1.6 to 4.9 mg/dL) and these patients tolerated a daily dose of 150 mg without unusual toxicity (299). Gefitinib has been given at a daily dose of 250 mg to two patients with CrCl of 24 and 26 mL/min and it was tolerated well (300).

Angiogenesis Inhibitors/Immunomodulators

Thalidomide is minimally metabolized by the liver but undergoes spontaneous hydrolysis into numerous metabolites which are renally excreted (301). A study of 40 patients with multiple myeloma and six patients on hemodialysis showed no influence of reduced renal function on the pharmacokinetics of thalidomide and the authors recommend not reducing the dose in patients with renal failure or on dialysis (302). Although thalidomide clearance was doubled during hemodialysis, it was recommended not to give a supplementary dose after dialysis. Similar findings were also described in a Japanese study (303).

Lenalidomide is used to treat patients with multiple myeloma (25 mg once daily for 21 days of a 28-day treatment cycle) or myelodysplastic syndrome (10 mg once daily). In contrast to thalidomide, lenalidomide undergoes extensive renal elimination (304). In one study of 30 patients with varying degrees of renal function (including six patients on hemodialysis), up to 80% of unchanged drug was recovered in the urine in those subjects with normal renal function (304). As expected, patients with decreased renal function and those on dialysis had decreased lenalidomide clearance resulting in drug retention and increased AUC. A four-hour dialysis resulted in the removal of 31% of lenalidomide. Based on these observations, the authors recommended proportional dose reductions according to the level of renal function and the disease being treated (304) (see Table 5.3).

Biphosphonates

All biphosphonates are excreted primarily by the kidney. Pharmacokinetic studies of pamidronate, zoledronic acid, and clodronate have shown slower elimination, higher drug concentrations, and increased systemic exposure (measured as AUC) in patients with impaired renal function (305–307). Despite these findings, one study found no evidence of drug accumulation

Table 5.3 Recommendations of dose adjustments of lenalidomide in patients with impaired renal function

CrCl	Multiple myeloma	Myelodysplastic syndrome
>50 mL/min	Full dose	full dose
30–49 mL/min	10 mg once daily*	5 mg once daily
<30 mL/min (not requiring dialysis)	15 mg every 48 hours	5 mg every 48 hours
<30 mL/min (requiring dialysis)	15 mg, 3 times a week**	5 mg, 3 times a week**

* The dose could be escalated to 15 mg, after two cycles if the patent does not respond to treatment and is tolerating the drug

** given after each dialysis

Adapted from Chen N, Lau H, Kong L, Kumar G, Zeldis JB, Knight R, et al. Pharmacokinetics of lenalidomide in subjects with various degrees of renal impairment and in subjects on hemodialysis. *J Clin Pharmacol* 2007 Dec; **47**(12):1466–75. Reprinted by permission of SAGE Publications.

after consecutive doses of zoledronic acid given every four weeks (306). Because successive doses of these drugs are usually separated by weeks, plasma accumulation is not expected to be clinically significant in patients with reduced renal function and two studies considered a dose reduction to be unnecessary (305–306). Because most of the patients studied had a creatinine clearance higher than 30 mL/min, the safety data is limited in patients with severe renal impairment (GFR less than 30 mL/min). We performed a retrospective study of 31 patients with underlying renal insufficiency (BUN 4.3–36 mmol/L (12–100 mg/dL) and serum creatinine 133–566 µmol/L (1.5–6.4 mg/dL)) who received 33 courses of pamidronate, in doses of 60–90 mg for the treatment of hypercalcemia of malignancy (308). A transient deterioration in renal function was observed in eight instances, but this was unrelated to pamidronate administration and no systemic ill effects that could be attributed to drug retention were observed (308). Thus, pamidronate appears to be a safe drug in patients with renal insufficiency. Zoledronic acid given as a rapid IV infusion can be nephrotoxic in patients with underlying renal disease and it is recommended that the dose be reduced. Biphosphonates have been given to patients on dialysis without untoward effects (309).

Chemotherapy in patients with urinary diversions

When the bladder is removed (either for cancer or other reasons) a variety of procedures are used to reconstruct the urinary tract and they include: the ileal conduit, orthotopic neo-bladders, and other continent urinary diversions such as the Indiana Pouch. It has been shown that drugs that are eliminated in the urine can be reabsorbed when they become in contact with the intestinal mucosa present in these urinary diversions (310–311).This unexpected phenomenon may have implications when these patients receive chemotherapy, especially those with continent diversions or orthotopic neo-bladders, when urine is in contact with the mucosa for prolonged periods of time (312–313). As a consequence of this recirculation, the elimination of drugs excreted in the urine may be delayed, necessitating a change in dose and possibly catheterization of the reservoir (314). There are two reports describing delayed clearance of methotrexate and increased systemic toxicity in patients with ileal conduits receiving this drug (312–313). In one study, patients with low CrCl, and those with a long ileal segment and/or an ileal conduit performed two years or less before chemotherapy, appeared to have been at a higher risk for this complication (313). Nonetheless, a prospective study conducted in 42 patients with urinary diversions (23 with a continent diversion and 19 with an ileal conduit) showed that, when compared to patients with native bladders, those with continent diversions did not exhibit increased toxicity from chemotherapy, even though none of these patients had an indwelling Foley catheter during treatment (315).

Radioactive materials in patients with impaired renal function

Case report
A chronic hemodialysis patient was found to have a thyroid carcinoma during neck exploration for secondary hyperparathyroidism and underwent a total thyroidectomy. The patient is now being considered for renal transplantation, but diagnosis and treatment of any remaining residual or metastatic disease is required as a prerequisite before transplantation.

Following total or near-total thyroidectomy, ablation of thyroid remnants or metastases with I^{131} is considered the treatment of choice for thyroid carcinoma. Renal excretion represents the main route of elimination of I^{131}, and in patients with renal insufficiency the renal clearance of I^{131} falls in parallel with the fall in GFR. Therefore, patients with thyroid cancer who have advanced renal failure present special problems for diagnosis and treatment, including the timing of dialysis after tracer administration given to detect residual thyroid tissue, the appropriate dose of I^{131} and radiation safety measures to avoid excessive radiation exposure to the patient and medical personnel.

There are at least 11 reports describing the use of I^{131} as treatment of hyperthyroidism (316) or thyroid cancer (317–321) in patients on dialysis. For scanning of thyroidal tissue, the tracer dose of I^{131} is given after the regular hemodialysis treatment. Hemodialysis effectively removes background radioactivity, and diagnostic image resolution is improved by obtaining the total body scan 24–48 hours later, after the next dialysis. Because renal excretion of I^{131} is practically nonexistent in patients on dialysis, bone marrow depression is a potential danger if excessive doses of radioiodine are utilized. Thus, two reports recommend reducing the dose of I^{131} (317–318). Nevertheless, other authors found that hemodialysis efficiently clears I^{131}, thus reducing the radiation exposure of non-thyroidal tissue (319–320). These studies reported 60–75% removal of I^{131} with dialysis, resulting in more rapid I^{131} clearance and reduced absorbed doses. Overall, the dose of I^{131} used in the studies reviewed ranged between 7–20 mCi in patients with hyperthyroidism (316) and 50–250 mCi in patients with thyroid carcinoma (317–321).

In contrast to hemodialysis, peritoneal dialysis is not as effective in removing radioactive iodine. In a study of ten patients receiving continuous ambulatory peritoneal dialysis, clearance rates of Na I^{131} were 20% of those in patients with normal renal function and serum radioiodine half-times were prolonged five-fold (322). Based on these findings, the authors treated two peritoneal dialysis patients with thyroid cancer with doses which were approximately 20% of the usual therapeutic dose (322).

References

1 Kintzel PE (2001). Anticancer drug-induced kidney disorders. *Drug Saf* **24**: 19–38.
2 Humphreys BD, Soiffer RJ, Magee CC (2005). Renal failure associated with cancer and its treatment: an update. *J Am Soc Nephrol* **16**: 151–61.
3 Sahni V, Choudhury D, Ahmed Z (2009). Chemotherapy-associated renal dysfunction. *Nat Rev Nephrol* **5**: 450–62.
4 Levey AS, Coresh J, Greene T, Stevens LA, Zhang YL, Hendriksen S, et al. (2006). Using standardized serum creatinine values in the modification of diet in renal disease study equation for estimating glomerular filtration rate. *Ann Intern Med* **145**: 247–54.
5 Cantrell Jr JE, Phillips TM, Schein PS (1985). Carcinoma-associated hemolytic-uremic syndrome: a complication of mitomycin C chemotherapy. *J Clin Oncol* **3**: 723–34.
6 Giroux L, Bettez P (1985). Mitomycin-C nephrotoxicity: a clinico-pathologic study of 17 cases. *Am J Kidney Dis* **6**: 28–39.
7 Lesesne JB, Rothschild N, Erickson B, Korec S, Sisk R, Keller J, et al. (1989). Cancer-associated hemolytic-uremic syndrome: analysis of 85 cases from a national registry. *J Clin Oncol* **7**: 781–9.
8 Valavaara R, Nordman E (1985). Renal complications of mitomycin C therapy with special reference to the total dose. *Cancer* **55**: 47–50.
9 Poch E, Gonzalez-Clemente JM, Torras A, Darnell A, Botey A, Revert L (1990). Silent renal microangiography after mitomycin C therapy. *Am J Nephrol* **10**: 514–7.
10 Cattell V (1985). Mitomycin-induced hemolytic uremic kidney. An experimental model in the rat. *Am J Pathol* **121**: 88–95.
11 Chow S, Roscoe J, Cattran DC (1986). Plasmapheresis and antiplatelet agents in the treatment of the hemolytic uremic syndrome secondary to mitomycin. *Am J Kidney Dis* **7**: 407–12.
12 Glezerman I, Kris MG, Miller V, Seshan S, Flombaum CD (2009). Gemcitabine nephrotoxicity and hemolytic uremic syndrome: report of 29 cases from a single institution. *Clin Nephrol* **71**: 130–9.

13 Fung MC, Storniolo AM, Nguyen B, Arning M, Brookfield W, Vigil J (1999). A review of hemolytic uremic syndrome in patients treated with gemcitabine therapy. *Cancer* **85**: 2023–32.

14 Izzedine H, Isnard-Bagnis C, Launay-Vacher V, Mercadal L, Tostivint I, Rixe O, et al. (2006). Gemcitabine-induced thrombotic microangiopathy: a systematic review. *Nephrol Dial Transplant* **21**: 3038–45.

15 Humphreys BD, Sharman JP, Henderson JM, Clark JW, Marks PW, Rennke HG, et al. (2004). Gemcitabine-associated thrombotic microangiopathy. *Cancer* **100**: 2664–70.

16 Green MR (1996). Gemcitabine safety overview. *Semin Oncol* **23**: 32–5.

17 Gore EM, Jones BS, Marques MB (2009). Is therapeutic plasma exchange indicated for patients with gemcitabine-induced hemolytic uremic syndrome? *J Clin Apher* **24**: 209–14.

18 Madias N, Harrington J (1987). Platinum nephrotoxicity. *Am J Med* **65**: 307–14.

19 Blachley JD, Hill JB (1981). Renal and electrolyte disturbances associated with cisplatin. *Ann Intern Med* **95**: 628–32.

20 Hayes DM, Cvitkovic E, Golbey RB, Scheiner E, Helson L, Krakoff IH (1977). High dose cis-platinum diammine dichloride: amelioration of renal toxicity by mannitol diuresis. *Cancer.* 1977 **39**: 1372–81.

21 Ostrow S, Egorin MJ, Hahn D, Markus S, Aisner J, Chang P, et al. (1981). High-dose cisplatin therapy using mannitol versus furosemide diuresis: comparative pharmacokinetics and toxicity. *Cancer Treat Rep* **65**: 73–8.

22 Dentino M, Luft FC, Yum MN, Williams SD, Einhorn LH (1978). Long term effect of cis-diamminedichloride platinum (CDDP) on renal function and structure in man. *Cancer* **41**: 1274–81.

23 Stark JJ, Howel SB (1978). Nephrotoxicity of cis-platinum (II) dichlorodiammine. *Clin Pharmacol Ther* **23**: 461–6.

24 Chiuten D, Vogl S, Kaplan B, Camacho F (1983). Is there cumulative or delayed toxicity from cis-platinum? *Cancer* **52**: 211–4.

25 Brock PR, Koliouskas DE, Barratt TM, Yeomans E, Pritchard J (1991). Partial reversibility of cisplatin nephrotoxicity in children. *J Pediatr* **118**: 531–4.

26 Hansen S, Groth S, Daugaard G, Rossing N, Rorth M (1998). Long-term effects on renal function and blood pressure of treatment with cisplatin, vinblastine, and bleomycin in patients with germ cell cancer. *J Clin Oncol* **6**: 1728–31.

27 Reed E, Jacob J, Brawley O (1991). Measures of renal function in patients with cisplatin-related chronic renal disease. *J Natl Med Assoc* **83**: 522–6.

28 Hamilton CR, Bliss JM, Horwich A (1989). The late effects of cis-platinum on renal function. *Eur J Cancer Clin Oncol* **25**: 185–9.

29 Donadio C, Lucchesi A, Gadducci A (1996). Prevention of cis-platinum nephrotoxicity in a high-risk patient. *Ren Fail* **18**: 691–5.

30 Wong DC, Deisseroth AB (1985). Successful continuation of cisplatin therapy after partial recovery from acute renal failure. *Cancer Treat Rep* **69**: 731–3.

31 Hrushesky WJ, Shimp W, Kennedy BJ (1984). Lack of age-dependent cisplatin nephrotoxicity. *Am J Med* **76**: 579–84.

32 Benisovich VI, Silverman L, Slifkin R, Stone N, Cohen E (1996). Cisplatin-based chemotherapy in renal transplant recipients. A case report and a review of the literature. *Cancer* **77**: 160–3.

33 Hutchison FN, Perez EA, Gandara DR, Lawrence HJ, Kaysen GA (1988). Renal salt wasting in patients treated with cisplatin. *Ann Intern Med* **108**: 21–5.

34 Schilsky RL, Anderson T (1979). Hypomagnesemia and renal magnesium wasting in patients receiving cisplatin. *Ann Intern Med* **90**: 929–31.

35 Vogelzang NJ, Bosl GJ, Johnson K, Kennedy BJ (1981). Raynaud's phenomenon: a common toxicity after combination chemotherapy for testicular cancer. *Ann Intern Med* **95**: 288–92.

36 Vogelzang NJ, Torkelson JL, Kennedy BJ (1985). Hypomagnesemia, renal dysfunction, and Raynaud's phenomenon in patients treated with cisplatin, vinblastine, and bleomycin. *Cancer* **56**: 2765–70.

37 Bosl GJ, Leitner SP, Atlas SA, Sealey JE, Preibisz JJ, Scheiner E (1986). Increased plasma renin and aldosterone in patients treated with cisplatin-based chemotherapy for metastatic germ-cell tumors. *J Clin Oncol* **4**: 1684–9.

38 Harrell RM, Sibley R, Vogelzang NJ (1982). Renal vascular lesions after chemotherapy with vinblastine, bleomycin, and cisplatin. *Am J Med* **73**: 429–33.

39 Vaughn DJ, Gignac GA, Meadows AT (2002). Long-term medical care of testicular *Cancer* survivors. *Ann Intern Med* **136**: 463–70.

40 McDonald BR, Kirmani S, Vasquez M, Mehta RL (1991). Acute renal failure associated with the use of intraperitoneal carboplatin: a report of two cases and review of the literature. *Am J Med* **90**: 386–91.

41 Reed E, Jacob J (1989). Carboplatin and renal dysfunction. *Ann Intern Med* **110**: 409.

42 Mulder PO, Sleijfer DT, de Vries EG, Uges DR, Mulder NH (1988). Renal dysfunction following high-dose carboplatin treatment. *J Cancer Res Clin Oncol* **114**: 212–4.

43 Sleijfer DT, Smit EF, Meijer S, Mulder NH, Postmus PE (1989). Acute and cumulative effects of carboplatin on renal function. *Br J Cancer* **60**: 116–20.

44 Tscherning C, Rubie H, Chancholle A, Claeyssens S, Robert A, Fabre J, et al. (1994). Recurrent renal salt wasting in a child treated with carboplatin and etoposide. *Cancer* **73**: 1761–3.

45 Shea TC, Storniolo AM, Mason JR, Newton B, Mullen M, Taetle R, et al. (1992). A dose-escalation study of carboplatin/cyclophosphamide/etoposide along with autologous bone marrow or peripheral blood stem cell rescue. *Semin Oncol* **19**: 139–44.

46 Beyer J, Rick O, Weinknecht S, Kingreen D, Lenz K, Siegert W (1997). Nephrotoxicity after high-dose carboplatin, etoposide and ifosfamide in germ-cell tumors: incidence and implications for hematologic recovery and clinical outcome. *Bone Marrow Transplant* **20**: 813–9.

47 Fields KK, Elfenbein GJ, Perkins JB, Janssen WE, Ballester OF, Hiemenz JW, et al. (1994). High-dose ifosfamide/carboplatin/etoposide: maximum tolerable doses, toxicities, and hematopoietic recovery after autologous stem cell reinfusion. *Semin Oncol* **21**: 86–92.

48 Grigg A, Szer J, Skov K, Barnett M (1996). Multi-organ dysfunction associated with high-dose carboplatin therapy prior to autologous transplantation. *Bone Marrow Transplant* **17**: 67–74.

49 Chollet P, Bensmaine MA, Brienza S, Deloche C, Cure H, Caillet H, et al. (1996). Single agent activity of oxaliplatin in heavily pretreated advanced epithelial ovarian cancer. *Ann Oncol* **7**: 1065–70.

50 Machover D, Delmas-Marsalet B, Misra SC, Gumus Y, Goldschmidt E, Schilf A, et al. (2001). Dexamethasone, high-dose cytarabine, and oxaliplatin (DHAOx) as salvage treatment for patients with initially refractory or relapsed non-Hodgkin's lymphoma. *Ann Oncol* **12**: 1439–43.

51 Condit PT, Chanes RE, Joel W (1969). Renal toxicity of methotrexate. *Cancer* **23**: 126–31.

52 Abelson HT, Fosburg MT, Beardsley GP, Goorin AM, Gorka C, Link M, et al. (1983). Methotrexate-induced renal impairment: clinical studies and rescue from systemic toxicity with high-dose leucovorin and thymidine. *J Clin Oncol* **1**: 208–16.

53 Widemann BC, Balis FM, Kempf-Bielack B, Bielack S, Pratt CB, Ferrari S, et al. (2004). High-dose methotrexate-induced nephrotoxicity in patients with osteosarcoma. *Cancer* **100**: 2222–32.

54 Widemann BC, Adamson PC (2006). Understanding and managing methotrexate nephrotoxicity. *Oncologist* **11**: 694–703.

55 Flombaum CD, Meyers PA (1999). High-dose leucovorin as sole therapy for methotrexate toxicity. *J Clin Oncol* **17**: 1589–94.

56 Goren MP, Wright RK, Horowitz ME, Meyer WH (1986). Enhancement of methotrexate nephrotoxicity after cisplatin therapy. *Cancer* **58**: 2617–21.

57 Crom WR, Pratt CB, Green AA, Champion JE, Crom DB, Stewart CF, et al. (1984). The effect of prior cisplatin therapy on the pharmacokinetics of high-dose methotrexate. *J Clin Oncol* **2**: 655–61.

58 Jolivet J, Cowan KH, Curt GA, Clendeninn NJ, Chabner BA (1983). The pharmacology and clinical use of methotrexate. *N Engl J Med* **309**: 1094–104.

59 Ackland SP, Schilsky RL (1987). High-dose methotrexate: a critical reappraisal. *J Clin Oncol* **5**: 2017–31.

60 Chu E, Allegra C (1996). Antifolates. In: *Cancer chemotherapy and biotherapy: principles and practice*. 2nd ed. (ed. B Chabner, DL Longo), 109–148. Lippincott-Raven, Philadelphia.

61 Molina R, Fabian C, Cowley Jr B. (1987). Use of charcoal hemoperfusion with sequential hemodialysis to reduce serum methotrexate levels in a patient with acute renal insufficiency. *Am J Med* **82**: 350–2.

62 Relling MV, Stapleton FB, Ochs J, Jones DP, Meyer W, Wainer IW, et al. (1988). Removal of methotrexate, leucovorin, and their metabolites by combined hemodialysis and hemoperfusion. *Cancer* **62**: 884–8.

63 Wall SM, Johansen MJ, Molony DA, DuBose Jr TD, Jaffe N, Madden T (1996). Effective clearance of methotrexate using high-flux hemodialysis membranes. *Am J Kidney Dis* **28**: 846–54.

64 Murashima M, Adamski J, Milone MC, Shaw L, Tsai DE, Bloom RD (2009). Methotrexate clearance by high-flux hemodialysis and peritoneal dialysis: a case report. *Am J Kidney Dis* **53**: 871–4.

65 Widemann BC, Balis FM, Murphy RF, Sorensen JM, Montello MJ, O'Brien M, et al. (1997). Carboxypeptidase-G2, thymidine, and leucovorin rescue in *Cancer* patients with methotrexate-induced renal dysfunction. *J Clin Oncol* **15**: 2125–34.

66 Buchen S, Ngampolo D, Melton RG, Hasan C, Zoubek A, Henze G, et al. (2005). Carboxypeptidase G2 rescue in patients with methotrexate intoxication and renal failure. *Br J Cancer* **92**: 480–7.

67 Schwartz S, Borner K, Muller K, Martus P, Fischer L, Korfel A, et al. (2007). Glucarpidase (carboxypeptidase g2) intervention in adult and elderly cancer patients with renal dysfunction and delayed methotrexate elimination after high-dose methotrexate therapy. *Oncologist* **12**: 1299–308.

68 Rinaldi DA, Kuhn JG, Burris HA, Dorr FA, Rodriguez G, Eckhardt SG, et al. (1999). A phase I evaluation of multitargeted antifolate (MTA, LY231514), administered every 21 days, utilizing the modified continual reassessment method for dose escalation. *Cancer Chemother Pharmacol* **44**: 372–80.

69 Vootukuru V, Liew YP, Nally Jr JV (2006). Pemetrexed-induced acute renal failure, nephrogenic diabetes insipidus, and renal tubular acidosis in a patient with non-small cell lung cancer. *Med Oncol* **23**: 419–22.

70 Castro M (2003). Thymidine rescue: an antidote for pemetrexed-related toxicity in the setting of acute renal failure. *Journal of Clinical Oncology* **2**: 4066.

71 Brandes JC, Grossman SA, Ahmad H (2006). Alteration of pemetrexed excretion in the presence of acute renal failure and effusions: presentation of a case and review of the literature. *Cancer Invest* **24**: 283–7.

72 Mita AC, Sweeney CJ, Baker SD, Goetz A, Hammond LA, Patnaik A, et al. (2006). Phase I and pharmacokinetic study of pemetrexed administered every 3 weeks to advanced *Cancer* patients with normal and impaired renal function. *J Clin Oncol* **24**: 552–62.

73 Skinner R, Sharkey IM, Pearson AD, Craft AW (1993). Ifosfamide, mesna, and nephrotoxicity in children. *J Clin Oncol* **11**: 173–90.

74 Goren MP, Wright RK, Horowitz ME, Pratt CB (1987). Ifosfamide-induced subclinical tubular nephrotoxicity despite mesna. *Cancer Treat Rep* **71**: 127–30.

75 Van Dyk JJ, Falkson HC, Van der Merwe AM, Falkson G (1972). Unexpected toxicity in patients treated with iphosphamide. *Cancer Res* **32**: 921–4.

76 Prasad VK, Lewis IJ, Aparicio SR, Heney D, Hale JP, Bailey CC, et al. (1996). Progressive glomerular toxicity of ifosfamide in children. *Med Pediatr Oncol* **27**: 149–55.

77 Cohen MH, Creaven PJ, Tejada F, Hansen HH, Muggia F, Mittelman A, et al. (1975). Phase I clinical trial of isophosphamide (NSC–109724). *Cancer Chemother Rep* **59**: 751–5.

78 Antman KH, Ryan L, Elias A, Sherman D, Grier HE (1989). Response to ifosfamide and mesna: 124 previously treated patients with metastatic or unresectable sarcoma. *J Clin Oncol* **7**: 126–31.

79 DeFronzo RA, Abeloff M, Braine H, Humphrey RL, Davis PJ (1974). Renal dysfunction after treatment with isophosphamide (NSC–109724). *Cancer Chemother Rep* **58**: 375–82.

80 Patterson WP, Khojasteh A (1989). Ifosfamide-induced renal tubular defects. *Cancer* **63**: 649–51.

81 Berns JS, Haghighat A, Staddon A, Cohen RM, Schmidt R, Fisher S, et al. (1995). Severe, irreversible renal failure after ifosfamide treatment. A clinicopathologic report of two patients. *Cancer* **76**: 497–500.

82 Goren MP, Wright RK, Pratt CB, Horowitz ME, Dodge RK, Viar MJ, et al. (1987). Potentiation of ifosfamide neurotoxicity, hematotoxicity, and tubular nephrotoxicity by prior cis-diamminedichloroplatinum(II) therapy. *Cancer Res* **47**: 1457–60.

83 Harmon WE, Cohen HJ, Schneeberger EE, Grupe WE (1979). Chronic renal failure in children treated with methyl CCNU. *N Engl J Med* **300**: 1200–3.

84 Ellis ME, Weiss RB, Kuperminc M (1985). Nephrotoxicity of lomustine. A case report and literature review. *Cancer Chemother Pharmacol* **15**: 174–5.

85 Schacht RG, Feiner HD, Gallo GR, Lieberman A, Baldwin DS (1981). Nephrotoxicity of nitrosoureas. *Cancer* **48**: 1328–34.

86 Micetich KC, Jensen-Akula M, Mandard JC, Fisher RI (1981). Nephrotoxicity of semustine (methyl-CCNU) in patients with malignant melanoma receiving adjuvant chemotherapy. *Am J Med* **71**: 967–72.

87 Sadoff L (1970). Nephrotoxicity of streptozotocin (NSC–85998). *Cancer Chemother Rep* **54**: 457–9.

88 Schein PS, O'Connell MJ, Blom J, Hubbard S, Magrath IT, Bergevin P, et al. (1974). Clinical antitumor activity and toxicity of streptozotocin (NSC–85998). *Cancer* **34**: 993–1000.

89 Hricik DE, Goldsmith GH (1988). Uric acid nephrolithiasis and acute renal failure secondary to streptozotocin nephrotoxicity. *Am J Med* **84**: 153–6.

90 O'Dwyer PJ, Wagner B, Leyland-Jones B, Wittes RE, Cheson BD, Hoth DF (1988). 2-Deoxycoformycin (pentostatin) for lymphoid malignancies. Rational development of an active new drug. *Ann Intern Med* **108**: 733–43.

91 Margolis J, Grever MR (2000). Pentostatin (Nipent): a review of potential toxicity and its management. *Semin Oncol* **27**: 9–14.

92 Leach JW, Pham T, Diamandidis D, George JN (1999). Thrombotic thrombocytopenic purpura-hemolytic uremic syndrome (TTP-HUS) following treatment with deoxycoformycin in a patient with cutaneous T-cell lymphoma (Sezary syndrome): A case report. *Am J Hematol* **61**: 268–70.

93 Peterson BA, Collins AJ, Vogelzang NJ, Bloomfield CD (1981). 5-Azacytidine and renal tubular dysfunction. *Blood* **57**: 182–5.

94 Peterson BA, Bloomfield CD, Gottlieb AJ, Coleman M, Greenberg MS (1982). 5-azactidine and zorubicin for patients with previously treated acute nonlymphocytic leukemia: a *Cancer* and Leukemia Group B pilot study. *Cancer Treat Rep* **66**: 563–6.

95 Leung N, Slezak JM, Bergstralh EJ, Dispenzieri A, Lacy MQ, Wolf RC, et al. (2005). Acute renal insufficiency after high-dose melphalan in patients with primary systemic amyloidosis during stem cell transplantation. *Am J Kidney Dis* **45**: 102–11.

96 Eskens FA, Verweij J (2006). The clinical toxicity profile of vascular endothelial growth factor (VEGF) and vascular endothelial growth factor receptor (VEGFR) targeting angiogenesis inhibitors; a review. *Eur J Cancer* **42**: 3127–39.

97 Izzedine H, Rixe O, Billemont B, Baumelou A, Deray G (2007). Angiogenesis inhibitor therapies: focus on kidney toxicity and hypertension. *Am J Kidney Dis* **50**: 203–18.

98 Zhu X, Wu S, Dahut WL, Parikh CR (2007). Risks of proteinuria and hypertension with bevacizumab, an antibody against vascular endothelial growth factor: systematic review and meta-analysis. *Am J Kidney Dis* **49**: 186–93.

99 Eremina V, Jefferson JA, Kowalewska J, Hochster H, Haas M, Weisstuch J, et al. (2008). VEGF inhibition and renal thrombotic microangiopathy. *N Engl J Med* **358**: 1129–36.

100 Riely GJ, Miller VA (2007). Vascular endothelial growth factor trap in non small cell lung cancer. *Clin Cancer Res* **13**: s4623–7.

101 Izzedine H, Brocheriou I, Deray G, Rixe O (2007). Thrombotic microangiopathy and anti-VEGF agents. *Nephrol Dial Transplant* **22**: 1481–2.

102 Zhu X, Stergiopoulos K, Wu S (2009). Risk of hypertension and renal dysfunction with an angiogenesis inhibitor sunitinib: systematic review and meta-analysis. *Acta Oncol* **48**: 9–17.

103 Bhojani N, Jeldres C, Patard JJ, Perrotte P, Suardi N, Hutterer G, et al. (2008). Toxicities associated with the administration of sorafenib, sunitinib, and temsirolimus and their management in patients with metastatic renal cell carcinoma. *Eur Urol* **53**: 917–30.

104 Azizi M, Chedid A, Oudard S (2008). Home blood-pressure monitoring in patients receiving sunitinib. *N Engl J Med* **358**: 95–7.

105 Choi MK, Hong JY, Jang JH, Lim HY (2008). TTP-HUS Associated with Sunitinib. *Cancer Res Treat* **40**: 211–3.

106 Patel TV, Morgan JA, Demetri GD, George S, Maki RG, Quigley M, et al. (2008). A preeclampsia-like syndrome characterized by reversible hypertension and proteinuria induced by the multitargeted kinase inhibitors sunitinib and sorafenib. *J Natl Cancer Inst* **100**: 282–4.

107 Launay-Vacher V, Deray G (2009). Hypertension and proteinuria: a class-effect of antiangiogenic therapies. *AntiCancer Drugs* **20**: 81–2.

108 Feldman DR, Baum MS, Ginsberg MS, Hassoun H, Flombaum CD, Velasco S, et al. (2009). Phase I trial of bevacizumab plus escalated doses of sunitinib in patients with metastatic renal cell carcinoma. *J Clin Oncol* **27**: 1432–9.

109 Azad NS, Posadas EM, Kwitkowski VE, Steinberg SM, Jain L, Annunziata CM, et al. (2008). Combination targeted therapy with sorafenib and bevacizumab results in enhanced toxicity and antitumor activity. *J Clin Oncol* **26**: 3709–14.

110 Soria JC, Massard C, Izzedine H (2009). From theoretical synergy to clinical supra-additive toxicity. *J Clin Oncol* **27**: 1359–61.

111 Hurwitz H, Saini S (2006). Bevacizumab in the treatment of metastatic colorectal *Cancer*: safety profile and management of adverse events. *Semin Oncol* **33**: S26–34.

112 Gordon MS, Cunningham D (2005). Managing patients treated with bevacizumab combination therapy. *Oncology* **69**: 25–33.

113 Izzedine H, Ederhy S, Goldwasser F, Soria JC, Milano G, Cohen A, et al. (2009). Management of hypertension in angiogenesis inhibitor-treated patients. *Ann Oncol* **20**: 807–15.

114 Schrag D, Chung KY, Flombaum C, Saltz L (2005). Cetuximab therapy and symptomatic hypomagnesemia. *J Natl Cancer Inst* **97**: 1221–4.

115 Tejpar S, Piessevaux H, Claes K, Piront P, Hoenderop JG, Verslype C, et al. (2007). Magnesium wasting associated with epidermal-growth-factor receptor-targeting antibodies in colorectal cancer: a prospective study. *Lancet Oncol* **8**: 387–94.

116 Ostro D, Lipton J (2007). Unusual fluid retention with imatinib therapy for chronic myeloid leukemia. *Leuk Lymphoma* **48**: 195–6.

117 Atallah E, Kantarjian H, Cortes J (2007). Emerging safety issues with imatinib and other Abl tyrosine kinase inhibitors. *Clin Lymphoma Myeloma* **7**: S105–12.

118 Zojer N, Keck AV, Pecherstorfer M (1999). Comparative tolerability of drug therapies for hypercalcaemia of malignancy. *Drug Saf* **21**: 389–406.

119 Markowitz GS, Fine PL, Stack JI, Kunis CL, Radhakrishnan J, Palecki W, et al. (2003). Toxic acute tubular necrosis following treatment with zoledronate (Zometa). *Kidney Int* **64**: 281–9.

120 Markowitz GS, Appel GB, Fine PL, Fenves AZ, Loon NR, Jagannath S, et al. (2001). Collapsing focal segmental glomerulosclerosis following treatment with high-dose pamidronate. *J Am Soc Nephrol* **12**: 1164–72.

121 Lockridge L, Papac RJ, Perazella MA (2002). Pamidronate-associated nephrotoxicity in a patient with Langerhans's histiocytosis. *Am J Kidney Dis* **40**: E2.

122 Willson RA (2002). Nephrotoxicity of interferon alfa-ribavirin therapy for chronic hepatitis C. *J Clin Gastroenterol* **35**: 89–92.

123 Nassar GM, Pedro P, Remmers RE, Mohanty LB, Smith W (1998). Reversible renal failure in a patient with the hypereosinophilia syndrome during therapy with alpha interferon. *Am J Kidney Dis* **31**: 121–6.

124 Coroneos E, Petrusevska G, Varghese F, Truong LD (1996). Focal segmental glomerulosclerosis with acute renal failure associated with alpha-interferon therapy. *Am J Kidney Dis* **28**: 888–92.

125 Hansen PB, Johnsen HE, Hippe E (1993). Hypereosinophilic syndrome treated with alpha-interferon and granulocyte colony-stimulating factor but complicated by nephrotoxicity. *Am J Hematol* **43**: 66–8.

126 Traynor A, Kuzel T, Samuelson E, Kanwar Y (1994). Minimal-change glomerulopathy and glomerular visceral epithelial hyperplasia associated with alpha-interferon therapy for cutaneous T-cell lymphoma. *Nephron* **67**: 94–100.

127 Ohta S, Yokoyama H, Wada T, Sakai N, Shimizu M, Kato T, et al. (1999). Exacerbation of glomerulonephritis in subjects with chronic hepatitis C virus infection after interferon therapy. *Am J Kidney Dis* **33**: 1040–8.

128 Quesada JR, Talpaz M, Rios A, Kurzrock R, Gutterman JU (1986). Clinical toxicity of interferons in cancer patients: a review. *J Clin Oncol* **4**: 234–43.

129 Kurschel E, Metz-Kurschel U, Niederle N, Aulbert E (1991). Investigations on the subclinical and clinical nephrotoxicity of interferon alpha–2B in patients with myeloproliferative syndromes. *Ren Fail* **13**: 87–93.

130 Zuber J, Martinez F, Droz D, Oksenhendler E, Legendre C (2002). Alpha-interferon-associated thrombotic microangiopathy: a clinicopathologic study of eight patients and review of the literature. *Medicine (Baltimore)* **81**: 321–31.

131 Baker GL, Kahl LE, Zee BC, Stolzer BL, Agarwal AK, Medsger Jr TA (1987). Malignancy following treatment of rheumatoid arthritis with cyclophosphamide. Long-term case-control follow-up study. *Am J Med* **83**: 1–9.

132 Leblond F, Guevin C, Demers C, Pellerin I, Gascon-Barre M, Pichette V (2001). Downregulation of hepatic cytochrome P450 in chronic renal failure. *J Am Soc Nephrol* **12**: 326–32.

133 Touchette MA, Slaughter RL (1991). The effect of renal failure on hepatic drug clearance. *DICP* **25**: 1214–24.

134 Dowling TC, Briglia AE, Fink JC, Hanes DS, Light PD, Stackiewicz L, et al. (2003). Characterization of hepatic cytochrome p4503A activity in patients with end-stage renal disease. *Clin Pharmacol Ther* **73**: 427–34.

135 Dreisbach AW, Lertora JJ (2008). The effect of chronic renal failure on drug metabolism and transport. *Expert Opin Drug Metab Toxicol* **4**: 1065–74.

136 Chabner BA (2001). *Cancer chemotherapy and biotherapy: Principles and practice*, 3 ed. Lippincott Williams and Wilkins, Philadelphia.

137 Balis FM, Holcenberg JS, Bleyer WA (1983). Clinical pharmacokinetics of commonly used anticancer drugs. *Clin Pharmacokinet* **8**: 202–32.

138 Kintzel PE, Dorr RT (1995). Anticancer drug renal toxicity and elimination: dosing guidelines for altered renal function. *Cancer Treat Rev* **21**: 33–64.

139 Powis G (1982). Effect of human renal and hepatic disease on the pharmacokinetics of anticancer drugs. *Cancer Treat Rev* **9**: 85–124.

140 Aronoff GR, Bennett WM (eds) (2007). *Drug prescribing in renal failure: dosing guidelines for adults*, 5 ed. ACP, Philadelphia.

141 Li YF, Fu S, Hu W, Liu JH, Finkel KW, Gershenson DM, et al. (2007). Systemic anticancer therapy in gynecological cancer patients with renal dysfunction. *Int J Gynecol Cancer* **17**: 739–63.

142 Lichtman SM, Wildiers H, Launay-Vacher V, Steer C, Chatelut E, Aapro M (2007). International Society of Geriatric Oncology (SIOG) recommendations for the adjustment of dosing in elderly *Cancer* patients with renal insufficiency. *Eur J Cancer* **43**: 14–34.

143 Tomita M, Aoki Y, Tanaka K (2004). Effect of haemodialysis on the pharmacokinetics of antineoplastic drugs. *Clin Pharmacokinet* **43**: 515–27.

144 Grochow LB, Colvin M (1983). Clinical pharmacokinetics of cyclophosphamide. In: *Pharmacokinetics of anticancer agents in humans* (ed. EA Ames), pp. 135–54. Elsevier, Amsterdam.

145 Bagley Jr CM, Bostick FW, DeVita Jr VT (1973). Clinical pharmacology of cyclophosphamide. *Cancer Res* **33**: 226–33.

146 Juma FD, Rogers HJ, Trounce JR (1981). Effect of renal insufficiency on the pharmacokinetics of cyclophosphamide and some of its metabolites. *Eur J Clin Pharmacol* **19**: 443–51.

147 Mouridsen HT, Jacobsen E (1975). Pharmacokinetics of cyclophosphamide in renal failure. *Acta Pharmacol Toxicol (Copenh)* **36**: 409–14.

148 Haubitz M, Bohnenstengel F, Brunkhorst R, Schwab M, Hofmann U, Busse D (2002). Cyclophosphamide pharmacokinetics and dose requirements in patients with renal insufficiency. *Kidney Int* **61**: 1495–501.

149 Bramwell V, Calvert RT, Edwards G, Scarffe H, Crowther D (1979). The disposition of cyclophosphamide in a group of myeloma patients. *Cancer Chemother Pharmacol* **3**: 253–9.

150 Humphrey RL, Kvols LK (1974). The influence of renal insufficiency on cyclophosphamide induced hematopoietic depression and recovery. *Proc Am Assoc Cancer Res* **15**: 84.

151 Tricot G, Alberts DS, Johnson C, Roe DJ, Dorr RT, Bracy D, et al. (1996). Safety of autotransplants with high-dose melphalan in renal failure: a pharmacokinetic and toxicity study. *Clin Cancer Res* **2**: 947–52.

152 Ballester OF, Tummala R, Janssen WE, Fields KK, Hiemenz JW, Goldstein SC, et al. (1997). High-dose chemotherapy and autologous peripheral blood stem cell transplantation in patients with multiple myeloma and renal insufficiency. *Bone Marrow Transplant* **20**: 653–6.

153 Perry JJ, Fleming RA, Rocco MV, Petros WP, Bleyer AJ, Radford Jr JE, et al. (1999). Administration and pharmacokinetics of high-dose cyclophosphamide with hemodialysis support for allogeneic bone marrow transplantation in acute leukemia and end-stage renal disease. *Bone Marrow Transplant* **23**: 839–42.

154 Bischoff ME, Blau W, Wagner T, Wagenmann W, Dorner O, Basara N, et al. (1998). Total body irradiation and cyclophosphamide is a conditioning regimen for unrelated bone marrow transplantation in a patient with chronic myelogenous leukemia and renal failure on hemodialysis. *Bone Marrow Transplant* **22**: 591–3.

155 Wang LH, Lee CS, Majeske BL, Marbury TC (1981). Clearance and recovery calculations in hemodialysis: application to plasma, red blood cells, and dialysate measurements for cyclophosphamide. *Clin Pharmacol Ther* **29**: 365–72.

156 McCune JS, Adams D, Homans AC, Guillot A, Iacono L, Stewart CF (2006). Cyclophosphamide disposition in an anephric child. *Pediatr Blood Cancer* **46**: 99–104.

157 Wagner T (1994). Ifosfamide clinical pharmacokinetics. *Clin Pharmacokinet* **26**: 439–56.

158 Carlson L, Goren MP, Bush DA, Griener JC, Quigley R, Tkaczewski I, et al. (1998). Toxicity, pharmacokinetics, and in vitro hemodialysis clearance of ifosfamide and metabolites in an anephric pediatric patient with Wilms' tumor. *Cancer Chemother Pharmacol* **41**: 140–6.

159 Alberts DS, Chen HG, Benz D, Mason NL (1981). Effect of renal dysfunction in dogs on the disposition and marrow toxicity of melphalan. *Br J Cancer* **43**: 330–4.

160 Cornwell 3rd GG, Pajak TF, McIntyre OR, Kochwa S, Dosik H (1982). Influence of renal failure on myelosuppressive effects of melphalan: *Cancer* and Leukemia Group B experience. *Cancer Treat Rep* **66**: 475–81.

161 Osterborg A, Ehrsson H, Eksborg S, Wallin I, Mellstedt H (1989). Pharmacokinetics of oral melphalan in relation to renal function in multiple myeloma patients. *Eur J Cancer Clin Oncol* **25**: 899–903.

162 Dhodapkar M, Rubin J, Reid JM, Burch PA, Pitot HC, Buckner JC, et al. (1997). Phase I trial of temozolomide (NSC 362856) in patients with advanced cancer. *Clin Cancer Res* **3**: 1093–100.

163 Jen JF, Cutler DL, Pai SM, Batra VK, Affrime MB, Zambas DN, et al. (2000). Population pharmacokinetics of temozolomide in cancer patients. *Pharm Res* **17**: 1284–9.

164 Chatham WW, Morgan SL, Alarcon GS (2000). Renal failure: a risk factor for methotrexate toxicity. *Arthritis Rheum* **43**: 1185–6.

165 Park GT, Jeon DW, Roh KH, Mun HS, Lee CH, Park CH, et al. (1999). A case of pancytopenia secondary to low-dose pulse methotrexate therapy in a patient with rheumatoid arthritis and renal insufficiency. *Korean J Intern Med* **14**: 85–7.

166 Nakamura M, Sakemi T, Nagasawa K (1999). Severe pancytopenia caused by a single administration of low dose methotrexate in a patient undergoing hemodialysis. *J Rheumatol* **26**: 1424–5.

167 Ellman MH, Ginsberg D (1990). Low-dose methotrexate and severe neutropenia in patients undergoing renal dialysis. *Arthritis Rheum* **33**: 1060–1.

168 Thomson AH, Daly M, Knepil J, Harden P, Symonds P (1996). Methotrexate removal during haemodialysis in a patient with advanced laryngeal carcinoma. *Cancer Chemother Pharmacol* **38**: 566–70.

169 Yokogi H, Yamasaki Y, Ishibe T (1993). [M-VAC therapy in a patient with ureteral carcinoma accompanied by chronic renal failure]. *Gan To Kagaku Ryoho* **20**: 2405–7.

170 Tokunaga J, Kikukawa H, Nishi K, Kitani K, Fujii J, Honda J, et al. (2000). [Pharmacokinetics of cisplatin and methotrexate in a patient suffering from advanced ureteral tumor accompanied by chronic renal failure, undergoing combined hemodialysis and systemic M-VAC chemotherapy]. *Gan To Kagaku Ryoho* **27**: 2079–85.

171 Rengelshausen J, Hull WE, Schwenger V, Goggelmann C, Walter-Sack I, Bommer J (2002). Pharmacokinetics of 5-fluorouracil and its catabolites determined by 19F nuclear magnetic resonance spectroscopy for a patient on chronic hemodialysis. *Am J Kidney Dis* **39**: E10.

172 Gusella M, Rebeschini M, Cartei G, Ferrazzi E, Ferrari M, Padrini R (2005). Effect c hemodialysis on the metabolic clearance of 5-Fluorouracil in a patient with end-sta renal failure. *Ther Drug Monit* **27**: 816–8.

173 Fleming GF, Schilsky RL, Schumm LP, Meyerson A, Hong AM, Vogelzang NJ, et ; (2003). Phase I and pharmacokinetic study of 24-hour infusion 5-fluorouracil and leucovorin in patients with organ dysfunction. *Ann Oncol* **14**: 1142–7.

174 Cassidy J, Twelves C, Van Cutsem E, Hoff P, Bajetta E, Boyer M, et al. (2002). First-line oral capecitabine therapy in metastatic colorectal cancer: a favorable safe profile compared with intravenous 5-fluorouracil/leucovorin. *Ann Oncol* **13**: 566–7

175 Katamura Y, Aikata H, Kimura Y, Azakami T, Kawaoka T, Takaki S, et al. (2009). Successful treatment of pulmonary metastases associated with advanced hepatocellu carcinoma by systemic 5-fluorouracil combined with interferon-alpha in a hemodialy patient. *Hepatol Res* **39**: 415–20.

176 Akiyama S, Nakayama H, Takami H, Gotoh H, Gotoh Y (2007). Pharmacodynamic study of the Saltz regimen for metastatic colorectal cancer in a hemodialyzed patien *Chemotherapy* **53**: 418–21.

177 Inauen R, Cathomas R, Boehm T, Koeberle D, Pestalozzi BC, Gillessen S, et al. (200 Feasibility of using cetuximab and bevacizumab in a patient with colorectal cancer and terminal renal failure. *Oncology* **72**: 209–10.

178 Stemmler J, Weise A, Hacker U, Heinemann V, Schalhorn A (2002). Weekly irinote in a patient with metastatic colorectal cancer on hemodialysis due to chronic rena failure. *Onkologie* **25**: 60–3.

179 Poole C, Gardiner J, Twelves C, Johnston P, Harper P, Cassidy J, et al. (2002). Eff of renal impairment on the pharmacokinetics and tolerability of capecitabine (Xeloda) in cancer patients. *Cancer Chemother Pharmacol* **49**: 225–34.

180 Smith GA, Damon LE, Rugo HS, Ries CA, Linker CA (1997). High-dose cytarabi dose modification reduces the incidence of neurotoxicity in patients with renal insufficiency. *J Clin Oncol* **15**: 833–9.

181 Poschl JM, Klaus G, Querfeld U, Ludwig R, Mehls O (1993). Chemotherapy wi cytosine arabinoside in a child with Burkitt's lymphoma on maintenance hemo and hemofiltration. *Ann Hematol* **67**: 37–9.

182 Nogue-Aliguer M, Carles J, Arrivi A, Juan O, Alonso L, Font A, et al. (2003). Gemcitabine and carboplatin in advanced transitional cell carcinoma of the uri tract: an alternative therapy. *Cancer* **97**: 2180–6.

183 Ricci S, Galli L, Chioni A, Iannopollo M, Antonuzzo A, Francesca F, et al. (2002 Gemcitabine plus epirubicin in patients with advanced urothelial carcinoma wh not eligible for platinum-based regimens. *Cancer* **95**: 1444–50.

184 Mir O, Alexandre J, Ropert S, Amsellem-Ouazana D, Flam T, Beuzeboc P, et al. (2005). Combination of gemcitabine and oxaliplatin in urothelial cancer patients with severe renal or cardiac comorbidities. *AntiCancer Drugs* **16**: 1017–21.

185 Delaloge S, Llombart A, Di Palma M, Tourani JM, Turpin F, Ni L, et al. (2004). Gemcitabine in patients with solid tumors and renal impairment: a pharmacokinetic phase I study. *Am J Clin Oncol* **27**: 289–93.

186 Venook AP, Egorin MJ, Rosner GL, Hollis D, Mani S, Hawkins M, et al. (2000). Phase I and pharmacokinetic trial of gemcitabine in patients with hepatic or renal dysfunction: *Cancer* and Leukemia Group B 9565. *J Clin Oncol* **18**: 2780–7.

187 Kiani A, Kohne CH, Franz T, Passauer J, Haufe T, Gross P, et al. (2003). Pharmacokinetics of gemcitabine in a patient with end-stage renal disease: effective clearance of its main metabolite by standard hemodialysis treatment. *Cancer Chemother Pharmacol* **51**: 266–70.

188 Masumori N, Kunishima Y, Hirobe M, Takeuchi M, Takayanagi A, Tsukamoto T, et al. (2008). Measurement of plasma concentration of gemcitabine and its metabolite dFdU in hemodialysis patients with advanced urothelial cancer. *Jpn J Clin Oncol* **38**: 182–5.

189 Koolen SL, Huitema AD, Jansen RS, van Voorthuizen T, Beijnen JH, Smit WM, et al. (2009). Pharmacokinetics of gemcitabine and metabolites in a patient with double-sided nephrectomy: a case report and review of the literature. *Oncologist* **14**: 944–8.

190 Odlind B, Hartvig P, Lindstrom B, Lonnerholm G, Tufveson G, Grefberg N (1986). Serum azathioprine and 6-mercaptopurine levels and immunosuppressive activity after azathioprine in uremic patients. *Int J Immunopharmacol* **8**: 1–11.

191 Chan GL, Canafax DM, Johnson CA (1987). The therapeutic use of azathioprine in renal transplantation. *Pharmacotherapy* **7**: 165–77.

192 Bach JF, Dardenne M (1971). The metabolism of azathioprine in renal failure. *Transplantation* **12**: 253–9.

193 Lathia C, Fleming GF, Meyer M, Ratain MJ, Whitfield L (2002). Pentostatin pharmacokinetics and dosing recommendations in patients with mild renal impairment. *Cancer Chemother Pharmacol* **50**: 121–6.

194 Malspeis L, Grever MR, Staubus AE, Young D (1990). Pharmacokinetics of 2-F-ara-A (9-beta-D-arabinofuranosyl–2-fluoroadenine) in cancer patients during the phase I clinical investigation of fludarabine phosphate. *Semin Oncol* **17**: 18–32.

195 Lichtman SM, Etcubanas E, Budman DR, Eisenberg P, Zervos G, D'Amico P, et al. (2002). The pharmacokinetics and pharmacodynamics of fludarabine phosphate in patients with renal impairment: a prospective dose adjustment study. *Cancer Invest* **20**: 904–13.

196 Tendas A, Cupelli L, Dentamaro T, Scaramucci L, Palumbo R, Niscola P, et al. (2009). Feasibility of a dose-adjusted fludarabine-melphalan conditioning prior autologous stem cell transplantation in a dialysis-dependent patient with mantle cell lymphoma. *Ann Hematol* **88**: 285–6.

197 Horwitz ME, Spasojevic I, Morris A, Telen M, Essell J, Gasparetto C, et al. (2007). Fludarabine-based nonmyeloablative stem cell transplantation for sickle cell disease with and without renal failure: clinical outcome and pharmacokinetics. *Biol Blood Marrow Transplant* **13**: 1422–6.

198 Liliemark J (1997). The clinical pharmacokinetics of cladribine. *Clin Pharmacokinet* **32**: 120–31.

199 D'Incalci M, Rossi C, Zucchetti M, Urso R, Cavalli F, Mangioni C, et al. (1986). Pharmacokinetics of etoposide in patients with abnormal renal and hepatic function. *Cancer Res* **46**: 2566–71.

200 Arbuck SG, Douglass HO, Crom WR, Goodwin P, Silk Y, Cooper C, et al. (1984). Etoposide pharmacokinetics in patients with normal and abnormal organ function. *J Clin Oncol* **4**: 1690–5.

201 Stewart CF (1994). Use of etoposide in patients with organ dysfunction: pharmacokinetic and pharmacodynamic considerations. *Cancer Chemother Pharmacol* **34**: S76–83.

202 Joel SP, Shah R, Clark PI, Slevin ML (1996). Predicting etoposide toxicity: relationship to organ function and protein binding. *J Clin Oncol* **14**: 257–67.

203 Holthuis JJ, Van de Vyver FL, van Oort WJ, Verleun H, Bakaert AB, De Broe ME (1985). Pharmacokinetic evaluation of increasing dosages of etoposide in a chronic hemodialysis patient. *Cancer Treat Rep* **69**: 1279–82.

204 Motzer RJ, Niedzwiecki D, Isaacs M, Menendez-Botet C, Tong WP, Flombaum C, et al. (1990). Carboplatin-based chemotherapy with pharmacokinetic analysis for patients with hemodialysis-dependent renal insufficiency. *Cancer Chemother Pharmacol* **27**: 234–8.

205 Canetta R, Benedetto P, Ehrlich C, McFadden, D., Motzer RJ, Florentine S. Administration of carboplatin followed by dialysis to anuric patients. *Eur Urol* 1990; **18**: 322.

206 Andes WA (1993). Case report: oat cell cancer and renal failure. *Am J Med Sci* **306**: 104.

207 English MW, Lowis SP, Peng B, Boddy A, Newell DR, Price L, et al. (1996). Pharmacokinetically guided dosing of carboplatin and etoposide during peritoneal dialysis and haemodialysis. *Br J Cancer* **73**: 776–80.

208 Dagher R, Kreissman S, Robertson KA, Provisor A, Bergstein J, Burke K, et al. (1998). High dose chemotherapy with autologous peripheral blood progenitor cell transplantation in an anephric child with multiply recurrent Wilms tumor. *J Pediatr Hematol Oncol* **20**: 357–60.

209 Farhangi M, Weinstein SH (1987). Carboplatin, etoposide, and bleomycin for treatment of stage IIC seminoma complicated by acute renal failure. *Cancer Treat Rep* **71**: 1123–4.

210 Suzuki S, Koide M, Sakamoto S, Matsuo T (1997). Pharmacokinetics of carboplatin and etoposide in a haemodialysis patient with Merkel-cell carcinoma. *Nephrol Dial Transplant* **12**: 137–40.

211 Bikfalvi A, Seiler KU, Schmitz N, Loffler H (1986). Cytotoxic chemotherapy with cisplatin in an anuric patient undergoing hemodialysis. *Tumor Diagnostik and Therapie* **7**: 42–3.

212 Yanagawa H, Takishita Y, Bando H, Sumitani H, Okada S (1996). Carboplatin-based chemotherapy in patients undergoing hemodialysis. *Anticancer Res* **16**: 533–5.

213 Sano F, Koike M, Ishibashi M, Tuji K, Katoh M, Hasegawa S, et al. (1996). [Chemotherapy for two patients with non-Hodgkin's lymphoma in hemodialysis]. *Rinsho Ketsueki* **37**: 688–93.

214 Sonnichsen DS, Relling MV (1994). Clinical pharmacokinetics of paclitaxel. *Clin Pharmacokinet* **27**: 256–69.

215 Vaughn DJ, Manola J, Dreicer R, See W, Levitt R, Wilding G (2002). Phase II study of paclitaxel plus carboplatin in patients with advanced carcinoma of the urothelium and renal dysfunction (E2896): a trial of the Eastern Cooperative Oncology Group. *Cancer* **95**: 1022–7.

216 Dreicer R, Gustin DM, See WA, Williams RD (1996). Paclitaxel in advanced urothelial carcinoma: its role in patients with renal insufficiency and as salvage therapy. *J Urol* **156**: 1606–8.

217 Bekele L, Vidal Vazquez M, Adjei AA (2001). Systemic chemotherapy in patients with renal failure. *Am J Clin Oncol* **24**: 382–4.

218 Balat O, Kudelka AP, Edwards CL, Verschraegen C, Mante R, Kavanagh JJ (1996). A case report of paclitaxel administered to a patient with platinum-refractory ovarian cancer on long-term hemodialysis. *Eur J Gynaecol Oncol* **17**: 232–3.

219 Woo MH, Gregornik D, Shearer PD, Meyer WH, Relling MV (1999). Pharmacokinetics of paclitaxel in an anephric patient. *Cancer Chemother Pharmacol* **43**: 92–6.

220 Melilli GA, Di Vagno G, Cormio G, Greco P, Fontana A, Carriero C, et al. (1999). La chemioterapia nel trattamento del carcinosarcoma dell'ovaio. *Minerva Ginecol* **51**: 445–8.

221 Dimopoulos MA, Deliveliotis C, Moulopoulos LA, Papadimitriou C, Mitropoulos D, Anagnostopoulos A, et al. (1998). Treatment of patients with metastatic urothelial carcinoma and impaired renal function with single-agent docetaxel. *Urology* **52**: 56–60.

222 Mencoboni M, Olivieri R, Vannozzi MO, Schettini G, Viazzi F, Ghio R (2006). Docetaxel pharmacokinetics with pre- and post-dialysis administration in a hemodyalized patient. *Chemotherapy* **52**: 147–50.

223 Hochegger K, Lhotta K, Mayer G, Czejka M, Hilbe W (2007). Pharmacokinetic analysis of docetaxel during haemodialysis in a patient with locally advanced non-small cell lung *Cancer Nephrol Dial Transplant* **22**: 289–90.

224 O'Reilly S, Rowinsky EK, Slichenmyer W, Donehower RC, Forastiere AA, Ettinger DS, et al. (1996). Phase I and pharmacologic study of topotecan in patients with impaired renal function. *J Clin Oncol* **14**: 3062–73.

225 O'Reilly S, Armstrong DK, Grochow LB (1997). Life-threatening myelosuppression in patients with occult renal impairment receiving topotecan. *Gynecol Oncol* **67**: 329–30.

226 Seiter K (2005). Toxicity of the topoisomerase I inhibitors. *Expert Opin Drug Saf* **4**: 45–53.

227 Armstrong DK (2004). Topotecan dosing guidelines in ovarian cancer: reduction and management of hematologic toxicity. *Oncologist* **9**: 33–42.

228 Herrington JD, Figueroa JA, Kirstein MN, Zamboni WC, Stewart CF (2001). Effect of hemodialysis on topotecan disposition in a patient with severe renal dysfunction. *Cancer Chemother Pharmacol* **47**: 89–93.

229 Iacono LC, Adams D, Homans AC, Guillot A, McCune JS, Stewart CF (2004). Topotecan disposition in an anephric child. *J Pediatr Hematol Oncol* **26**: 596–600.

230 Lugtenberg RT, Cransberg K, Loos WJ, Wagner A, Alders M, van den Heuvel-Eibrink MM (2008). Topotecan distribution in an anephric infant with therapy-resistant bilateral Wilms tumor with a novel germline WT1 gene mutation. *Cancer Chemother Pharmacol* **62**: 1039–44.

231 Chabot GG, Abigerges D, Catimel G, Culine S, de Forni M, Extra JM, et al. (1995). Population pharmacokinetics and pharmacodynamics of irinotecan (CPT–11) and active metabolite SN–38 during phase I trials. *Ann Oncol* **6**: 141–51.

232 Slatter JG, Schaaf LJ, Sams JP, Feenstra KL, Johnson MG, Bombardt PA, et al. (2000). Pharmacokinetics, metabolism, and excretion of irinotecan (CPT–11) following I.V. infusion of [C]CPT–11 in cancer patients. *Drug Metab Dispos* **28**: 423–33.

233 Sparreboom A, de Jonge MJ, de Bruijn P, Brouwer E, Nooter K, Loos WJ, et al. (1998). Irinotecan (CPT–11) metabolism and disposition in cancer patients. *Clin Cancer Res* **4**: 2747–54.

234 Venook AP, Enders Klein C, Fleming G, Hollis D, Leichman CG, Hohl R, et al. (2003). A phase I and pharmacokinetic study of irinotecan in patients with hepatic or renal dysfunction or with prior pelvic radiation: CALGB 9863. *Ann Oncol* **14**: 1783–90.

235 de Jong FA, van der Bol JM, Mathijssen RH, van Gelder T, Wiemer EA, Sparreboom A, et al. (2008). Renal function as a predictor of irinotecan-induced neutropenia. *Clin Pharmacol Ther* **84**: 254–62.

236 Czock D, Rasche FM, Boesler B, Shipkova M, Keller F (2009). Irinotecan in Cancer patients with end-stage renal failure. *Ann Pharmacother* **43**: 363–9.

237 Budakoglu B, Abali H, Uncu D, Yildirim N, Oksuzoglu B, Zengin N (2005). Good tolerance of weekly irinotecan in a patient with metastatic colorectal Cancer on chronic hemodialysis. *J Chemother* **17**: 452–3.

238 Kim DM, Kim HL, Chung CH, Park CY (2009). Successful treatment of small-cell lung cancer with irinotecan in a hemodialysis patient with end-stage renal disease. *Korean J Intern Med* **24**: 73–5.

239 Venat-Bouvet L, Saint-Marcoux F, Lagarde C, Peyronnet P, Lebrun-Ly V, Tubiana-Mathieu N (2007). Irinotecan-based chemotherapy in a metastatic colorectal cancer patient under haemodialysis for chronic renal dysfunction: two cases considered. *Anticancer Drugs* **18**: 977–80.

240 Galsky MD, Iasonos A, Mironov S, Scattergood J, Boyle MG, Bajorin DF (2007). Phase II trial of dose-dense doxorubicin plus gemcitabine followed by paclitaxel plus carboplatin in patients with advanced urothelial carcinoma and impaired renal function. *Cancer* **109**: 549–55.

241 Yoshida H, Goto M, Honda A, Nabeshima T, Kumazawa T, Inagaki J, et al. (1994). Pharmacokinetics of doxorubicin and its active metabolite in patients with normal renal function and in patients on hemodialysis. *Cancer Chemother Pharmacol* **33**: 450–4.

242 Alberts DS, Chen HS, Liu R, Himmelstein KJ, Mayersohn M, Perrier D, et al. (1978). Bleomycin pharmacokinetics in man. I. Intravenous administration. *Cancer Chemother Pharmacol* **1**: 177–81.

243 Crooke ST, Comis RL, Einhorn LH, Strong JE, Broughton A, Prestayko AW (1977). Effects of variations in renal function on the clinical pharmacology of bleomycin administered as an iv bolus. *Cancer Treat Rep* **61**: 1631–6.

244 Crooke ST, Luft F, Broughton A, Strong J, Casson K, Einhorn L (1977). Bleomycin serum pharmacokinetics as determined by a radioimmunoassay and a microbiologic assay in a patient with compromised renal function. *Cancer* **39**: 1430–4.

245 Yee GC, Crom WR, Champion JE, Brodeur GM, Evans WM (1993). Cisplatin-induced changes in bleomycin elimination. *Cancer Treat Rep* **67**: 587–9.

246 Bennett WM, Pastore L, Houghton DC (1980). Fatal pulmonary bleomycin toxicity in cisplatin-induced acute renal failure. *Cancer Treat Rep* **64**: 921–4.

247 van Barneveld PW, Sleijfer DT, van der Mark TW, Mulder NH, Donker AJ, Meijer S, et al. (1984). Influence of platinum-induced renal toxicity on bleomycin-induced pulmonary toxicity in patients with disseminated testicular carcinoma. *Oncology* **41**: 4–7.

248 Dalgleish AG, Woods RL, Levi JA (1984). Bleomycin pulmonary toxicity: its relationship to renal dysfunction. *Med Pediatr Oncol* **12**: 313–7.

249 Chang AY, Kuebler JP, Tormey DC, Anderson S, Pandya KJ, Borden EC, et al. (1986). Phase II evaluation of a combination of mitomycin C, vincristine, and cisplatin in advanced non-small cell lung cancer. *Cancer* **57**: 54–9.

250 Yoshida T, Ohsawa K, Goto T, Chiba S, Nakamura Y, Kondoh K, et al. (1990). [A case of hepatocellular carcinoma treated by intrahepatic arterial administration of anticancer agents: serial determination of the concentration of the chemotherapeutic agents in serum and dialysate during hemodialysis]. *Gan To Kagaku Ryoho* **17**: 2257–60.

251 Kamidono S, Fujii A, Hamami G, Nakano Y, Umezu K, Oda Y, et al. (1984). New preoperative chemotherapy for bladder cancer using combination hemodialysis and direct hemoperfusion: preliminary report. *J Urol* **131**: 36–40.

252 Rostaing L, Chatelut E, Payen JL, Izopet J, Thalamas C, Ton-That H, et al. (1998). Pharmacokinetics of alphaIFN–2b in chronic hepatitis C virus patients undergoing chronic hemodialysis or with normal renal function: clinical implications. *J Am Soc Nephrol* **9**: 2344–8.

253 Pol S, Zylberberg H, Fontaine H, Brechot C (1999). Treatment of chronic hepatitis C in special groups. *J Hepatol* **31**: 205–9.

254 Huraib S, Tanimu D, Romeh SA, Quadri K, Al Ghamdi G, Iqbal A, et al. (1999). Interferon-alpha in chronic hepatitis C infection in dialysis patients. *Am J Kidney Dis* **34**: 55–60.

255 Ellis ME, Alfurayh O, Halim MA, Sieck JO, Ali MA, Bernvil SS, et al. (1993). Chronic non-A, non-B hepatitis complicated by end-stage renal failure treated with recombinant interferon alpha. *J Hepatol* **18**: 210–6.

256 Ozyilkan E, Simsek H, Uzunalimoglu B, Telatar H (1995). Interferon treatment of chronic active hepatitis C in patients with end-stage chronic renal failure. *Nephron* **71**: 156–9.

257 Kamar N, Kany M, Bories P, Ribes D, Izopet J, Durand D, et al. (2001). Reversible posterior leukoencephalopathy syndrome in hepatitis C virus-positive long-term hemodialysis patients. *Am J Kidney Dis* **37**: E29.

258 Janssen HL, Berk L, Vermeulen M, Schalm SW (1990). Seizures associated with low-dose alpha-interferon. *Lancet* **336**: 1580.

259 Prestayko AW, Luft FC, Einhorn L, Crooke ST (1978). Cisplatin pharmacokinetics in a patient with renal dysfunction. *Med Pediatr Oncol* **5**: 183–8.

260 Rebibou JM, Chauffert B, Dumas M, Mousson C, Bone MC, Tanter Y, et al. (1996). Combined chemotherapy and radiotherapy for esophageal carcinoma in a hemodialyzed patient. Long-term survival. *Nephron* **74**: 611–2.

261 Fox JG, Kerr DJ, Soukop M, Farmer JG, Allison ME (1991). Successful use of cisplatin to treat metastatic seminoma during cisplatin-induced acute renal failure. *Cancer* **68**: 1720–3.

262 Gorodetsky R, Vexler A, Bar-Khaim Y, Biran H (1995). Plasma platinum elimination in a hemodialysis patient treated with cisplatin. *Ther Drug Monit* **17**: 203–6.

263 Ribrag V, Droz JP, Morizet J, Leclercq B, Gouyette A, Chabot GG (1993). Test dose-guided administration of cisplatin in an anephric patient: a case report. *Ann Oncol* **4**: 679–82.

264 Gouyette A, Lemoine R, Adhemar JP, Kleinknecht D, Man NK, Droz JP, et al. (1981). Kinetics of cisplatin in an anuric patient undergoing hemofiltration dialysis. *Cancer Treat Rep* **65**: 665–8.

265 Giudicelli CP, Ricordel I, Josipovici JJ, Falcot J, Renaudeau G, Bassoulet J, et al. (1981). [Kinetic study of cis-diamminedichloroplatinum in a case of serous cystadenocarcinoma of ovary with severe renal insufficiency (author's transl)]. *Therapie* **36**: 653–8.

266 Miyakawa M, Sugimoto K, Ohe Y, Masuoka H, Miyahara T (1987). [Pharmacokinetics of cis-dichlorodiammine platinum (II) in patients undergoing hemodialysis]. *Gan To Kagaku Ryoho* **14**: 2491–5.

267 Suwata J, Hiraga S, Hida M, Takamiya T, Iida T, Sato T (1988). [Study on changes in plasma platinum concentrations after administration of CDDP to maintenance hemodialysis patients]. *Gan To Kagaku Ryoho* **15**: 243–8.

268 Sturn W, Sanwald R, Ehninger G (1989). [Pharmacokinetics of cisplatin in long-term hemodialysis treatment]. *Dtsch Med Wochenschr* **114**: 337–9.

269 Ayabe H, Uchikawa T, Kimino K, Tagawa Y, Kawahara K, Tomita M (1989). [Pharmacokinetics of cisplatin and vindesine in a patient with chronic renal failure undergoing hemodialysis]. *Gan To Kagaku Ryoho* **16**: 3283–5.

270 Berland Y, Bues-Charbit M, Merzouk T, Boutin C, Cano JP, Olmer M (1990). Kinetics of cisplatin in a patient with lung carcinoma on continuous ambulatory peritoneal dialysis. *Nephron* **54**: 105–6.

271 Ono S, Miyazaki T, Nishikawa K, Watanabe K, Hisanaga S (1992). [Etoposide and cisplatin combination chemotherapy in a patient with small cell lung carcinoma under artificial hemodialysis]. *Gan To Kagaku Ryoho* **19**: 115–8.

272 Dahl O, Vagstad G, Iversen B (1996). Cisplatin-based chemotherapy in a renal transplant recipient with metastatic germ cell testicular cancer. *Acta Oncol* **35**: 759–61.

273 Viddeleer AC, Lycklama a Nijeholt GA, Beekhuis-Brussee JA (1992). A late manifestation of testicular seminoma in the bladder in a renal transplant recipient: a case report. *J Urol* **148**: 401–2.

274 Egorin MJ, Van Echo DA, Tipping SJ, Olman EA, Whitacre MY, Thompson BW, et al. (1984). Pharmacokinetics and dosage reduction of cis-diammine(1,1-cyclobutanedi-carboxylato)platinum in patients with impaired renal function. *Cancer Res* **44**: 5432–8.

275 Calvert AH, Newell DR, Gumbrell LA, O'Reilly S, Burnell M, Boxall FE, et al. (1989). Carboplatin dosage: prospective evaluation of a simple formula based on renal function. *J Clin Oncol* **7**: 1748–56.

276 Chatelut E, Rostaing L, Gualano V, Vissac T, De Forni M, Ton-That H, et al. (1994). Pharmacokinetics of carboplatin in a patient suffering from advanced ovarian carcinoma with hemodialysis-dependent renal insufficiency. *Nephron* **66**: 157–61.

277 Koren G, Weitzman S, Klein J, Moselhy G (1993). Comparison of carboplatin pharmacokinetics between an anephric child and two children with normal renal function. *Med Pediatr Oncol* **21**: 368–72.

278 Massari C, Brienza S, Rotarski M, Gastiaburu J, Misset JL, Cupissol D, et al. (2000). Pharmacokinetics of oxaliplatin in patients with normal versus impaired renal function. *Cancer Chemother Pharmacol* **45**: 157–64.

279 Levi F, Metzger G, Massari C, Milano G (2000). Oxaliplatin: pharmacokinetics and chronopharmacological aspects. *Clin Pharmacokinet* **38**: 1–21.

280 Takimoto CH, Remick SC, Sharma S, Mani S, Ramanathan RK, Doroshow J, et al. (2003). Dose-escalating and pharmacological study of oxaliplatin in adult cancer patients with impaired renal function: a National Cancer Institute Organ Dysfunction Working Group Study. *J Clin Oncol* **21**: 2664–72.

281 Ohnishi T, Kanoh T, Shiozaki K, Kimura Y, Iwazawa T, Tono T, et al. (2007). [FOLFOX 4 in a patient with metastatic colorectal cancer on hemodialysis due to chronic renal failure]. *Gan To Kagaku Ryoho* **34**: 1299–302.

282 Fujita M, Koide T, Katayama T, Matsuda H, Yamagishi Y, Okuda M, et al. (2009). [The pharmacokinetics and safety of oxaliplatin in a hemodialysis patient treated with mFOLFOX6 therapy]. *Gan To Kagaku Ryoho* **36**: 1379–82.

283 Matoba S, Sawada T, Toda Sea (2008). Modified FOLFOX 6 in a patient on hemodialysis with metastatic colorectal cancer. *Jpn J Cancer Chemother* **35**: 673–5.

284 Shitara K, Munakata M, Muto O, Okada R, Mitobe S, Mino M, et al. Hepatic arterial infusion of oxaliplatin for a patient with hepatic metastases from colon cancer undergoing hemodialysis. *Jpn J Clin Oncol* 2007 **37**: 540–3.

285 Garnier-Viougeat N, Rixe O, Paintaud G, Ternant D, Degenne D, Mouawad R, et al. (2007). Pharmacokinetics of bevacizumab in haemodialysis. *Nephrol Dial Transplant* **22**: 975.

286 Thariat J, Azzopardi N, Peyrade F, Launay-Vacher V, Santini J, Lecomte T, et al. (2008). Cetuximab pharmacokinetics in end-stage kidney disease under hemodialysis. *J Clin Oncol* **26**: 4223–5.

287 Lainakis G, Bamias A, Psimenou E, Fountzilas G, Dimopoulos MA (2009). Sunitinib treatment in patients with severe renal function impairment: a report of four cases by the Hellenic Cooperative Oncology Group. *Clin Nephrol* **72**: 73–8.

288 Izzedine H, Etienne-Grimaldi MC, Renee N, Vignot S, Milano G (2009). Pharmacokinetics of sunitinib in hemodialysis. *Ann Oncol* **20**: 190–2.

289 Reckova M, Kakalejcik M, Beniak J (2009). Treatment of hemodialyzed patient with sunitinib. *Ann Oncol* **20**: 392–3.

290 Zastrow S, Froehner M, Platzek I, Novotny V, Wirth MP (2009). Treatment of metastatic renal cell cancer with sunitinib during chronic hemodialysis. *Urology* **73**: 868–70.

291 Park CY (2009). Successful sunitinib treatment of metastatic renal cell carcinoma in a patient with end stage renal disease on hemodialysis. *Anticancer Drugs* **20**: 848–9.

292 Miller AA, Murry DJ, Owzar K, Hollis DR, Kennedy EB, Abou-Alfa G, et al. (2009). Phase I and pharmacokinetic study of sorafenib in patients with hepatic or renal dysfunction: CALGB 60301. *J Clin Oncol* **27**: 1800–5.

293 Rey PM, Villavicencio H (2008). Sorafenib: tolerance in patients on chronic hemodialysis: a single-center experience. *Oncology* **74**: 245–6.

294 Hilger RA, Richly H, Grubert M, Kredtke S, Thyssen D, Eberhardt W, et al. (2009). Pharmacokinetics of sorafenib in patients with renal impairment undergoing hemodialysis. *Int J Clin Pharmacol Ther* **47**: 61–4.

295 Gibbons J, Egorin MJ, Ramanathan RK, Fu P, Mulkerin DL, Shibata S, et al. (2008). Phase I and pharmacokinetic study of imatinib mesylate in patients with advanced malignancies and varying degrees of renal dysfunction: a study by the National Cancer Institute Organ Dysfunction Working Group. *J Clin Oncol* **26**: 570–6.

296 Ozdemir E, Koc Y, Kansu E (2006). Successful treatment of chronic myeloid leukemia with imatinib mesylate in a patient with chronic renal failure on hemodialysis. *Am J Hematol* **81**: 474.

297 Pappas P, Karavasilis V, Briasoulis E, Pavlidis N, Marselos M (2005). Pharmacokinetics of imatinib mesylate in end stage renal disease. A case study. *Cancer Chemother Pharmacol* **56**: 358–60.

298 Sonmez M, Cobanoglu U, Ovali E, Omay SB (2008). Use of dasatinib in the patient with Philadelphia chromosome-positive acute lymphoblastic leukaemia with resistance to imatinib and renal failure. *J Clin Pharm Ther* **33**: 329–30.

299 Miller AA, Murry DJ, Owzar K, Hollis DR, Lewis LD, Kindler HL, et al. (2007). Phase I and pharmacokinetic study of erlotinib for solid tumors in patients with hepatic or renal dysfunction: CALGB 60101. *J Clin Oncol* **25**: 3055–60.

300 Rossi A, Maione P, Del Gaizo F, Guerriero C, Castaldo V, Gridelli C (2005). Safety profile of gefitinib in advanced non-small cell lung cancer elderly patients with chronic renal failure: two clinical cases. *Lung Cancer* **47**: 421–3.

301 Breitkreutz I, Anderson KC (2008). Thalidomide in multiple myeloma—clinical trials and aspects of drug metabolism and toxicity. *Expert Opin Drug Metab Toxicol* **4**: 973–85.

302 Eriksson T, Hoglund P, Turesson I, Waage A, Don BR, Vu J, et al. (2003). Pharmacokinetics of thalidomide in patients with impaired renal function and while on and off dialysis. *J Pharm Pharmacol* **55**: 1701–6.

303 Arai A, Hirota A, Fukuda T, Tohda S, Mori Y, Terada Y, et al. (2009). [Analysis of plasma concentration of thalidomide in Japanese patients of multiple myeloma with renal dysfunction]. *Rinsho Ketsueki* **50**: 295–9.

304 Chen N, Lau H, Kong L, Kumar G, Zeldis JB, Knight R, et al. (2007). Pharmacokinetics of lenalidomide in subjects with various degrees of renal impairment and in subjects on hemodialysis. *J Clin Pharmacol* **47**: 1466–75.

305 Berenson JR, Rosen L, Vescio R, Lau HS, Woo M, Sioufi A, et al. (1997). Pharmacokinetics of pamidronate disodium in patients with cancer with normal or impaired renal function. *J Clin Pharmacol* **37**: 285–90.

306 Skerjanec A, Berenson J, Hsu C, Major P, Miller WH, Jr., Ravera C, et al. (2003). The pharmacokinetics and pharmacodynamics of zoledronic acid in cancer patients with varying degrees of renal function. *J Clin Pharmacol* **43**: 154–62.

307 Saha H, Castren-Kortekangas P, Ojanen S, Juhakoski A, Tuominen J, Tokola O, et al. (1994). Pharmacokinetics of clodronate in renal failure. *J Bone Miner Res* **9**: 1953–8.

308 Machado CE, Flombaum CD (1996). Safety of pamidronate in patients with renal failure and hypercalcemia. *Clin Nephrol* **45**: 175–9.

309 Ala-Houhala I, Saha H, Liukko-Sipi S, Ylitalo P, Pasternack A (1999). Pharmacokinetics of clodronate in haemodialysis patients. *Nephrol Dial Transplant* **14**: 699–705.

310 Mattioli F, Tognoni P, Manfredi V, Gosmar M, Corbu C, Garbero C, et al. (2006). Interindividual variability in the absorption of ciprofloxacin and hydrocortisone from continent ileal reservoir for urine. *Eur J Clin Pharmacol* **62**: 119–21.

311 Ekman I, Mansson W, Nyberg L (1989). Absorption of drugs from continent caecal reservoir for urine. *Br J Urol* **64**: 412–6.

312 Bowyer GW, Davies TW (1987). Methotrexate toxicity associated with an ileal conduit. *Br J Urol* **60**: 592.

313 Fossa SD, Heilo A, Bormer O (1990). Unexpectedly high serum methotrexate levels in cystectomized bladder cancer patients with an ileal conduit treated with intermediate doses of the drug. *J Urol* **143**: 498–501.

314 Broderick GA, Stone AR, deVere White R (1990). Neobladders: clinical management and considerations for patients receiving chemotherapy. *Semin Oncol* **17**: 598–605.

315 Srinivas S, Mahalati K, Freiha FS (1998). Methotrexate tolerance in patients with ileal conduits and continent diversions. *Cancer* **82**: 1134–6.

316 Miyasaka Y, Yoshimura M, Tabata S, Shozu A, Nishikawa M, Iwasaka T, et al. (1997). Successful treatment of a patient with Graves' disease on hemodialysis complicated by antithyroid drug-induced granulocytopenia and angina pectoris. *Thyroid* **7**: 621–4.

317 Howard N, Glasser M (1981). Iodine 131 ablation therapy for a patient on maintenance haemodialysis. *Br J Radiol* **54**: 259.

318 Daumerie C, Vynckier S, Caussin J, Jadoul M, Squifflet JP, de Patoul N, et al. (1996). Radioiodine treatment of thyroid carcinoma in patients on maintenance hemodialysis. *Thyroid* **6**: 301–4.

319 Morrish DW, Filipow LJ, McEwan AJ, Schmidt R, Murland KR, von Westarp C, et al. (1990). 131I treatment of thyroid papillary carcinoma in a patient with renal failure. *Cancer* **66**: 2509–13.

320 Culpepper RM, Hirsch JI, Fratkin MJ (1992). Clearance of 131I by hemodialysis. *Clin Nephrol* **38**: 110–4.

321 Mello AM, Isaacs R, Petersen J, Kronenberger S, McDougall IR (1994). Management of thyroid papillary carcinoma with radioiodine in a patient with end stage renal disease on hemodialysis. *Clin Nucl Med* **19**: 776–81.

322 Kaptein EM, Levenson H, Siegel ME, Gadallah M, Akmal M (2000). Radioiodine dosimetry in patients with end-stage renal disease receiving continuous ambulatory peritoneal dialysis therapy. *J Clin Endocrinol Metab* **85**: 3058–64.

Chapter 6

Biological cancer therapies and the kidney

Vincent Launay-Vacher

Case report

A 47-year-old woman was diagnosed with metastatic lung cancer. In June 2009, she was started on chemotherapy along with bevacizumab, an anti-angiogenic monoclonal antibody. Due to the potential renal and vascular effects of bevacizumab, the patient was closely monitored with periodic serum creatinine determination, calculation of her renal function with the aMDRD formula (abbreviated modification of diet in renal disease formula), urinary dipstick, and blood pressure testing, at each cycle of treatment.

In October 2009, renal deterioration occurred; her serum creatinine increased from 78 µmol/L to 105 µmol/L. Her corresponding aMDRD estimated glomerular filtration rate (GFR) had declined by one-third, from 73 to 52 mL/min/1.73m². There was no proteinuria, no sign of thrombotic microangiopathy (TMA), and no hypertension.

Further examinations confirmed normal blood pressure, the absence of proteinuria, and the absence of other signs of TMA (no anemia, and no thrombocytopenia). Renal imaging showed two kidneys of a normal shape and size. A careful medication and medical history revealed that she had started to take an over-the-counter non-steroidal anti-inflammatory drug (NSAID) for recurrent headaches. The NSAID was stopped, and renal function recovered.

This case emphasizes the monitoring of the renovascular tolerance of anti-angiogenic drugs but also illustrates that common medication toxicities may also occur. In this case, we could continue bevacizumab treatment.

Introduction

There are several kinds of biological therapies of cancer. The common characteristic of those drugs remains in their origin, which is biological rather than chemical. Among them can be found monoclonal antibodies and growth factors. Other drugs which share the same mechanisms of action are also commonly considered as biological therapies given that they share the same mechanism of action or have similar targets. This is the case for a number of tyrosine kinase inhibitors.

Monoclonal antibodies in the treatment of cancer include rituximab, which is directed towards the CD20 protein present at the surface of lymphocytes; bevacizumab, whose target is the vascular endothelial growth factor (VEGF); trastuzumab, which targets the human epidermal growth factor receptor 2 (HER–2); and cetuximab, which targets the epidermal growth factor receptor (eGFR). Several other monoclonal antibodies are currently under phase two or three studies such as panitumumab (EGFR), or pertuzumab (HER–2, with a different binding site on the receptor as compared to trastuzumab). In addition, erlotinib targets the eGFR and lapatinib the HER–2. Growth factors mainly include white blood cell growth factors such as filgrastim or red blood cell growth factors such as erythropoetins, alpha or beta. Numerous tyrosine kinase inhibitors (TKIs) have been or are currently developed in cancer. They act by inhibiting the intracellular tyrosine kinase of growth factor receptors. VEGF receptor TKIs include sunitinib, sorafenib, pazopanib, axitinib, mosetanib, and others that are under development.

This chapter focuses on the interactions of those biological therapies with the kidney. We focus on the effects of anti-VEGF drugs, both monoclonal antibodies and TKIs, since their mode of action on the VEGF pathway results in significant effects on blood vessels which may lead to renal and vascular side effects. Those side effects mainly manifest as arterial hypertension (HTN), proteinuria (Pu), and in some cases renal impairment (RI).

Anti-VEGF drugs

In recent years, the therapeutic armamentarium for the treatment of the most common cancers (cancer of the colon, breast, lung, liver, and kidney) has been extended by the addition of a new therapeutic class known as 'anti-angiogenics' or 'anti-VEGF'. This has come about as the result of improved understanding of tumoral growth, which requires the development of a network of neovessels. Tumoral angiogenesis is a complex process involving an imbalance between proangiogenic factors (chiefly vascular endothelial growth factor (VEGF) and basic fibroblast growth factor (bFGF)) and anti-angiogenic factors (angiostatin, endostatin, and thrombospondin) in favour of the former. (1). The growth factor VEGF and its receptors (VEGF receptor (VEGFR)-1, VEGFR-2 and VEGFR-3) are key factors for the survival of endothelial cells and are essential in the process of tumor angiogenesis (2).

Inhibition of the VEGF pathway is achieved either by direct binding of VEGF by a monoclonal antibody or by inhibition of the tyrosine kinase function of VEGF receptors by small molecule tyrosine kinase inhibitors (TKIs) (3). The monoclonal antibody bevacizumab is highly specific to an epitope present on the target and interacts solely with the extracellular circulating growth factor, while the small molecules interact with several intracellular targets in a less selective fashion.

Bevacizumab is a humanized immunoglobulin-G1 monoclonal antibody that binds selectively to human VEGF and thus neutralizes its biological activity (4). It has a strong affinity for an epitope that is present on all VEGF isoforms, and it partially straddles the VEGFR-1 and VEGFR-2 binding sites. As a result, the binding of VEGF to these endothelial cell receptors is inhibited (5). Bevacizumab therefore inhibits endothelial proliferation and consequently blocks the neo-vascularization necessary for tumoral growth and dissemination. Bevacizumab has an additive, even synergistic effect, with 'standard' cytotoxic drugs (6). Bevacizumab is approved in first- and second-line treatment of metastatic colorectal cancer, in first-line treatment of advanced pulmonary adenocarcinoma, in the treatment of advanced breast cancer, and in advanced clear cell renal cell carcinoma (CCRCC).

Sorafenib is a multitargeted TKI that targets VEGFR-2, VEGFR-3, platelet derived growth factor receptor-β (PDGFR-β), fms-related tyrosine kinase 3 (FLT3), the Ras/Raf/MEK (mitogen-activated protein kinase)/ERK (extracellular-signal-regulated kinase) pathway, and (stem-cell growth factor receptor) KIT (7) (see Fig. 6.1). It is indicated for the treatment of advanced cancers of the kidney and liver (8, 9). Sunitinib is also a multitargeted TKI. It targets colony-stimulating factor 1 receptor (CSF1R), and also all receptors targeted by sorafenib (3). It is indicated in the treatment of advanced CCRCC; in the first-line setting, and as second-line treatment of gastrointestinal stromal tumors.

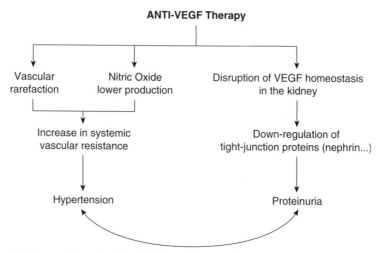

Fig. 6.1 Suggested mechanisms linking anti-VEGF therapy, proteinuria, and hypertension.

Anti-VEGF renovascular tolerance

Hypertension and proteinuria

Clinical experience shows a similar tolerance profile among anti-angiogenic drugs, consisting of vascular and renal toxicity. Hypertension and proteinuria have been well described with bevacizumab, the first-in-class drug of this class.

In the normal kidney, VEGF is produced by the podocytes and plays an essential autocrine role in the normal functioning of the fenestrated endothelium of the glomerular capillaries, via binding on endothelial cells. Podocytes normally express VEGF at high levels. Too little or too much VEGF expression may induce proteinuria. Eremina et al. (10) showed that podocyte-specific heterozygosity for VEGF resulted in renal disease by 2.5 weeks of age in mice. Renal disease was characterized by nephrotic-range proteinuria, endotheliosis, and hyaline deposits that resemble the pathological lesions seen in renal biopsy specimens from patients with preeclampsia (11), the development of which can be predicted by increased levels of soluble VEGFR-1 protein (soluble FLT1) and decreased levels of placenta growth factor (12).

A meta-analysis by Zhu et al. reported that the relative risk (RR) for proteinuria was 1.4 with bevacizumab at doses of 3, 5, or 7.5 mg/kg/dose and 2.2 at doses of 10 or 15 mg/kg/dose, as compared to patients not receiving bevacizumab (13). The RR for hypertension were 3.0 and 7.5, for the same ranges of doses. Low molecular weight (LMW) molecules that directly inhibit the tyrosine kinases on VEGF receptors (VEGFR) show similar tolerance profiles. Sunitinib was the first to be released. In clinical trials, as compared to placebo, it has been reported to induce hypertension in 30% vs. 4% of metastatic renal cell carcinoma patients, and in 15% vs. 11% of gastrointestinal stromal tumor patients (14). A recent publication reported seven cases of proteinuria and hypertension in patients who received either sunitinib alone (four patients) or sorafenib followed by sunitinib (two patients). One patient was treated with sorafenib alone and developed proteinuria but no hypertension (15). A potential class-effect has been suggested by those authors, and others (12, 16, 17). According to in vitro and in vivo animal studies, there is evidence that those side effects most probably result from the inhibition of the VEGF pathway. This is a mechanism which is similar to that proposed for preeclampsia (18). This disease is characterized by hypertension and proteinuria and renal thrombotic microangiopathy. It is also associated with high circulating levels of an endogenous inhibitor of VEGF signaling (sFlt1) (19). The toxicity profile of anti-angiogenic drugs is thus dependent on their pharmacological activity on the VEGF pathway, and is not related to their target (circulating VEGF or

VEGF receptor). Moreover, the nature of the molecule, either large or small, monoclonal antibody or TKI, has no influence on its toxicity, and clinical evidence for similar toxicities is emerging with all anti-angiogenic drugs: bevacizumab, sunitinib, sorafenib, axitinib, or the more recent aflibercept (VEGF-Trap) (13), a soluble recombinant decoy that binds to circulating VEGF (20) (Table 6.1).

Several hypertension-related clinical complications have been reported in patients receiving anti-angiogenic agents, including malignant hypertension, severe refractory hypertension, and reversible posterior leucoencephalopathy syndrome associated with severe hypertension (21). Iatrogenic hypertension can generally be effectively controlled by anti-hypertensive therapy and only in

Table 6.1 Renovascular side effects of antiangiogenic therapies

Drug	Renal side effect	Prevalence relative risk	References
Bevacizumab	Proteinuria	23–64% / 1.4–2.2	(13)
	Proteinuria > 3.5 g/day	6.5%	(32)
	Cryoglobulinemic glomerulonephritis or membranoproliferative glomerulonephritis (confirmed on renal biopsy)	2 cases	(33, 34)
	Hypertension	11 to 36% / 3.0–7.5	(13, 30, 35)
	Acute interstitial nephritis	1 case	(36)
	Thrombotic microangiopathy	2 cases	(30, 37)
	Thrombotic microangiopathy + IgA nephropathy	1 case	(38)
Sunitinib	Hypertension	18%	(39)
	Hypertension	15 cases	(40, 41)
	Thrombotic microangiopathy	4 cases	(21, 30, 42, 43)
	Proteinuria	7 cases	(15)
	Acute interstitial nephritis	1 case	(44)
	Acute nephritic syndrome	1 case	(45)
Sorafenib	Hypertension	43–75 %	(46, 25)
	Acute interstitial nephritis	1 case	(31)
	Proteinuria	1 case	
Axitinib	Hypertension	50–100 %	
	Proteinuria	23–70 %	

very rare cases necessitates discontinuation of the anti-angiogenic treatment. More rarely, short-term consequences have been observed. Long-term consequences of anti-angiogenic-induced hypertension have not been well studied yet but may become more important as survival times increase (22).

The pathophysiology of high blood pressure linked to anti-angiogenic therapy is linked to the neutralization of the major physiological effects of VEGF. Indeed, perfusion of exogenous VEGF is accompanied by hypotension caused by the activation of endothelial NO synthase and the production of NO (23). Thus, iatrogenic hypertension is thought to be due to inhibition of endothelial NO synthase with reduced release of NO by the endothelial cells in response to different stimuli, leading in turn to endothelium-dependent deterioration of endothelial vasodilation, sympathetic adrenergic activity, and even structural damage with arterial and capillary rarefaction (24, 25). Facemire et al. reported that the administration of a specific antibody against the major VEGF receptor, VEGFR-2, to normal mice caused hypertension (26). Compared with vehicle-treated controls, administration of the anti-VEGFR-2 antibody caused a rapid and sustained increase in blood pressure (BP) of 10 mm Hg. Treatment with the anti-VEGFR-2 antibody also caused a marked reduction in the expression of endothelial and neuronal NO synthases in the kidney. To examine the role of NO in the hypertension caused by blocking VEGFR-2, mice were treated with N(omega)-nitro-L-arginine methyl ester (L-NAME), an inhibitor of NO production. L-NAME administration abolished the difference in BP between the vehicle- and anti-VEGFR-2-treated groups. This suggests that VEGF and VEGFR-2 play a critical role in BP control by promoting NO synthase expression and NO activity. Interfering with this pathway is likely to be one mechanism underlying hypertension caused by anti-angiogenic agents targeting VEGF (23).

Proteinuria also occurs in patients receiving an anti-angiogenic agent. Proteinuria may develop at any time point after the beginning of anti-angiogenic treatment. It is frequently associated with hypertension. Like hypertension, iatrogenic proteinuria is also usually reversible on discontinuation of anti-angiogenic treatment. However, iatrogenic proteinuria is not usually a cause for discontinuation of anti-angiogenic treatment and does not indicate any clinically significant adverse effects on renal function.

An apparent association between hypertension and proteinuria was noted in the bevacizumab arm of the study of Miller et al. (27): patients who developed proteinuria were more likely to become hypertensive (47.1% versus 16.9%; P <0.001) than patients who did not develop proteinuria. A recent publication of a phase II study of cediranib also showed that development of hypertension and proteinuria may occur early during the course of the treatment with anti-angiogenics (28). A simplified Figure for potential mechanisms by which anti-VEGF therapies can induce hypertension and proteinuria has been suggested by Izzedine et al. and synthesized in Fig. 6.1 (29).

Glomerular lesions in thrombotic microangiopathy (TMA) after high-dose treatment with an anti-angiogenic agent are easily distinguishable from other glomerular lesions. There is endotheliosis with turgid endothelial cells swelling into the capillary lumen, and mesangiolysis occurs, with swollen endothelial cells and an extracellular matrix which is edematous, fibrillary and accompanied by the loss of mesangial nuclei. Capillary walls show 'double contours' with a clear space and the lumens are reduced. Moreover, the capillary lumens are congested with red blood cells and platelet thrombi obstruct the capillary lumens or the preglomerular arterioles. Immunofluorescence shows few or no fibrin and C3 deposits in the glomerular or arteriolar thromboses.

Table 6.1 summarizes the renal adverse events in patients receiving anti-angiogenic treatment (30, 31).

Hypertension could be a biomarker of anti-angiogenic activity/efficacy. It was first suggested for Sunitinib (48). In this study of 40 patients treated for a metastatic renal cell carcinoma, the authors retrospectively analyzed the incidence of hypertension in relation to the response to the treatment including sunitinib. Among the 14 patients who were considered as responding to the treatment according to RECIST criteria, 43% had grade 3 hypertension and the remaining 57% had less than grade 3 hypertension (no data shown on Grade 2, 1, and no hypertension in the article). Among the non-responders, 12% had grade 3 and 88% had less than grade 3 hypertension. The authors reported that multivariate analysis showed that worsening or appearing grade 2 or more hypertension was the only single independent predictor of clinical response. However, the data presented in this article do not support this assumption. Another retrospective study performed in patients treated with bevacizumab for metastatic colorectal cancer suggested that patients who developed hypertension under anti-angiogenic therapy had more often reached remission than patients who did not develop grade 2 or 3 hypertension (49). However, no data are available on whether patients had hypertension at baseline and what anti-hypertensive drugs they were eventually treated with.

Azizi M et al. (40) provide some evidence for hypertension as a biomarker for anti-angiogenic drugs activity. In their study, the authors demonstrated that all patients receiving sunitinib for metastatic renal cell carcinoma experienced an elevation in their blood pressure (home-monitored), both patients with pre-existing hypertension and patients with normal blood pressure at baseline. The elevation in blood pressure can thus be considered as a marker of the anti-angiogenic activity on the VEGF pathway. However, there is a lack of evidence on whether this biomarker could predict the clinical response to treatment, and further studies are mandatory, based on clear and well-designed studies (50).

Renal impairment

Most oncologists consider their cancer patients as having a 'normal' renal function. As a result, the renal tolerance of anti-angiogenics is given less importance than it may deserve since those drugs do not induce acute renal failure, but most often a subtle decline in renal function. However, most cancer patients with solid tumor often present with abnormal renal function. The first IRMA (*Insuffisance Rénale et Médicaments Anticancéreux*) study (51) reported a high prevalence of abnormal renal function in a cohort of 4684 patients with solid tumors. In this cohort, the estimated glomerular filtration rate (eGFR) was calculated with the abbreviated MDRD formula (52) and the international definition was used to define renal insufficiency, as per K/DOQI (53) and KDIGO (54). In IRMA-1, the prevalence of an eGFR below 90 mL/min/1.73m^2 was high, occurring in 53% of the patients, and that of an eGFR lower than 60 mL/min/1.73m^2 was 12%. This high prevalence was confirmed on another cohort of 4945 solid tumor patients in the IRMA-2 study, where 50% of the patients had an eGFR lower than 90 mL/min/1.73m^2, and 12% an eGFR lower than 60 mL/min/1.73m^2 (55).

In those two cohorts, none of them was receiving any anti-angiogenic since those drugs were not available at the time the study was performed. In the IRMA-2 study, patients with an eGFR lower than 60 mL/min/1.73m^2 at time of inclusion had a reduced survival as compared to patients with an eGFR greater than 60 mL/min/1.73m^2 with a median survival of 16 vs. 25 months (p <0.0001) and a hazard ratio in a Cox-model analysis adjusted for sex and age of 1.27 (1.12–1.44) (p = 0.0002) (56). This observation was observed on the whole cohort of IRMA-2 patients, whatever the type of solid tumor, but also within specific tumors, such as for breast cancer patients (57). These findings suggest that cancer patients with a reduced GFR have more toxicity of medications or do not get the medications that they need. Either way, it is a strong effect of decreased GFR. It is worth stating as such, independently of anti-angiogenics. Perhaps if biologics give us less toxic drugs, we can use them in subjects with kidney disease, and achieve better remission rates. The findings also warn us that even before anti-angiogenics, cancer patients may have reduced GFR. They are thus at risk.

Due to the renal effects of anti-angiogenic drugs, the question of their long-term impact on GFR was raised. We reported on the evolution of renal function in patients treated with anti-angiogenic drugs (sunitinib and sorafenib) for renal cell carcinoma (58) (see Chapter 12). The median age was 59 years.

Fifty-two patients were treated with sunitinib and 15 with sorafenib. The mean baseline GFR before initiation of anti-angiogenic therapy was 63 mL/min/1.73m^2. Thirty-eight patients (52%) had a baseline aMDRD GFR ranging from 60 to 90 mL/min/1.73m^2, and 29 (40%) had a aMDRD GFR<60 mL/min/1.73m^2. Eighteen patients had pre-existing hypertension (HTN). GFR in the whole population of patients decreased under anti-angiogenic therapy with a yearly loss of 1.2 to 2.5 mL/min/1.73m^2/year, depending on the method used, either using the slope of the linear regression over the whole follow-up or by calculating the absolute difference in GFR at the end of follow-up minus that at the beginning. Considering the age of the patients, such a decline is faster than the physiological reduction in renal function according to Hemmelgarn et al. who reported a mean decline in aMDRD eGFR of 0.8 and 1.4 mL/min/1.73m^2/year in women and men without diabetes mellitus, respectively (59). The decline in GFR was similar whatever the anti-angiogenic therapy used. Indeed, it was 1.0 to 2.1 mL/min/1.73m^2/year in the 52 patients who were treated with sunitinib and 0.7 to 3.4 mL/min/1.73m^2/year in those treated with sorafenib (15 patients). However, when analyzing the subgroup of patients who presented with HTN at baseline (18 patients), ie. before the anti-angiogenic therapy was started, a dramatically higher decrease in renal function was observed: −13.3 and −12.1 mL/min/1.73m^2/year, depending on the method used to evaluate the evolution of renal function. This was even more marked for patients with baseline HTN and receiving sunitinib (ten patients, mean baseline GFR 58 mL/min/1.73m^2) with a decrease in GFR of −26.2 and −30.3 mL/min/1.73m^2/year. Meanwhile, patients with no HTN at baseline (55 patients) had a stable, even increasing, renal function with an evolution of +2.7 to +0.6 mL/min/1.73m^2/year, whatever the anti-angiogenic drug used.

Those results demonstrated that anti-angiogenic therapy in patients with cancer and pre-existing hypertension may result in dramatic decreases in renal function, leading to renal insufficiency which may be severe.

Other biological therapies

Epidermal growth factor/epidermal growth factor receptor (EGF/EGFR) inhibitors

Cetuximab and erlotinib

Cetuximab was well tolerated in clinical development studies. The most frequently occurring adverse events did not include hypertension or proteinuria. However in one study, it is reported that 13 of 633 patients (2%) developed kidney failure (60). Another concern regarding the renal tolerance of cetuximab is hypomagnesemia, which can be problematic in patients with or without kidney disease (see Chapter 5). In two studies, the authors showed that both from a pharmacokinetic point of view and a biological tolerance point of view, the use of cetuximab appeared to be safe, even in patients with end-stage renal disease undergoing hemodialysis (61, 62). There are no data in the literature reporting any renal side effect related to erlotinib. In one study, there was no impact of renal dysfunction on the pharmacokinetics of erlotinib, while hepatic dysfunction was suggested to require dose reduction of that drug (63).

Drugs targeting the HER-2 receptor: trastuzumab and lapatinib

Trastuzumab, a recombinant humanized monoclonal antibody directed against the extracellular domain of the HER–2 (human epidermal growth factor receptor 2) has not been reported to induce hypertension or proteinuria. However, cardiorenal syndrome can occur with the use of this agent in combination with anthracyclines (64), although recent data suggest that the cardiac tolerance of trastuzumab in combination with epirubicine could be of an acceptable range (65). The same pattern of renal tolerance is expected for lapatinib, although clinical experience is reduced as compared to trastuzumab. The cardiac tolerance of lapatinib in combination with anthracyclines or other chemotherapy still has to be properly investigated.

Conclusion

Anti-angiogenic agents have a broadly favorable risk/benefit ratio in patients with advanced cancer. These encouraging results have prompted evaluation of anti-angiogenic drugs earlier in the disease course, at the adjuvant stage. The management of adverse effects appears to be critical at this stage. Long-term toxicity from treatment with anti-angiogenic agents may become apparent only after several years or decades, making long-term effects of significant concern in patients who have received these agents earlier in their disease course. Maintenance treatment following a treatment response or, better still, disease remission could avoid or slow down further tumoral growth. These indications are currently being studied. However, in the absence of structured and appropriate patient care, the risk/benefit ratio of anti-angiogenic treatment could invert because of the risk of iatrogenic cardiovascular and iatrogenic renal complications. The early appearance of hypertension and proteinuria may be easy-to-use predictors of anti-tumoral activity by the anti-angiogenics, but still require further validation to be recommended as routine indicators for efficacy.

Many pathways for intracellular and extracellular signaling have been identified to date and include potential targets for new targeted therapies aiming at receptors or mediators (see Fig. 6.2). It is now thought that acting on one pathway may not be enough and that several targeted therapies, with different

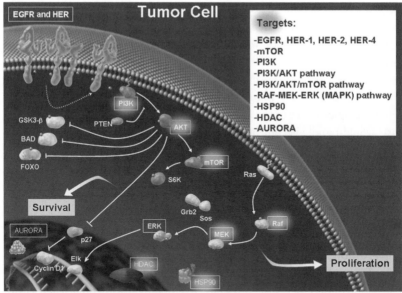

(a)

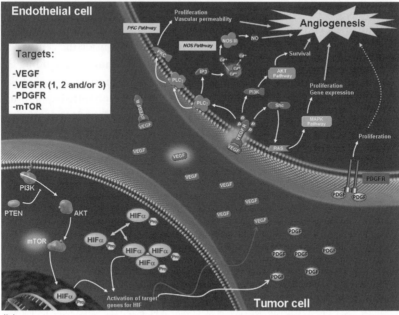

(b)

Fig. 6.2 Signaling pathways involved in tumor development, growth, and dissemination.

With permission from Vincent Launay-Vacher and Jean-Baptiste Rey, ASCOPharma®
2009, available online at www.efp-online.org, European Fellowship for Pharmacists,
Paris, 2009.

targets, should or could be associated. Anti-angiogenics for instance, should be used in association with chemotherapy, but they have also shown some interesting results in association with other targeted therapies such as trastuzumab in HER-2 breast cancer. One could suggest that when a tumor cell proliferation is blocked through one pathway, the tumor uses other pathways to bypass this blockade and grow and/or disseminate. While we may have several targeted therapies to act on several pathways in the near future, the treatment costs would rapidly become a concern and associating several targeted therapies may not be feasible in every country (66). Another way of seeing the future would be to apply the knowledge developed with research on targeted therapies to improve the tolerance, and potentially the efficacy, of cytotoxic agents. Two recent drugs may illustrate this. The first one is nab-paclitaxel which consists of albumin-bound paclitaxel nanoparticules. This drug is not a targeted therapy as such, but binding paclitaxel to nanoparticules of albumin makes its delivery more specific to tumor cells and may improve the benefit/risk balance. The second drug is trastuzumab-DM1 (T-DM1) which consists of an association of the efficacy of both a targeted therapy (trastuzumab) and a cytotoxic (DM1) which is grafted on the antibody. T-DM1 binds to the HER-2 receptor at the surface of cancer cells, and acts as trastuzumab does. When the receptor-drug complex is internalized by the cell, DM1 is released from the antibody inside the cell and acts as a cytotoxic, directly inside the cancer cell. Nab-paclitaxel has already been approved in several countries, including the USA and Europe. T-DM1 has demonstrated promising results at the last San Antonio Breast Cancer Symposium (67), and should be submitted for approval in the USA and in Europe very soon. The question of the tolerance of those drugs however remains, with limited clinical experience.

References

1 Risau W (1997). Mechanisms of angiogenesis. *Nature* **386**: 671–4.

2 Ferrara N (2004). Vascular endothelial growth factor: basic science and clinical progress. *Endocrine Reviews* **4**: 581–611.

3 Rini BI, Rathmell WK (2007). Biological aspects and binding strategies of vascular endothelial growth factor in renal cell carcinoma. *Clin Cancer Res* **13**: 741s–6s.

4 Presta LG, Chen H, O'Connor SJ, et al. (1997). Humanization of an antivascular endothelial growth factor monoclonal antibody for the therapy of solid tumors and other disorders. *Cancer Res* **57**: 4593–9.

5 Muller YA, Chen Y, Christinger HW, et al. (1998). VEGF and the Fab fragment of a humanized neutralizing antibody: crystal structure of the complex at 2.4 A resolution and mutational analysis of the interface. *Structure* **6**: 1153–67.

6 Gerber HP, Ferrara N (2005). Pharmacology and pharmacodynamics of bevacizumab as monotherapy or in combination with cytotoxic therapy in preclinical studies. *Cancer Res* **65**: 671–80.

7 Le Tourneau C, Faivre S, Raymond E (2008). New developments in multitargeted therapy for patients with solid tumours. *Cancer Treat Rev* **34**: 37–48.

8 Escudier B, Eisen T, Stadler WM, et al. (2007) Sorafenib in Advanced Clear-Cell Renal-Cell Carcinoma. *N Engl J Med 2007*, **356**, 125–34.

9 Llovet JM, Ricci S, Mazzaferro V, et al. (2007). Sorafenib improves survival in advanced hepatocellular carcinoma: Results of a Phase III randomized placebo-controlled trial (SHARP study). *J Clin Oncol* **25**: LBA1.

10 Eremina V, Jefferson JA, Kowalewska J, et al. (2008). VEGF inhibition and renal thrombotic microangiopathy. *N Engl J Med* **358**: 1129–36.

11 Kincaid-Smith P (1991). The renal lesion of preeclampsia revisited. *Am J Kidney Dis* **17**: 144–8.

12 Levine RJ, Maynard SE, Qian C, et al. (2004). Circulating angiogenic factors and the risk of preeclampsia. *N Engl J Med* **350**: 672–83.

13 Zhu X, Wu S, Dahut WL, Parikh CR (2007). Risks of proteinuria and hypertension with bevacizumab, an antibody against vascular endothelial growth factor: systematic review and meta-analysis. *Am J Kidney Dis* **49**: 186–93.

14 SUTENT(R), sunitinib malate oral capsules. Full Prescribing Information, Pfizer, Inc, New York, NY, 2007, http://www.fda.gov/cder/foi/label/2007/021968s005lbl.pdf, accessed 03/18/2008.

15 Patel TV, Morgan JA, Demetri GD, et al. (2008). A preeclampsia-like syndrome characterized by reversible hypertension and proteinuria induced by the multitargeted kinase inhibitors sunitinib and sorafenib. *J Natl Cancer Inst* **100**: 282–4.

16 Riely GJ, Miller VA (2007). Vascular endothelial growth factor trap in non small cell lung cancer. *Clin Cancer Res* **13**: s4623–4627.

17 Launay-Vacher V, Deray G (2009). Hypertension and proteinuria: a class-effect of antiangiogenic therapies. *Anticancer Drugs* **20**: 81–2.

18 Patel TV, Morgan JA, Demetri GD, et al. (2008). A preeclampsia-like syndrome characterized by reversible hypertension and proteinuria induced by the multitargeted kinase inhibitors sunitinib and sorafenib. *J Natl Cancer Inst* **100**: 282–4.

19 Maynard SE, Min JY, Merchan J, et al. (2003). Excess placental soluble fms-like tyrosine kinase 1 (sFlt1) may contribute to endothelial dysfunction, Hypertension and proteinuria in preeclampsia. *J Clin Invest* **111**: 649–58.

20 Rudge JS, Thurston G, Davis S, et al. (2005). VEGF trap as a novel antiangiogenic treatment currently in clinical trials for cancer and eye diseases, and VelociGene-based discovery of the next generation of angiogenesis targets. *Cold Spring Harb Symp Quant Biol* **70**: 411–18.

21 Kapiteijn E, Brand A, Kroep J, Gelderblom H (2007). Sunitinib induced Hypertension thrombotic microangiopathy and reversible posterior leukencephalopathy syndrome. *Ann Oncol* **18**: 1745–7.

22 Glusker P, Larry Recht L, Lane L (2006). Reversible posterior leukoencephalopathy syndrome and bevacizumab. *N Engl J Med* **354**: 980–1.

23 Henry TD, Annex BH, McKendall GR, et al. (2003). The VIVA trial: vascular endothelial growth factor in Ischemia for Vascular Angiogenesis. *Circulation* **107**: 1359–65.

24 Mourad JJ, des Guetz G, Debbabi H, Levy BI (2008). Blood pressure rise following angiogenesis inhibition by bevacizumab. A crucial role for microcirculation. *Ann Oncol* **19**: 927–34.

25 Veronese ML, Mosenkis A, Flaherty KT, et al. (2006). Mechanisms of hypertension associated with BAY 43–9006. *J Clin Oncol* **24**: 1363–9.

26 Facemire CS, Nixon AB, Griffiths R, Hurwitz H, Coffman TM (2009). Vascular endothelial growth factor receptor 2 controls blood pressure by regulating nitric oxide synthase expression. *Hypertension* **54**: 652–8.

27 Miller KD, Chap LI, Holmes FA (2005). Randomized phase III trial of capecitabine compared with bevacizumab plus capecitabine in patients with previously treated metastatic breast cancer. *J Clin Oncol* **23**: 792–9.

28 Robinson ES, Matulonis UA, Ivy P, et al. (2010). Rapid development of hypertension and proteinuria with cediranib, an oral vascular endothelial growth factor receptor inhibitor. *Clin J Am Soc Nephrol* **5**: 477–83.

29 Izzedine H, Rixe O, Billemont B, Baumelou A, Deray G (2007). Angiogenesis inhibitor therapies: focus on kidney toxicity and hypertension. *Am J Kidney Dis* **50**: 203–18.

30 Frangié C, Lefaucheur C, Medioni J, Jacquot C, Hill GS, Nochy D (2007). Renal thrombotic microangiopathy caused by anti-VEGF-antibody treatment for metastatic renal-cell carcinoma. *Lancet Oncol* **8**: 177–8.

31 Izzedine H, Brocheriou I, Rixe O, Deray G (2007). Interstitial nephritis in a patient taking sorafenib. *Nephrol Dial Transplant* **22**: 2411.

32 Yang JC, Haworth L, Sherry RM, et al. (2003). A randomized trial of bevacizumab, an anti-vascular endothelial growth factor antibody, for metastatic renal cancer. *N Engl J Med* **349**: 427–34.

33 Johnson DH, Fehrenbacher L, Novotny WF, et al. (2004). Randomized phase II trial comparing bevacizumab plus carboplatin and paclitaxel with carboplatin and paclitaxel alone in previously untreated locally advanced or metastatic non-small-cell lung cancer. *J Clin Oncol* **22**: 2184–91.

34 George BA, Zhou XJ, Toto R (2007). Nephrotic syndrome after bevacizumab: case report and literature review. *Am J Kidney Dis* **49**: e23–e29.

35 Dincer M, Altundag K (2006). Angiotensin-converting enzyme inhibitors for bevacizumab-induced hypertension. *Ann Pharmacother* **40**: 2278–9.

36 Barakat RK, Singh N, Lal R, Verani RR, Finkel KW, Foringer JR (2007). Interstitial nephritis secondary to bevacizumab treatment in metastatic leiomyosarcoma. *Ann Pharmacother* **41**: 707–10.

37 Uy AL, Simper NB, Champeaux AL, Perkins RM (2009). Progressive bevacizumab-associated renal thrombotic microangiopathy. *NDT Plus* **2**: 36–9.

38 Roncone D, Satoskar A, Nadasdy T, Monk JP, Rovin BH (2007). Proteinuria in a patient receiving anti-VEGF therapy for metastatic renal cell carcinoma. *Nat Clin Pract Nephrol* **3**: 287–93.

39 Faivre S, Delbaldo C, Vera K, et al. (2006). Safety, pharmacokinetic, and antitumor activity of SU11248, a novel oral multitarget tyrosine kinase inhibitor, in patients with cancer. *J Clin Oncol* **24**: 25–35.

40 Azizi M, Chedid A, Oudard S (2008). Home blood-pressure monitoring in patients receiving sunitinib. *N Engl J Med* **358**: 95–7.

41 Obhrai JS, Patel TV, Humphreys BD (2008). The case/progressive hypertension and proteinuria on anti-angiogenic therapy. *Kidney Int* **74**: 685–6.

42 Bollée G, Patey N, Cazajous G, et al. (2009). Thrombotic microangiopathy secondary to VEGF pathway inhibition by sunitinib. *Nephrol Dial Transplant* **24**: 682–5.

43 Levey SA, Bajwa RS, Picken MM, Clark JI, Barton K, Leehey DJ (2008). Thrombotic microangiopathy associated with sunitinib, a VEGF inhibitor, in a patient with factor V Leiden mutation. *NDT Plus* **3**: 154–6.

44 Winn SK, Ellis S, Savage P, Sampson S, Marsh JE (2009). Biopsy-proven acute interstitial nephritis associated with the tyrosine kinase inhibitor sunitinib: a class effect? *Nephrol Dial Transplant* **24**: 673–5.

45 Rolleman EJ, Weening J, Betjes MG (2009). Acute nephritic syndrome after anti-VEGF therapy for renal cell carcinoma. *Nephrol Dial Transplant* **24**: 2002–3.

46 Ratain MJ, Eisen T, Stadler WM, et al. (2006). Phase II placebo-controlled randomized discontinuation trial of sorafenib in patients with metastatic renal cell carcinoma. *J Clin Oncol* **24**: 2505–12.

47 Rugo HS, Herbst RS, Liu G, et al. (2005). Phase I trial of the oral antiangiogenesis agent AG–013736 in patients with advanced solid tumors: pharmacokinetic and clinical results. *J Clin Oncol* **23**: 5474–83.

48 Rixe O, Billemont B, Izzedine H (2007). Hypertension as a predictive factor of Sunitinib activity. *Ann Oncol* **18**: 1117.

49 Scartozzi M, Galizia E, Chiorrini S, et al. (2009). Arterial hypertension correlates with clinical outcome in colorectal cancer patients treated with first-line bevacizumab. *Ann Oncol* **20**: 227–30.

50 Humphreys BD, Atkins MB (2009). Rapid development of hypertension by sorafenib: toxicity or target? *Clin Cancer Res* **15**: 5947–9.

51 Launay-Vacher V, Oudard S, Janus N, et al. (2007). Prevalence of Renal Insufficiency in cancer patients and implications for anticancer drug management: the renal insufficiency and anticancer medications (IRMA) study. *Cancer* **110**: 1376–84.

52 Levey AS, Bosch JP, Lewis JB, Greene T, Rogers N, Roth D (1999). A more accurate method to estimate glomerular filtration rate from serum creatinine: a new prediction equation. Modification of Diet in Renal Disease Study Group. *Ann Intern Med* **130**: 461–70.

53 National Kidney Foundation (2002). K/DOQI clinical practice guidelines for chronic kidney disease: evaluation, classification, and stratification. *Am J Kidney Dis* **39**: S1–S266.

54 Levey AS, Eckardt KU, Tsukamoto Y, et al. (2005). Definition and classification of chronic kidney disease: a position statement from Kidney Disease: Improving Global Outcomes (KDIGO). *Kidney Int* **67**: 2089–100.

55 Janus N, Oudard S, Beuzeboc P, et al. (2009). Prevalence of renal insufficiency in cancer patients: Data from the IRMA-2 study. *J Clin Oncol* **27**: 15s (suppl; abstr 9559).

56 Launay-Vacher V, Janus N, Spano J, et al. (2009) Impact of renal insufficiency on cancer survival: Results of the IRMA-2 study. *J Clin Oncol* **27**: 15s (suppl; abstr 9585).

57 Launay-Vacher V, Janus N, Gligorov J, et al. (2009). Renal Insufficiency in Breast Cancer Patients: High Prevalence and Reduced Survival. *Cancer Res* (suppl.: 609S–610S; abstr. 2054).

58 Launay-Vacher V, Ayllon J, Janus N, et al. (2009). Evolution of renal function in patients treated with antiangiogenics after nephrectomy for renal cell carcinoma. *Urol Oncol* (Epub ahead of print).

59 Hemmelgarn BR, Zhang J, Manns BJ, et al. (2006). Progression of kidney dysfunction in the community-dwelling elderly. *Kidney Int* **69**: 2155–61.

60 Harari PM (2004). Epidermal growth factor receptor inhibition strategies in oncology. *Endocr Relat Cancer* **11**: 689–708.

61 Thariat J, Launay-Vacher V, Italiano A, Santini J, Peyrade F (2008). Impact of cetuximab conventional dosing on cetuximab-induced magnesium concentration under haemodialysis in head and neck cancer. *NDT Plus* **3**: 196–7.

62 Thariat J, Azzopardi N, Peyrade F, et al. (2008) Cetuximab pharmacokinetics in end-stage kidney disease under hemodialysis. *J Clin Oncol* **26**: 4223–5.

63 Miller AA, Murry DJ, Owzar K, et al. (2007). Phase I and pharmacokinetic study of erlotinib for solid tumors in patients with hepatic or renal dysfunction: CALGB 60101. *J Clin Oncol* **25**: 3055–60.

64 Jensen BV (2006). Cardiotoxic consequences of anthracycline-containing therapy in patients with breast cancer. *Semin Oncol* **33**: S15–S21.

65 Untch M, Muscholl M, Tjulandin S, et al. (2010). First-line trastuzumab plus epirubicin and cyclophosphamide therapy in patients with human epidermal growth factor receptor 2-positive metastatic breast cancer: cardiac safety and efficacy data from the herceptin, cyclophosphamide, and epirubicin (HERCULES) trial. *J Clin Oncol* **28**: 1473–80.

66 Cressey D (2009). Health economics: Life in the balance. *Nature* **461**: 336–9.

67 Krop I, LoRusso P, Miller KD, et al. (2009). A Phase II study of trastuzumab-DM1 (T-DM1), a novel HER2 antibody-drug conjugate, in patients previously treated with lapatinib, trastuzumab, and chemotherapy. *San Antonio Breast Cancer Symposium 2009*, abstract 5090.

Chapter 7

Radiation nephropathy

Eric P. Cohen and John E. Moulder

Case report

A 32-year-old man underwent an allogeneic bone marrow transplantation (BMT) for refractory Hodgkin's disease in November 1987. The BMT was preceded by a chemo-irradiation 'conditioning' regimen that included cytarabine, cyclophosphamide, and 1400 cGy fractionated total body irradiation. At discharge, the serum creatinine level was 114 µmol/L. By September 1989, it had reached 290 µmol/L and there were 560 mg protein in a 24-hour urine collection. A kidney biopsy was done, which showed capillary dilatation, extreme subendothelial space widening, hyalinization of afferent arterioles, and tubular atrophy with interstitial fibrosis. Antihypertensive treatment was started, including minoxidil and the angiotensin-converting-enzyme inhibitor lisinopril. Hyperkalemia occurred in 1992 and lisinopril was stopped. Sodium polystyrene sulfonate was started. Anemia was observed and erythropoietin was started. Hypothyroidism occurred in 1994 and levothyroxine was started. Metabolic acidosis was treated with sodium bicarbonate supplements. By 2001, the parathyroid hormone (PTH) level rose to 436 pg/mL (normal 10–65) and there was osteopenia with foot pain. Oral calcitriol was initiated. Since the uric acid level was 468 µmol/L, allopurinol was started. As of March 2002, even though the foot pain persisted, the patient could still walk and drive. His medication included levothyroxine, calcitriol, minoxidil, sodium bicarbonate, erythropoietin, allopurinol, and sodium polystyrene sulfonate. The urea level was 18 µmol/L. The serum creatinine was 317 µmol/L. The hematocrit was 32%, the serum calcium was 2.3 mmol/L, and the PTH level, 185 pg/mL. The evolution of his kidney function portrayed as 100/serum creatinine is shown in Fig. 7.1. He has since undergone successful kidney transplantation, from his marrow donor.

Definition

Radiation nephropathy is renal injury and loss of function caused by ionizing radiation.

Occurrence

Kidney damage from ionizing radiation was recognized a decade after the discovery of X-ray (1). By the early 1950s, the dose tolerance of kidneys to

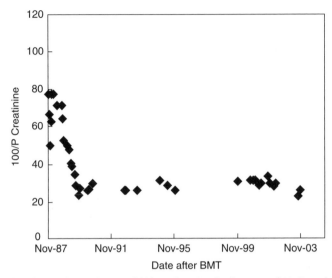

Fig. 7.1 This shows the evolution of kidney function in the case of BMT nephropathy presented for this chapter. Despite an initial and substantial loss of kidney function, there was long-term stabilization of the kidney function, shown here as the 100/plasma creatinine quotient.

irradiation had been worked out, based on clinical experience (2). Subsequently, clinical radiation nephropathy has become less common. This was not only because the kidneys were shielded during therapeutic irradiation, but also because of the development of more effective chemotherapy, which displaced radiation therapy in the care of many cancer patients (3).

In the past 25 years, however, radiation nephropathy has resurfaced as a clinical problem. This is because, first, chronic renal failure occurs as a delayed complication of an allogeneic bone marrow transplantation, so-called bone marrow transplant nephropathy (4, 5). Second, it occurs as a syndrome of chronic renal failure in patients treated with parenteral isotope radiotherapy (6, 7).

Pathogenesis

The studies of Luxton and colleagues established the dose threshold beyond which therapeutic irradiation was likely to cause radiation nephropathy. This was 2300 cGy or more, given in multiple fractions over five weeks. Experience of the BMT patients showed that a lesser dose of ionizing radiation, 1000 cGy, as a single fraction, was sufficient to cause radiation nephropathy (8, 9). At our center, the total body irradiation (TBI) regimen that precedes most allogeneic

BMTs was given at a total dose of 14 Gy, in three fractions per day, over three days. This regimen was associated with a 20% actuarial incidence of chronic renal failure (10), which has led to the use of partial kidney shielding during the TBI. As a result, the total kidney dose that our BMT patients now receive is 9.8 Gy and there was a significant reduction in the occurrence of BMT nephropathy at our center with this TBI dose reduction (11) (Fig. 7.2). A similar dose-response relationship was described by Miralbell and colleagues (12).

That radiation injury in BMT occurs at doses of irradiation less than half of the 'classical' limit of 23 Gy is related to dose per fraction, dose rate, fractionation interval, and use of chemotherapy. Thus, a 14 Gy total dose in nine fractions over three days could pose a similar risk of renal radiation injury to that of a 23 Gy total dose in 20 fractions over four weeks. In addition, the use of cytotoxic chemotherapy, both previous to the BMT and concurrently with the TBI just before the BMT, could potentiate the radiation injury (13).

In the case of nephrotoxicity caused by parenteral radioisotopes, the exact radiation dose delivered to the kidneys is not well-known, or is difficult to measure (14). But, it is known that for yttrium 90, conjugated to the somatostatin analogue dota-D-phe-tyr-octreotide (DOTATOC), there is filtration at the glomeruli and reabsorption of the isotope conjugate by the proximal tubules. The amount of isotope given was 200 millicuries per meter squared of the body surface area or higher in the cases reported by Moll et al. (6).

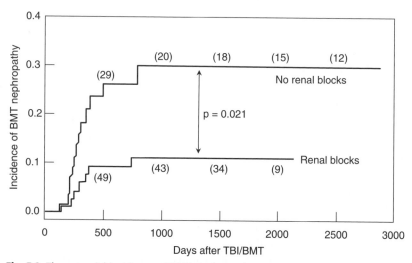

Fig. 7.2 The actuarial incidence of BMT nephropathy at our center is shown. Without renal shielding, this reaches 30% by three years after BMT. In the combined group of patients having either 15% or 30% renal radiation dose reduction, there is a significant reduction in the occurrence of BMT nephropathy.

In the case of rhenium 188 conjugated to an antibody against CD 66, there is probably no appreciable glomerular filtration of the conjugate. This isotope is a beta as well as a gamma emitter, and its external dosimetry suggests an average kidney dose of 700 cGy, when 10 GBq (270 millicurie) of the rhenium conjugate are infused intravenously (15).

In a cohort analysis of 83 patients receiving [166]Ho-DOTMP as internal radioisotope therapy for multiple myeloma, seven patients developed thrombotic microangiopathy with renal insufficiency. In these patients, the median dose to the kidneys was calculated at 710 cGy (16). Thus, irradiation of the kidneys at less than the traditional limit of 2000 cGy is capable of causing renal injury.

Total body or radioisotope exposures are to both kidneys, i.e. the entire kidney volume. Partial kidney exposures could include a single kidney and cause unilateral injury with subsequent hypertension that could be relieved by nephrectomy of the irradiated kidney (17). Exposures to lesser amounts of the renal parenchyma may also cause injury. Definition of that injury depends on the chosen endpoint and also on the timing of the endpoint. Using the endpoint of tolerance dose in 5% of subjects at 5 years ('TD 5/5'), it is reported that clinical nephritis will be evident after 50 Gy exposure of one-third of kidney volume, and after 30 Gy to two-thirds of the kidney volume (18). It is likely that such partial kidney irradiation cases will combine the effects of radiation-induced parenchymal loss with the effects of a scarred kidney that causes renin-mediated hypertension.

At the tissue and the cellular levels, the pathogenesis of radiation nephropathy is understood only in general terms. Ionizing radiation causes injury either to cancer cells or to normal cells by radiochemical injury to the DNA of the cells. Either apoptotic death or death in mitosis can follow. This simple cellular mechanism is several steps short of what happens on a tissue and on a whole organ level. On a morphological level, the earliest cellular injury appears to be to the glomerular endothelial cell (19), and, on a tissue level, glomerular injury precedes a tubular injury (20). The importance of an endothelial injury is underlined clinically by the more severe variants of BMT nephropathy, which have features of thrombotic microangiopathy. Mesangiolysis is a typical histological feature.

The renal tubular epithelium is also involved in radiation nephropathy. In the laboratory rat, tubular epithelial proliferation is detected at three weeks after 17 Gy fractionated irradiation (21). An additional study has found apoptosis of mouse renal proximal tubular epithelial cells after 5 Gy single fraction in vivo irradiation (22). Conceivably, there is an early apoptotic response to irradiation, followed by compensatory cell proliferation. The proliferative response could be damaging, because the irradiated cells harbor DNA injury that could lead to their death in mitosis. The inhibition of renal tubular cell proliferation, using angiotensin II blockers, has been associated with the preservation of the renal function in experimental radiation nephropathy (21).

The renin–angiotensin system does appear to play a role in experimental radiation nephropathy, in as much as either the angiotensin-converting-enzyme (ACE) inhibitors or the angiotensin II blockers are effective in both treatment and prevention of experimental radiation nephropathy (5). Yet, activation of the renin–angiotensin system, either systemically or within the kidney, has thus far not been found in radiation nephropathy (23).

Presentation

Classical radiation nephropathy occurred in an acute and a chronic form (2). Acute radiation nephropathy presented at six months after irradiation, with azotemia, hypertension, and anemia. Chronic radiation nephropathy had a longer latent period of a year or more. A generally unfavorable evolution to renal failure was described, and, as recently as 1987, treatment was felt to be ineffective (24).

BMT nephropathy was first described in 1978 in a child who had undergone a BMT proceeded by 1000 cGy TBI given in a single fraction (8). In that case, six months after the BMT, there was microhematuria, proteinuria, azotemia, and hypertension, followed by rapid death. Similar presentations in children, as well as adults, were described over the ensuing decade, and in 1988, the relation to irradiation was acknowledged (4).

In our initial series, the average latency from the time of BMT to the diagnosis of BMT nephropathy was eight months, which is analogous to acute radiation nephropathy (25). The clinical features are of azotemia, hypertension, and proteinuria. The more severe cases have presentations similar to the hemolytic uremic syndrome or thrombotic thrombocytopenic purpura (HUS/TTP). The laboratory features not only include azotemia, but also disproportionately severe anemia. Hyperkalemia can occur, with or without the use of ACE inhibitors, as in the case presented at the beginning of this chapter. A transient rise in serum levels of lactate dehydrogenase (LDH) is often found, and that rise correlates with a drop in platelet count that can occur even in the absence of frank HUS/TTP.

Although the diagnosis of BMT nephropathy can be made without using a kidney biopsy, the histological appearance of the biopsies are striking and are unlike other kidney diseases (Fig. 7.3). As is the case for a classical radiation nephropathy, BMT nephropathy is not an inflammatory condition—there are few inflammatory cells in the affected kidneys—hence the use of 'nephropathy' instead of 'nephritis'. The glomeruli show the distinctive changes of

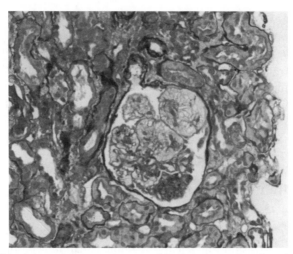

Fig. 7.3 Light microscopic image of a case of BMT nephropathy. There is extreme subendothelial expansion of the glomerular tufts by a cellular 'fluffy' appearing matrix. Cellular proliferation is not visible. There is minimal inflammatory infiltrate in the interstitium.

mesangiolysis, which is a dissolution of the mesangial cells, and there is extreme widening between the endothelium and the glomerular basement membrane. This morphology is very similar to that of classical radiation nephropathy. The loss of kidney function in a BMT nephropathy can be very rapid. Fig. 7.4 shows a typical case, graphed as 100/serum creatinine vs. time, in which there is a rapid decline in kidney function within a year of BMT, then stabilization, which occurred in this, as in other cases, in association with control of the blood pressure. The rate of loss of function in the rapid phase is up to five times more rapid when compared to the other forms of renal failure, such as chronic glomerulonephritis.

The clinical presentations of radiation nephropathy after yttrium 90-DOTATOC exposure appear to be similar to, if not a little more severe than, those of BMT nephropathy. That is, they are similar to what Luxton termed acute radiation nephritis (2). In the five cases reported by Moll and colleagues (6), renal failure developed within three months after the last yttrium 90 dose, and in three of the five who required hemodialysis, within six months. In three cases undergoing kidney biopsy, there was thrombotic micro-angiopathy, as in the five cases reported by Giralt et al. (16), and in the single case reported by Fonck and colleagues (26).

It is possible that less severe variants of radiation nephropathy after radioiso-tope exposure may be recognized in the future. Recognition of such cases will

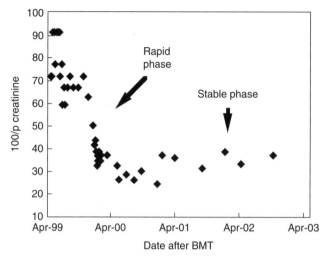

Fig. 7.4 This shows the evolution of kidney function over time in a case of BMT nephropathy. There is an initial, rapid phase that starts at about six months after the BMT. During this phase, there is a steep decline in kidney function, shown as 100/plasma or serum creatinine, from approximately 70% of normal to 30% of normal. Thereafter, and for the ensuing two years, there has been stabilization of the kidney function in association with good control of the blood pressure (BP). In this case, at the most recent office visit, the sitting BP was 130/80 mmHg. This man has been lost to follow-up since November 2002.

depend on the knowledge of exposure to the therapeutic doses of a radioisotope with pharmacokinetics that are consistent with nephrotoxicity.

Management

In BMT nephropathy, as in any other hypertensive kidney disease, the control of blood pressure to the normal range is advised. Experimental data strongly support the use of ACE inhibitors or angiotensin II blockers in the treatment and prevention of experimental radiation nephropathy (5), but there are no comparative clinical data on the relative merits of one or the other type of anti-hypertensive drug in BMT nephropathy. Diuretic drugs are needed in about three-quarters of the cases. In one case of radiation nephropathy occurring as a consequence of local renal irradiation in the treatment for kidney transplant rejection, there was a clear-cut stabilization of kidney function with the use of an angiotensin II blocker (27).

The anemia of BMT nephropathy may be relatively more severe than expected for the degree of azotemia (25). When measured, the blood erythropoietin levels have been low, and, correspondingly, treatment with parenteral erythropoietin, successful.

Hyperkalemia may occur, with or without the use of ACE inhibitors or angiotensin II blockers. This indicates a tubular defect, but that has not been studied in detail. Sodium polystyrene sulfonate resin (Kayexalate®) may be needed to lower the potassium level, as for the case presented in this chapter.

In cases with a dramatic HUS/TTP presentation, plasmapheresis has sometimes been used. But although there may be hematologic improvement with plasmapheresis in this syndrome, there does not seem to be any renal benefit (28).

It is likely that the principles of management thus outlined would be the same for radiation nephropathy as they are for BMT nephropathy, whether caused by external beam radiation or use of parenteral radioisotopes.

Outcome

Classical radiation nephropathy had been more common in an era when antihypertensive therapy was less effective and when dialysis was not available. Thus, progressive radiation nephropathy was formerly felt to be untreatable.

The first decade of reports of BMT nephropathy emphasized the severity and high mortality of the syndrome. As reported in 1988, four of eight of Chappell's cases died, and one required dialysis (4). Six of the 19 of our case series reported in 1993 have died, and nine of the series eventually required dialysis or kidney transplant. But only three of our 18 cases since 1995 have died, and only three required dialysis or a kidney transplant.

Of the cases evolving to the need for dialysis, our clinical impression was that they had unfavorable courses. Indeed, a case-control analysis of our single-center data showed that survival on chronic dialysis of patients with BMT nephropathy as the cause of end-stage renal disease (ESRD) was worse than that of patients with diabetes, matched for age and start-date of dialysis (29) (Fig. 7.5). This emphasizes the importance of an early diagnosis and treatment, which may be the reason why our recent experiences with BMT nephropathy have been more optimistic.

The use of kidney transplantation as treatment for ESRD after a BMT was first reported in two cases in 1991 (30) and we have reported six cases from our center (31). Fifty-three cases have been identified by searching the United Network for Organ Sharing (UNOS) database from 1994–2001. Of our six cases, three received a kidney from their marrow donor. In this special situation, as had been first reported in 1991, and as for the case reported at the start of this chapter, immunosuppressive medication is not needed to prevent kidney transplant rejection. That is because the recipient's immune system is identical to that of the donor.

In a single case of classical radiation nephropathy at our center, kidney transplantation from a living donor was performed in 1998.

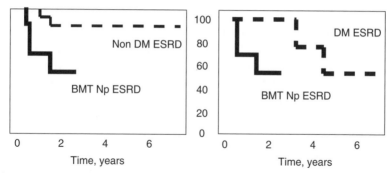

Fig. 7.5 These graphs show the actuarial survival of subjects with BMT nephropathy who have developed chronic renal failure requiring dialysis. The left-hand panel shows their survival compared to that of matched subjects with non-diabetic renal failure. The right-hand panel shows their survival compared to that of matched subjects with diabetic renal failure. Both comparisons show significantly decreased survival for BMT nephropathy, compared to other causes of ESRD, p < 0.03 by log-rank test. Reproduced with permission from Cohen EP et al (1998) End-Stage Renal Disease (ESRD) after Bone Marrow Transplantation: Poor survival compared to other causes of ESRD. *Nephron*, **79**; 408–12. Published by S. Karger AG, Basel.

Mitigation and treatment

In the case of classical radiation nephropathy, avoidance of renal irradiation is the most obvious preventive measure. Use of therapeutic irradiation of the upper abdomen could irradiate 50% of the entire kidney volume or an entire kidney, leaving the remaining volume unirradiated, with only a small risk of subsequent renal failure. There would still be a risk of hypertension in such cases, because of ischemia and scarring in the irradiated kidney (32).

At our center, the TBI that precedes BMT includes a 30% shielding of both kidneys, such that the absorbed dose to the kidneys is only 9.8 Gy. This has resulted in a significant reduction in the occurrence of BMT nephropathy, although cases still occur (Fig. 7.2).

It is in part because of this persistent problem, but also because of the favorable experimental studies (5), that we performed a study of mitigation of BMT nephropathy using the ACE inhibitor captopril. In 55 adults and children undergoing a TBI-based BMT at our center, captopril or placebo was given from the time of the new marrow engraftment, up to one year after the BMT. Importantly, captopril was given starting at engraftment, well after irradiation. This use is so-called mitigation, as it takes place after the inciting injury but before there is evidence of that injury. Outcomes, including BMT nephropathy and kidney function, were compared between those given captopril and those given placebo. Subjects on captopril had less occurrence of BMT nephropathy, and less occurrence of chronic renal failure. Patient survival was better in subjects on captopril compared to those on placebo, but these endpoints did not reach statistical significance (33). An extended analysis of this study increased the placebo group by adding to it those subjects who were eligible for the study but did not enroll, the 'non-study cohort'. Comparison of the captopril group to the no-drug group (placebo plus the non-study cohort) showed a significantly better patient survival for the subjects on captopril (p = 0.03). This favorable outcome justifies further study of the mitigation of radiation injury, in kidney or other organs. Generally, if captopril mitigates clinical radiation nephropathy, then further use of captopril and congeners may be planned for the protection of other normal tissues in radiation therapy.

Use of lysine infusions has been advocated to reduce the potential nephrotoxicity of yttrium 90-DOTATOC internal radiotherapy (6). The principle of this maneuver is that the infused lysine would reduce the tubular reabsorption of the filtered radioisotope, thereby enhancing its excretion in urine and reducing its nephrotoxicity. Use of albumin fragments and bovine gelatin have also been reported (34). This intervention, which would only affect tubular reabsorption, would probably not be effective in preventing injury due to rhenium 188 conjugated to an antibody.

Future trends

It is unlikely that classical radiation nephropathy from external beam radiation will be a major problem in future. Use of TBI-based BMT did increase steadily from the early 1980s to the 1990s, but there has been a slowing down of the increase in recent years (www.ibmtr.org). This is perhaps related to better chemotherapies, including newer drugs such as imatinib mesylate (Gleevec®), which is effective in the treatment of chronic myeloid leukemia. It is also related to the use of conditioning regimens that do not include radiation. Low-dose TBI, for instance 200 cGy at time of conditioning, is used for non-myeloablative BMT, but this radiation dose is not likely to cause radiation-related renal injury.

Parenteral radioisotope radiotherapies remain a potential problem. Given the 'right' mix of pharmacokinetics and isotope half-life, nephrotoxicities such as that seen with yttrium 90-DOTATOC are possible, and will require clinical vigilance.

Radionuclear exposures as might occur in accidents or by terrorism are a modern threat. Total body single fraction doses of 5 Gy or more could be survivable with proper medical care to overcome the hematological effects of radiation; subjects might then evolve to develop chronic kidney disease in months to years following. Mitigation of kidney and other normal tissue radiation injuries is an area of ongoing research (35).

References

1 Edsall DL (1906). The attitude of the clinician in regard to exposing patients to the X-ray. *J Am Med Assoc* **47**: 1425–9.

2 Luxton RW (1953). Radiation nephritis. *QJ Med* **22**: 215–42.

3 Duchesne GM, Stenning SP, Aass N, et al. (1997). Radiotherapy after chemotherapy for metastatic seminoma—a diminishing role. *Eur J Cancer* **33**: 829–35.

4 Chappell ME, Keeling DM, Prentice HG, Sweny P (1988). Haemolytic uraemic syndrome after bone marrow transplantation: an adverse effect of total body irradiation. *Bone Marrow Transplant* **3**: 339–47.

5 Cohen EP (2000). Radiation nephropathy after bone marrow transplantation. *Kidney Int* **58**: 903–18.

6 Moll S, Nickeleit V, Mueller-Brand J, Brunner FP, Maecke HR, Mihatsch MJ (2001). A new cause of renal thrombotic microangiopathy: Yttrium 90-DOTATOC internal radiotherapy. *Am J Kidney Dis* **37**: 847–51.

7 Lambert B, Cybulla M, Weiner SM, Van De Wiele C, Ham H, Dierckx RA, Otte A. (2004). Renal toxicity after radionuclide therapy. *Radiat Res* **161**: 607–11.

8 Kamil ES, Latta H, Johnston WH, Feig SA, Bergstein JM (1978). Radiation nephritis following bone marrow transplantation [abstract]. *Kidney Int* **14**: 713.

9 Antignac C, Gubler MC, Leverger G, Broyer M, Habib R (1989). Delayed renal failure with extensive mesangiolysis following bone marrow transplantation. *Kidney Int* **35**: 1336–44.

10 Lawton CA, Cohen EP, Barber-Derus SW, et al. (1991). Late renal dysfunction in adult survivors of bone marrow transplantation. *Cancer* **67**: 2795–800.

11 Lawton CA, Cohen EP, Murray KJ, Derus SW, Moulder JE (1997). Long-term results of selective renal shielding in patients undergoing total body irradiation in preparation for bone marrow transplantation. *Bone Marrow Transplant* **12**: 1069–74.

12 Miralbell R, Bieri S, Mermillod B, et al. (1996). Renal toxicity after allogeneic bone marrow transplantation: The combined effects of total-body irradiation and graft-versus-host disease. *J Clin Oncol* **14**: 579–85.

13 Phillips TL, Wharam MD, and Margolis LW (1975). Modification of radiation injury to normal tissues by chemotherapeutic agents. *Cancer* **35**: 1678–84.

14 Behr TM, Béhé M, Kluge G, et al. (2002). Nephrotoxicity versus anti-tumor efficacy in radiopeptide therapy: facts and myths about the Scylla and Charybdis. *Eur J Nucl Med* **29**: 277–9.

15 Bunjes D (2002). [188]Re labeled anti-CD66 monoclonal antibody in stem cell trans-plantation for patients with high-risk acute myeloid leukemia. *Leuk Lymphoma* **43**: 2125–31.

16 Giralt S, Bensinger W, Goodman M, et al. (2003). [166]Ho-DOTMP plus melphalan followed by peripheral blood stem cell transplantation in patients with multiple myeloma: results of two phase 1/2 trials. *Blood* **102**: 2684–91.

17 Salvi S, Green DM, Brecher ML, et al. (1983). Renal artery stenosis and hypertension after abdominal irradiation for Hodgkin disease-successful treatment with nephrectomy. *Urology* **21**: 611–15.

18 Emami B, Lyman J, Brown A, et al. (1991). Tolerance of normal tissue to therapeutic irradiation. *Int J Radiat Oncol Biol Phys* **21**: 109–22.

19 Jaenke RS, Robbins MEC, Bywaters T, Whitehouse E, Rezvani M, Hopewell JW (1993). Capillary endothelium: Target site of renal radiation injury. *Lab Invest* **68**: 396–405.

20 Glatstein E, Fajardo LF, Brown JM (1977). Radiation injury in the mouse kidney— I sequential light microscopic study. *Int J Radiat Oncol Biol Phys* **2**: 933–43.

21 Moulder JE, Fish BL, Regner KR, Cohen EP (2002). Angiotensin II blockade reduces radiation-induced proliferation in experimental radiation nephropathy. *Radiat Res* **157**: 393–401.

22 Ghassah M, Labejof L, Berry JP, Galle P (1997). Early ultrastructural lesions of apoptosis induced in vivo in two varieties of tissues (thymus and kidneys) after a single whole-body-gamma irradiation of adult mice. *Cell Mol Biol* **43**: 1197–204.

23 Cohen EP, Fish BL, Moulder JE (2002). The renin-angiotensin system in experimental radiation nephropathy. *J Lab Clin Med* **139**: 251–7.

24 Asscher AW (1987). Interstitial nephritis and urinary tract infections. In: *Oxford Textbook of Medicine* (ed. DJ Weatherall, JGG Ledingham, DA Warrell), pp. 18.67–18.80. Oxford University Press, Oxford.

25 Cohen EP, Lawton CA, Moulder JE, Becker CG, Ash RC (1993). Clinical course of late-onset bone marrow transplant nephropathy. *Nephron* **64**: 626–35.

26 Fonck C, Cosyns JP, Goffin E, et al. (2000). Glomerulopathie après radiotherapie métabolique pour insulinome métastatique. *Néphrologie* **21**: 206.

27 Cohen EP, Hussain S, Moulder JE (2003). Successful treatment of radiation nephropathy with angiotensin II blockade. *Int J Radiat Oncol Biol Phys* **55**: 190–3.

28 Sarode R, McFarland JG, Flomenberg N, et al. (1995). Therapeutic serum exchange does not appear to be effective in the management of thrombotic thrombocytopenic purpura/hemolytic uremic syndrome following bone marrow transplantation. *Bone Marrow Transplant* **16**: 271–5.

29 Cohen EP, Piering WF, Kabler-Babbitt C, Moulder JE (1998). End-stage renal disease (ESRD) after bone marrow transplantation: Poor survival compared to other causes of ESRD. *Nephron* **79**: 408–12.

30 Sayegh MH, Fine NA, Smith JL, Rennke HG, Milford EL, Tilney NL (1991). Immunologic tolerance to renal allografts after bone marrow transplants from the same donors. *Ann Intern Med* **114**: 954–5.

31 Butcher JA, Hariharan S, Adams MB, Johnson CP, Roza AM, Cohen EP (1999). Renal transplantation for end-stage renal disease following bone marrow transplantation: A report of six cases, with and without immunosuppression. *Clin Transplant* **13**: 330–5.

32 Crummy WE, Hellman S, Stansel HC, Hakill PB (1965). Renal hypertension secondary to unilateral radiation damage relieved by nephrectomy. *Radiology* **84**: 108–11.

33 Cohen EP, Irving AA, Drobyski WR, Klein JP, Passweg J, Talano J, et al. (2008). Captopril to mitigate chronic renal failure after hematopoietic stem cell transplantation: a randomized controlled trial. *Int J Radiat Oncol Biol Phys* **70**: 1546–51.

34 Rolleman EJ, Melis M, Valkema R, et al. (2010). Kidney protection during peptide receptor radionuclide therapy with somatostatin analogues. *Eur J Nucl Med Imaging*, **37**: 1018–31.

35 Moulder JE, Cohen EP (2007). Future strategies for mitigation and treatment of chronic radiation-induced normal tissue injury. *Sem Rad Onc* **17**: 141–8.

Chapter 8

Renal complications of hematopoietic stem cell transplantation

Benjamin D. Humphreys

Hematopoietic stem cell transplantation (HSCT) offers a cure for both malignant and non-malignant hematologic disease. Despite advances in the procedure leading to rapid growth in number of HSCTs performed over the last two decades, renal complications remain a very important cause of morbidity and mortality. Peri-transplant acute kidney injury (AKI) is common and severe cases are associated with very high mortality. The risk of AKI depends on the type of conditioning (myeloablative or non-myeloablative) and the source of stem cells (autologous or allogeneic). Glomerular disease in HSCT recipients is more common than in the general population, and is associated with graft vs. host disease (GVHD). With increasing numbers of HSCT survivors many years out from transplant, long-term morbidity such as chronic kidney disease (CKD) and end-stage renal disease (ESRD) represent a growing problem.

Overview of HSCT protocols

The HSCT procedure consists of three components. First, intensive conditioning is administered consisting of irradiation and/or chemotherapy for the purpose of immunoablation and disease eradication. Second, donor hematopoietic cells are infused to rescue the patient from myeloablation. Third, post-graft immunosuppression is given to control graft vs. host disease (GVHD) and to establish graft–host tolerance.

Myeloablative conditioning regimens employ otherwise lethal doses of irradiation and chemotherapy. These protocols may be associated with significant morbidity during the cytopenic interval, and for this reason myeloablative HSCT has traditionally been limited to younger patients without co-morbidities. Non-myeloablative allogeneic transplants utilize reduced intensity conditioning designed to allow engraftment of donor stem cells without myeloablation. These 'mini-allo' transplants take advantage of the graft vs. tumor effect seen in many of the more indolent cancers such as chronic myelogenous leukemia and chronic lymphocytic leukemia.

The source of hematopoietic stem cells is from either a donor (allogeneic) or from the patient (autologous). Allogeneic cells are harvested from marrow, peripheral blood, or cord blood. The establishment of large registries for bone marrow donors and typed cord blood has greatly increased the chance of finding a match in allogeneic transplants. In autologous HSCT, cells are harvested from either the marrow or peripheral blood of the patient to be transplanted, then cryo-preserved until needed.

Immunosuppression is administered to promote tolerance of the graft and reduce GVHD. Standard regimens include calcineurin inhibitors such as cyclosporine given for the first three months post transplant. These regimens are associated with a 25% incidence of moderate to severe acute GVHD. While many transplant recipients are on calcineurin inhibitors for a relatively short time, roughly 50% of HSCT survivors develop chronic GVHD and are maintained on calcineurin for years with attendant risks of nephrotoxicity (1).

Case report

A 45-year-old man underwent myeloablative allogeneic hematopoietic stem cell transplantation (HSCT) for acute myelogenous leukemia. Conditioning consisted of total body irradiation and cyclophosphamide. Beginning on day 3 after stem cell infusion, progressive edema and weight gain developed followed by right upper quadrant tenderness and hyperbilirubinemia. Liver ultrasound disclosed ascites and reversal of flow in the portal vein. The serum creatinine rose progressively, beginning on day 8 with a low fractional excretion of sodium and bland sediment. Liver biopsy showed occlusion of hepatic venules with concentric intimal thickening and centrilobular sinusoidal congestion. Veno-occlusive disease was diagnosed and high-dose intravenous diuretics prescribed to treat fluid overload. The serum creatinine continued to rise and respiratory failure developed, requiring intiation of renal replacement therapy and mechanical ventilation. Increasing pressors were required and on day 30 care was withdrawn and the patient died.

Epidemiology of acute kidney injury after hematopoietic stem cell transplantation

The risk of AKI after HSCT varies according to the type of transplant (Table 8.1). In myeloablative allogeneic HSCT, Zager originally reported that 53% of patients developed ARF (defined as >50% reduction in GFR), with half of these patients requiring dialysis (2). Today, a similar percentage of patients develop AKI but only about a quarter of these require renal replacement therapy, presumably due to better supportive care and the availability of less nephrotoxic antibiotic alternatives (3,4). An important factor that may be driving the sustained rates of AKI over time despite advances in HSCT

Table 8.1 Rates of AKI according to type of HSCT (2, 3, 62)

HSCT Type	Mod-severe AKI[a]	AKI requiring RRT[b]	Mortality if RRT
Allogeneic			
Myeloablative	59%	17%	>80%
Non-myeloablative	39%	4%	>80%
Autologous	18%	4%	70%

[a]Moderate to severe AKI is defined as at least a doubling of the serum creatinine whether or not renal replacement therapy was required
[b]RRT, renal replacement therapy

protocol and supportive care is the age at time of transplant, which is steadily increasing. The most rapidly growing group of patients receiving either autologous or allogeneic HSCT are patients over the age of 60 (Fig. 8.1). Age is a well-known risk factor for AKI (5).

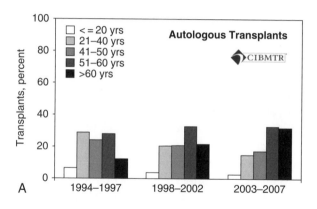

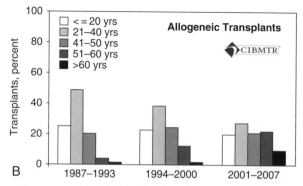

Fig. 8.1 Increasing age at time of HSCT. (a) Age at time of autologous HSCT for AML, ALL, CML, MM, NHL, CLL, MDS. (b) Age at time of allogeneic HSCT. Note that in both cases the fastest growing subgroup is patients over 60 years old.
Reprinted with permission from Center for International Blood and Marrow Transplant Research, 2009.

The incidence of AKI after autologous HSCT is lower than after allogeneic HSCT, ranging between 15–21% in recent studies (3, 6–8). Two factors likely explain the lower incidence of ARF in autologous HSCT. First, GVHD does not occur in autologous HSCT and so nephrotoxic calcineurin inhibitors are not required. Second, most autologous HSCTs are performed with peripheral blood stem cells: these engraft sooner than marrow or cord-derived stem cells, shortening the cytopenic interval and reducing the risk of bleeding, sepsis, and nephrotoxic antibiotic exposure.

Existing data indicates that the incidence of AKI after non-myeloablative allogeneic HSCT is substantially lower than after myeloablative HSCT. Parikh et al. found a cumulative incidence of AKI (defined as doubling of Scr at four months) in non-myeloablative HSCT of 40.4%, but only 4.4% of all patients required dialysis (9). In distinction from myeloablative HSCT, veno-occlusive disease was not a major cause of AKI. The timing of AKI in non-myeloablative HSCT is distributed over the first three months post-HSCT, whereas in myeloablative HSCT, AKI occurs primarily in the first three weeks. Similarly, Kersting and colleagues performed a retrospective cohort study on 150 adults receiving non-myeloablative HSCT and found a 33% rate of AKI (defined as doubling of serum creatinine) with no patients requiring renal replacement therapy (10). But when dialysis is needed for AKI after non-myeloablative HSCT, it is associated with 80% patient mortality (3).

Regardless of the setting in which AKI occurs, the degree of renal failure correlates with short-term mortality. A meta-analysis reviewing 1,211 HSCT recipients found that AKI was independently associated with a greater than twofold increased risk of death (11) and AKI requiring renal replacement therapy carries a mortality in excess of 80%, at least in part because of concurrent multi-organ failure (12, 13). More recent studies suggest that the occurrence of AKI within the first 100 days of HSCT is also an independent predictor of long-term mortality, at least in non-myeloablative HSCT. In a cohort of patients receiving non-myeloablative HSCT between 1997 and 2006, the adjusted hazards ratio of overall mortality was 1.57 (95% CI 1.2–2.3; P = .0006) among the group of patients developing AKI in the first 100 days after transplant (14).

Acute kidney injury after hematopoietic stem cell transplantation

AKI during the HSCT itself is most frequently a consequence of sepsis, hypotension, or nephrotoxins received during the cytopenic interval (15, 16). Occasionally, tumor lysis syndrome may cause AKI as a consequence of the conditioning regimen. A pre-renal state during the transplant is common, resulting from vomiting and diarrhea, the consequence of conditioning or acute GVHD. Exposure to potentially nephrotoxic agents including methotrexate, amphotericin B, acyclovir, aminoglycosides, angiotensin-converting enzyme inhibitors, intravenous contrast, and calcineurin inhibitors predisposes to the development of acute tubular necrosis. Thrombocytopenia and neutropenia predispose to hemorrhagic or septic shock, respectively, and may lead to acute tubular necrosis.

Veno-occlusive disease

Hepatorenal syndrome is a relatively common and serious renal complication after myeloablative HSCT, usually due to veno-occlusive disease (VOD) (2). VOD, also known as sinusoidal obstruction syndrome, is a conditioning-related toxicity most commonly associated with regimens including cyclophosphamide, busulfan, and/or total body irradiation (17). The pathophysiology of VOD involves damage to hepatic sinusoidal endothelial cells causing sinusoidal obstruction, portal hypertension and microvascular intrahepatic portosystemic shunting (Fig. 8.2). The incidence of VOD varies according to the diagnostic criteria used and ranges between 5% and 70% in myeloablative HSCT, with the rate of clinically significant VOD at 15–25% (18). This rate has been falling with the advent of less intensive conditioning regimens in

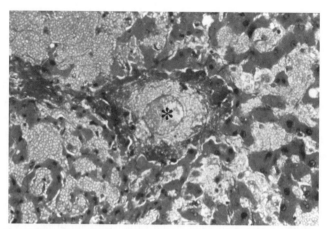

Fig. 8.2 Liver biopsy showing typical changes seen in veno-occlusive disease (VOD). Note occlusion of central hepatic vein (*) with surrounding intimal thickening and fibrosis. Centrilobular hemorrhagic necrosis is present with hepatocyte dropout. Micrograph provided by Paul Richardson, MD.

myeloablative HSCT. Although severe cases with multi-organ failure are uncommon, they are associated with a mortality in excess of 80% (19, 20).

Clinical features of VOD include weight gain, painful hepatomegaly and jaundice. Conditions that mimic VOD includes acute hepatic GVHD, sepsis or drug-induced cholestasis, calcineurin inhibitor toxicity, gall bladder disease, and use of total parenteral nutrition (20). Timing of symptom onset aids in diagnosis: VOD generally appears during the first 30 days post-HSCT. Sodium retention predominates in the early stages with consequent weight gain, edema, and ascites. Jaundice and right upper quadrant pain follow. Abdominal ultrasound with Doppler may show reversal of flow in the portal vein. Acute renal failure often arises, precipitated by renal insults such as sepsis or nephrotoxins. Roughly 50% of those with VOD develop AKI, but some degree of renal insufficiency exists in every patient (12, 21). The severity of disease varies. In mild to moderate cases hepatic injury is self-limited and symptoms may be treated with analgesia and diuresis and the syndrome eventually resolves completely. Severe VOD is characterized by advanced hepatic failure with the cause of death generally from progressive multi-organ failure rather than liver failure itself (18, 22).

VOD-associated acute kidney injury is clinically indistinguishable from hepatorenal syndrome. Patients are oliguric with very low fractional excretion of sodium. Total body sodium and water overload are common. Patients generally have low blood pressures, may have hyponatremia and usually have a bland sediment, although later in the course of the disease tubular damage with granular casts may result from hypotension or nephrotoxin exposure. Biopsy and autopsy studies have confirmed that kidneys do not have structural lesions in VOD, consistent with the notion that the renal injury in hepatorenal syndrome is hemodynamic (23).

Treatment of severe VOD and AKI is primarily supportive. Maintenance of intravascular volume is of paramount importance. The hematocrit should be maintained above 35% and intravenous albumin should be avoided as it accumulates in the extravascular space. Sodium restriction and diuretics are necessary, the latter often as a continuous infusion. Paracentesis for ascites and lactulose for encephalopathy may be required. When renal replacement is indicated, continuous therapies are advantageous due to the very high daily obligate fluid intake in HSCT patients. Defibrotide, a single stranded polydeoxyribonucleotide (24, 25) that has fibrinolytic, anti-thrombotic, and anti-ischemic properties, is being evaluated for the treatment of established VOD. Initial results are very promising, and prospective trials are under way to confirm its efficacy in the prophylaxis and treatment of VOD (26).

Case report

A 64-year-old man with myelodysplasia underwent two successive non-myeloablative allogeneic HSCTs and each failed. Ultimately he underwent myeloablative allogeneic HSCT with success, and developed chronic GVHD of his eyes and mouth. Five years after transplant he developed new dependent edema and was found to have new hypoalbuminemia and a urine protein to creatinine ratio of 20. Serum creatinine was unchanged. Renal biopsy revealed membranous nephropathy.

Glomerular disease after hematopoietic stem cell transplantation

Nephrotic syndrome is a well described but unusual complication of HSCT. Membranous nephropathy is the most frequent form of immune-complex glomerulonephritis, occurring in about 75% of all cases of HSCT-associated nephrotic syndrome (27–29). Srinivasan et al. reported seven cases of nephrotic syndrome in a consecutive series of non-myeloablative HSCT recipients, and four of these patients had membranous nephropathy on biopsy (30). Most cases did not respond to increased immunosuppression and three went on to ESRD. Because non-myeloablative transplants result in host/donor marrow chimerism, the persistence of host lymphocytes surviving conditioning is one factor that could increase susceptibility to nephrotic syndrome in these patients. The overall incidence of 4% in this case series, however, contrasts with other centers where the incidence is less than 1% among non-myeloablative HSCT recipients, pointing to the possible role of different conditioning regimens in susceptibility to nephrotic syndrome (31). The two largest series describing nephrotic syndrome after allogeneic HSCT are from Reddy and Terrier, comprising 14 cases between them (32, 33). Reddy and colleagues also report an overall incidence of 1% of nephrotic syndrome after allogeneic HSCT, with membranous nephropathy the most common finding on biopsy (Fig. 8.3). The pathophysiology of idiopathic membranous nephropathy has recently been linked to podocyte-expressed phospholiase A2 receptor (34), and antenatal allo-immune glomerulopathy is linked to podocyte neutral endopeptidase (35), but whether these antigens are relevant to HSCT-associated membranous nephropathy is unknown. Minimal change nephrotic syndrome is also reported after HSCT and comprises about 25% of all reported cases of nephrotic syndrome (28, 36, 37). It is important to rule out lymphoma relapse in this setting, as minimal change disease is associated with lymphoma by unknown mechanisms (38).

Intriguingly, most patients with HSCT-associated nephrotic syndrome had manifestations of chronic GVHD (cGVHD) around the time of diagnosis,

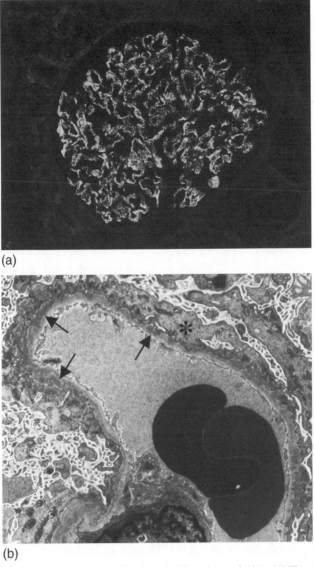

Fig. 8.3 Renal biopsy showing early membranous nephropathy in a HSCT recipient. (a) Immunofluorescence showing strong IgG reactivity throughout glomerulus in a diffuse, finely granular pattern along the capillary wall, reflecting subepithelial immune complexes. (b) Electron micrograph of capillary loop revealing electron-dense subepithelial deposits corresponding to granular IgG deposits detected by immunofluorescence (arrows) with complete effacement of podocyte foot processes (*). Courtesy of Vanesa Bijol, MD.

raising the possibility that membranous nephropathy represents a form of renal GVHD. In support of this possibility, animal models of GVHD show disease manifestation in the kidney, even though the kidney is not classically considered a site of GVHD activity in humans (39). Moreover, Brukamp and colleagues reported that nephrotic syndrome has typically been diagnosed after cessation of immunosuppression in 63% of patients reported in the literature (37). Currently, no firm conclusions can be drawn based on available evidence, and more research is needed in this area. Treatment of HSCT-associated nephrotic syndrome is controversial, and in the absence of any clinical trial evidence, most clinicians use disease-specific therapy as they would for idiopathic membranous nephropathy or minimal change disease.

Case report

A 33-year-old female presented to renal clinic for chronic kidney disease. She had been healthy until three years before, when she developed aplastic anemia. She was treated with immunosuppression including anti-thymocyte globulin, but required increasing transfusion support. One year before she had undergone myeloablative umbilical cord blood HSCT including TBI conditioning. One month after transplant she was readmitted for shortness of breath and rapidly decompensated, requiring ventilatory support. She had thrombocytopenia and microangiopathic hemolysis, and received plasmapheresis for presumed hemolytic uremic syndrome, a pericardial window for cardiac effusion, as well as ultrafiltration for volume overload. She eventually recovered, and serum creatinine was 110 µMol/L. Six months later her creatinine rose to 186 µMol/L. In clinic, she had 1 gram proteinuria, a bland sediment and a normal haptoglobin. Blood pressure was 125/82, which was higher than the patient's previous baseline of 100/60. Over the next three months creatinine rose to 240 µMol/L and renal biopsy revealed severe thrombotic microangiopathy. Her serum creatinine continued to rise over the next six months to 397 µMol/L, and plans were made for renal transplantation.

Chronic kidney disease after HSCT

Chronic kidney disease (CKD) is an increasingly recognized and important long-term complication of HSCT. In one single-institution cohort study of 1635 HSCT recipients surviving at least three months, CKD was identified in 23% (40). With more than 100,000 survivors of HSCT alive today, the overall burden of CKD in survivors of allogeneic HSCT represents a growing public health problem (41). The growth in non-myeloablative protocols may actually increase the incidence of CKD in HSCT survivors despite its milder conditioning regimen, because of older age and increased baseline co-morbidities in this population. Weiss and colleagues recently performed a retrospective cohort study of 122 patients who underwent non-myeloablative HSCT. They determined that 66% of patients had CKD within one year of transplant, as defined by a 25% or greater reduction in baseline GFR as estimated by the modification of diet in renal disease equation. Twenty-two percent had a 50% or greater reduction in GFR at six months. Independent risk factors for development of CKD included AKI in the first 100 days, previous autologous HSCT, calcineurin inhibitor use, and chronic GVHD (42). Similarly, Hingorani and colleagues identified AKI and GVHD as independent risk factors for development of CKD in their larger cohort study (40).

In contrast, with non-myeloablative HSCT, the majority of cases of CKD after myeloablative allogeneic HSCT are caused by a low-grade renal TMA. This syndrome has also been called bone marrow transplant nephropathy or radiation nephropathy and resembles hemolytic uremic syndrome (41, 43). Characteristic clinical features include slowly rising plasma creatinine, hypertension, and disproportionate anemia. Some cases have a more fulminant presentation, however (Fig. 8.4). Urinalysis shows variable proteinuria and hematuria. This chronic TMA may manifest as low-grade microangiopathic hemolysis with elevated plasma lactate dehydrogenase, low serum haptoglobin, thrombocytopenia, anemia, and sometimes schistocytosis. Renal imaging is usually unremarkable. Kidney biopsy is rarely required—unless the presentation is very atypical. The lab features are often suggestive and biopsy findings are unlikely to significantly alter management. Typical histology includes mesangiolysis, basement membrane duplication, glomerular endothelial cell swelling and tubular injury with interstitial fibrosis (44).

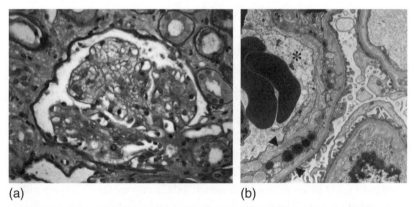

(a)   (b)

Fig. 8.4 Renal biopsy showing severe thrombotic microangiopathy in a HSCT recipient. (a) PAS stained section reveals severe mesangiolysis, with occlusion of the capillary lumens. (b) Electron micrograph shows loss of endothelial fenestrae and endotheliosis causing narrowing of the capillary lumen (*), with double contour formation (arrowheads).
Courtesy of Helmut Rennke, MD.

The pathogenesis of thrombotic microangiopathy after HSCT is poorly understood but renal endothelial damage plays a central role. The conditioning regimen—particularly the irradiation—is a primary cause of renal endothelial damage with post-HSCT factors such as GVHD, infections, and medications (such as the calcineurin inhibitors) playing a later modulatory role (45). Risk factors for development of TMA syndromes post-HSCT include dose of radiotherapy and use of concurrent cytotoxic chemotherapy (46). Sirolimus, when added to calcineurin inhibitor therapy for GVHD prophylaxis, is associated with a higher incidence of TMA but fortunately this is often reversible (47). Partial renal shielding during TBI may reduce the occurrence of CKD after HSCT (48). Preclinical evidence indicates that angiotensin converting enzyme inhibition is useful in the treatment of HSCT-related TMA (44, 49).

Chronic CNI toxicity

Moderate to severe graft vs. host disease carries a mortality of 10–50% (50) but methotrexate, cyclosporine, and tacrolimus reduce the incidence of both acute and chronic graft vs. host disease after allogeneic HSCT. In patients who do not develop GVHD, the CNIs are discontinued six months after HSCT and are therefore unlikely to play any role in promoting CKD. Fifty percent of transplant recipients do develop chronic GVHD, however, and require long-term immunosuppression (average of 23 months) (1). Long-term use of calcineurin inhibitors after HSCT in this setting certainly contributes to CKD as has been well described in non-renal solid organ transplantation and autoimmune disease (51). It is likely that in some cases calcineurin inhibitors also exacerbate the TMA which can arise after HSCT (calcineurin inhibitor induced TMA has been well described after kidney transplantation, for example) or perhaps contribute to development of focal and segmental glomerulosclerosis (52, 53).

Management of HSCT-related chronic kidney disease

Important aspects of the patient's history include the type of HSCT, the conditioning regimen (in particular, was total body irradiation used and at what dose?) and the degree of exposure to nephrotoxins (for example, prolonged treatment with amphotericin). Physical examination frequently shows hypertension, hypervolemia, and skin GVHD. Blood tests should be carefully reviewed and repeated to assess for TMA—it should be noted that laboratory features are often intermittent and not florid. Renal ultrasound is often used to exclude post-renal causes but other imaging studies are rarely required.

General treatment should be as recommended for any CKD patient (4, 54). Control of hypertension is especially important in patients with a TMA syndrome to reduce endothelial damage. Angiotensin converting enzyme or angiotensin receptor blockade slows progression in animal models of radiation nephropathy, which supports use in humans (49). In a randomized controlled trial of ACE inhibitorS for prevention of HSCT-associated TMA syndromes, patients received either placebo or captopril beginning at engraftment. Fifty-five patients were enrolled, and the captopril group showed a favorable trend (p = 0.07, for GFR) toward protection against CKD in those patients receiving allogeneic HSCT that used TBI-based conditioning (55). Hyperkalemia may be more common in this setting than in patients with other forms of CKD and requires treatment with a low potassium diet, diuretics, and sodium polystyrene (56). Diuretics are frequently required. Anemia may be more severe than expected for the degree of renal insufficiency and can be treated with erythropoietin. It is worthwhile minimizing calcineurin inhibitor dosage—if possible—as is sometimes done in solid organ transplantation (51). There is no evidence that plasma-exchange is beneficial, though it is occasionally used in very severe cases of TMA after HSCT (57).

End-stage renal disease after HSCT

A subset of patients progress to end-stage renal disease, and overall these patients have worse survival on hemodialysis than patients with end-stage renal disease from other causes. In one single center retrospective analysis of 1341 HSCT carried out between 1985 and 2007 determined that 19 patients (1.4%) developed ESRD at a median of seven years after HSCT—a rate 16 times higher than the expected age-adjusted rate (58). There are very few studies addressing outcomes in these patients, but in one study patients starting dialysis after HSCT had a higher mortality than patients with diabetes after matching for age and start-date of dialysis (59). Renal transplantation is a good option for eligible patients, and those who receive a renal allograft from the same donor as their original HSCT require minimal or no immunosuppression due to immunologic tolerance of the allograft (60, 61).

Future trends

Advances in transplant protocols and supportive care over the last two decades have driven an impressive growth in HSCT. In the future, the growing fraction of older patients with increased comorbidities at transplant mean that both AKI and CKD in this population will remain important complications of the procedure. Further research aimed at defining the pathophysiologic link between HSCT, GVHD and glomerular disease, particularly TMA, is required. Understanding the mechanisms of CKD among HSCT-recipients is an important first step toward identifying new treatment protocols aimed at reducing the burden of kidney disease in this patient population.

References

1 Stewart BL, Storer B, Storek J, Deeg HJ, Storb R, Hansen JA, et al. (2004). Duration of immunosuppressive treatment for chronic graft-versus-host disease. *Blood* **104**: 3501–6.

2 Zager RA, O'Quigley J, Zager BK, Alpers CE, Shulman HM, Gamelin LM, et al. (1989). Acute renal failure following bone marrow transplantation: a retrospective study of 272 patients. *Am J Kidney Dis* **13**: 210–16.

3 Parikh CR, Coca SG (2006). Acute renal failure in hematopoietic cell transplantation. *Kidney Int* **69**: 430–5.

4 Humphreys BD, Soiffer RJ, Magee CC (2005). Renal failure associated with cancer and its treatment: an update. *J Am Soc Nephrol* **16**: 151–61.

5 Xue JL, Daniels F, Star RA, Kimmel PL, Eggers PW, Molitoris BA, et al. (2006). Incidence and mortality of acute renal failure in Medicare beneficiaries, 1992 to 2001. *J Am Soc Nephrol* **17**: 1135–42.

6 Merouani A, Shpall EJ, Jones RB, Archer PG, Schrier RW (1996). Renal function in high dose chemotherapy and autologous hematopoietic cell support treatment for breast cancer. *Kidney Int* **50**: 1026–31.

7 Fadia A, Casserly LF, Sanchorawala V, Seldin DC, Wright DG, Skinner M, et al. (2003). Incidence and outcome of acute renal failure complicating autologous stem cell transplantation for AL amyloidosis. *Kidney Int* **63**: 1868–73.

8 Hingorani SR, Guthrie K, Batchelder A, Schoch G, Aboulhosn N, Manchion J, et al. (2005). Acute renal failure after myeloablative hematopoietic cell transplant: incidence and risk factors. *Kidney Int* **67**: 272–7.

9 Parikh CR, Sandmaier BM, Storb RF, Blume KG, Sahebi F, Maloney DG, et al. (2004). Acute renal failure after nonmyeloablative hematopoietic cell transplantation. *J Am Soc Nephrol* **15**: 1868–76.

10 Kersting S, Dorp SV, Theobald M, Verdonck LF (2008). Acute renal failure after nonmyeloablative stem cell transplantation in adults. *Biol Blood Marrow Transplant* **14**: 125–31.

11 Parikh CR, McSweeney P, Schrier RW (2005). Acute renal failure independently predicts mortality after myeloablative allogeneic hematopoietic cell transplant. *Kidney Int* **67**: 1999–2005.

12 Hahn T, Rondeau C, Shaukat A, Jupudy V, Miller A, Alam AR, et al. (2003). Acute renal failure requiring dialysis after allogeneic blood and marrow transplantation identifies very poor prognosis patients. *Bone Marrow Transplant* **32**: 405–10.

13 Parikh CR, McSweeney PA, Korular D, Ecder T, Merouani A, Taylor J, et al. (2002). Renal dysfunction in allogeneic hematopoietic cell transplantation. *Kidney Int* **62**: 566–73.

14 Parikh CR, Yarlagadda SG, Storer B, Sorror M, Storb R, Sandmaier B (2008). Impact of acute kidney injury on long-term mortality after nonmyeloablative hematopoietic cell transplantation. *Biol Blood Marrow Transplant* **14**: 309–15.

15 Noel C, Hazzan M, Noel-Walter MP, Jouet JP (1998). Renal failure and bone marrow transplantation. *Nephrol Dial Transplant* **13**: 2464–6.

16 Zager RA (1994). Acute renal failure in the setting of bone marrow transplantation. *Kidney Int* **46**: 1443–58.

17 McDonald GB, Hinds MS, Fisher LD, Schoch HG, Wolford JL, Banaji M, et al. (1993). Veno-occlusive disease of the liver and multiorgan failure after bone marrow transplantation: a cohort study of 355 patients. *Ann Intern Med* **118**: 255–67.

18 Coppell JA, Richardson PG, Soiffer R, Martin PL, Kernan NA, Chen A, et al. (2009). Hepatic veno-occlusive disease following stem cell transplantation: incidence, clinical course and outcome. *Biol Blood Marrow Transplant* **15**: 157–68.

19 Kumar S, DeLeve LD, Kamath PS, Tefferi A (2003). Hepatic veno-occlusive disease (sinusoidal obstruction syndrome) after hematopoietic stem cell transplantation. *Mayo Clin Proc* **78**: 589–98.

20 Wadleigh M, Ho V, Momtaz P, Richardson P (2003). Hepatic veno-occlusive disease: pathogenesis, diagnosis and treatment. *Curr Opin Hematol* **10**: 451–62.

21 Fink JC, Cooper MA, Burkhart KM, McDonald GB, Zager RA (1995). Marked enzymuria after bone marrow transplantation: a correlate of veno-occlusive disease-induced 'hepatorenal syndrome'. *J Am Soc Nephrol* **6**: 1655–60.

22 Carreras E, Bertz H, Arcese W, Vernant JP, Tomas JF, Hagglund H, et al. (1998). Incidence and outcome of hepatic veno-occlusive disease after blood or marrow transplantation: a prospective cohort study of the European Group for Blood and Marrow Transplantation. European Group for Blood and Marrow Transplantation Chronic Leukemia Working Party. *Blood* **92**: 3599–604.

23 El-Seisi S, Gupta R, Clase CM, Forrest DL, Milandinovic M, Couban S (2003). Renal pathology at autopsy in patients who died after hematopoietic stem cell transplantation. *Biol Blood Marrow Transplant* **9**: 683–8.

24 Richardson PG, Murakami C, Jin Z, Warren D, Momtaz P, Hoppensteadt D, et al. (2002). Multi-institutional use of defibrotide in 88 patients after stem cell transplantation with severe veno-occlusive disease and multisystem organ failure: response without significant toxicity in a high-risk population and factors predictive of outcome. *Blood* **100**: 4337–43.

25 Chopra R, Eaton JD, Grassi A, Potter M, Shaw B, Salat C, et al. (2000). Defibrotide for the treatment of hepatic veno-occlusive disease: results of the European compassionate-use study. *Br J Haematol* **111**: 1122–9.

26 Ho VT, Linden E, Revta C, Richardson PG (2007). Hepatic veno-occlusive disease after hematopoietic stem cell transplantation: review and update on the use of defibrotide. *Semin Thromb Hemost* **33**: 373–88.

27 Lin J, Markowitz GS, Nicolaides M, Hesdorffer CS, Appel GB, D'Agati VD, et al. (2001). Membranous glomerulopathy associated with graft-versus-host disease following allogeneic stem cell transplantation. Report of 2 cases and review of the literature. *Am J Nephrol* **21**: 351–6.

28 Rao PS (2005). Nephrotic syndrome in patients with peripheral blood stem cell transplant. *Am J Kidney Dis* **45**: 780–85.

29 Chang A, Hingorani S, Kowalewska J, Flowers ME, Aneja T, Smith KD, et al. (2007). Spectrum of renal pathology in hematopoietic cell transplantation: a series of 20 patients and review of the literature. *Clin J Am Soc Nephrol* **2**: 1014–23.

30 Srinivasan R, Balow JE, Sabnis S, Lundqvist A, Igarashi T, Takahashi Y, et al. (2005). Nephrotic syndrome: an under-recognised immune-mediated complication of non-myeloablative allogeneic haematopoietic cell transplantation. *Br J Haematol* **131**: 74–9.

31 Ruiz-Arguelles GJ, Gomez-Almaguer D (2006). Nephrotic syndrome after non-myeloablative stem cell transplantation. *Br J Haematol* **132**: 801–2; author reply 802–3.

32 Reddy P, Johnson K, Uberti JP, Reynolds C, Silver S, Ayash L, et al. (2006). Nephrotic syndrome associated with chronic graft-versus-host disease after allogeneic hematopoietic stem cell transplantation. *Bone Marrow Transplant* **38**: 351–7.

33 Terrier B, Delmas Y, Hummel A, Presne C, Glowacki F, Knebelmann B, et al. (2007). Post-allogeneic haematopoietic stem cell transplantation membranous nephropathy: clinical presentation, outcome and pathogenic aspects. *Nephrol Dial Transplant* **22**: 1369–76.

34 Beck Jr LH, Bonegio RG, Lambeau G, Beck DM, Powell DW, Cummins TD, et al. (2009). M-type phospholipase A2 receptor as target antigen in idiopathic membranous nephropathy. *N Engl J Med* **361**: 11–21.

35 Debiec H, Guigonis V, Mougenot B, Decobert F, Haymann JP, Bensman A, et al. (2002). Antenatal membranous glomerulonephritis due to anti-neutral endopeptidase antibodies. *N Engl J Med* **346**: 2053–60.

36 Romagnani P, Lazzeri E, Mazzinghi B, Lasagni L, Guidi S, Bosi A, et al. (2005). Nephrotic syndrome and renal failure after allogeneic stem cell transplantation: novel molecular diagnostic tools for a challenging differential diagnosis. *Am J Kidney Dis* **46**: 550–6.

37 Brukamp K, Doyle AM, Bloom RD, Bunin N, Tomaszewski JE, Cizman B (2006). Nephrotic syndrome after hematopoietic cell transplantation: do glomerular lesions represent renal graft-versus-host disease? *Clin J Am Soc Nephrol* **1**: 685–94.

38 Alpers CE, Cotran RS (1986). Neoplasia and glomerular injury. *Kidney Int* **30**: 465–73.

39 Murphy WJ (2000). Revisiting graft-versus-host disease models of autoimmunity: new insights in immune regulatory processes. *J Clin Invest* **106**: 745–7.

40 Hingorani S, Guthrie KA, Schoch G, Weiss NS, McDonald GB (2007). Chronic kidney disease in long-term survivors of hematopoietic cell transplant. *Bone Marrow Transplant* **39**: 223–9.

41 Cohen EP (2001). Renal failure after bone-marrow transplantation. *Lancet* **357**: 6–7.

42 Weiss AS, Sandmaier BM, Storer B, Storb R, McSweeney PA, Parikh CR (2006). Chronic kidney disease following non-myeloablative hematopoietic cell transplantation. *Am J Transplant* **6**: 89–94.

43 Cohen EP, Moulder JE (2005). Radiation nephropathy. In: *Cancer and the Kidney* (ed. EP Cohen), pp. 169–80. Oxford University Press, Oxford.

44 Cohen EP, Hussain S, Moulder JE (2003). Successful treatment of radiation nephropathy with angiotensin II blockade. *Int J Radiat Oncol Biol Phys* **55**: 190–3.

45 Cutler C, Kim HT, Hochberg E, Ho V, Alyea E, Lee SJ, et al. (2004). Sirolimus and tacrolimus without methotrexate as graft-versus-host disease prophylaxis after matched related donor peripheral blood stem cell transplantation. *Biol Blood Marrow Transplant* **10**: 328–36.

46 Miralbell R, Bieri S, Mermillod B, Helg C, Sancho G, Pastoors B, et al (1996). Renal toxicity after allogeneic bone marrow transplantation: the combined effects of total-body irradiation and graft-versus-host disease. *J Clin Oncol* **14**: 579–85.

47 Cutler C, Henry NL, Magee C, Li S, Kim HT, Alyea E, et al (2005). Sirolimus and thrombotic microangiopathy after allogeneic hematopoietic stem cell transplantation. *Biol Blood Marrow Transplant* **11**: 551–7.

48 Lawton CA, Barber-Derus SW, Murray KJ, Cohen EP, Ash RC, Moulder JE (1992). Influence of renal shielding on the incidence of late renal dysfunction associated with T-lymphocyte deplete bone marrow transplantation in adult patients. *Int J Radiat Oncol Biol Phys* **23**: 681–6.

49 Cohen EP (2000). Radiation nephropathy after bone marrow transplantation. *Kidney Int* **58**: 903–18.

50 Couriel D, Caldera H, Champlin R, Komanduri K (2004). Acute graft-versus-host disease: Pathophysiology, clinical manifestations, and management. *Cancer* **101**: 1936–46.

51 Magee C, Pascual M (2003). The growing problem of chronic renal failure after transplantation of a nonrenal organ. *N Engl J Med* **349**: 994–6.

52 Zarifian A, Meleg-Smith S, O'Donovan R, Tesi RJ, Batuman V (1999). Cyclosporine-associated thrombotic microangiopathy in renal allografts. *Kidney Int* **55**: 2457–66.

53 Young BA, Marsh CL, Alpers CE, Davis CL (1996). Cyclosporine-associated thrombotic microangiopathy/hemolytic uremic syndrome following kidney and kidney-pancreas transplantation. *Am J Kidney Dis* **28**: 561–71.

54 Eknoyan G (2003). Meeting the challenges of the new K/DOQI guidelines. *Am J Kidney Dis* **41**: 3–10.

55 Cohen EP, Irving AA, Drobyski WR, Klein JP, Passweg J, Talano JA, et al (2008). Captopril to mitigate chronic renal failure after hematopoietic stem cell transplantation: a randomized controlled trial. *Int J Radiat Oncol Biol Phys* **70**: 1546–51.

56 Palmer BF (2004). Managing hyperkalemia caused by inhibitors of the renin-angiotensin-aldosterone system. *N Engl J Med* **351**: 585–92.

57 George JN, Li X, McMinn JR, Terrell DR, Vesely SK, Selby GB (2004). Thrombotic thrombocytopenic purpura-hemolytic uremic syndrome following allogeneic HPC transplantation: a diagnostic dilemma. *Transfusion* **44**: 294–304.

58 Cohen EP, Drobyski WR, Moulder JE (2007). Significant increase in end-stage renal disease after hematopoietic stem cell transplantation. *Bone Marrow Transplant* **39**: 571–2.

59 Cohen EP, Piering WF, Kabler-Babbitt C, Moulder JE (1998). End-stage renal disease (ESRD) after bone marrow transplantation: poor survival compared to other causes of ESRD. *Nephron* **79**: 408–12.

60 Hamawi K, De Magalhaes-Silverman M, Bertolatus JA (2003). Outcomes of renal transplantation following bone marrow transplantation. *Am J Transplant* **3**: 301–5.

61 Butcher JA, Hariharan S, Adams MB, Johnson CP, Roza AM, Cohen EP (1999). Renal transplantation for end-stage renal disease following bone marrow transplantation: a report of six cases, with and without immunosuppression. *Clin Transplant* **13**: 330–5.

62 Gruss E, Bernis C, Tomas JF, Garcia-Canton C, Figuera A, Motellon JL, et al (1995). Acute renal failure in patients following bone marrow transplantation: prevalence, risk factors and outcome. *Am J Nephrol* **15**: 473–9.

Chapter 9

Acute renal failure in cancer patients*

Jasmin Levallois and Martine Leblanc

Case report

A 66-year-old man presented in our emergency room in November 2008 for marked fatigue and nausea. Initial laboratory findings showed a serum creatinine of 1236 µmol/L and a serum urea of 30.8 mmol/L. Electrolytes were as follows: K+ 5.8 mmol/L, corrected total calcium 2.38 mmol/L, phosphate 2.35 mmol/L. On the complete blood count, the hemoglobin was 126 g/L and a mild eosinophilia was noticed. He had no significant past medical history besides mild chronic obstructive pulmonary disease (COPD) and controlled hypertension. He mentioned loss of appetite and a weight reduction of 15 pounds over the last six weeks. The work-up found a monoclonal gammopathy and a bone marrow biopsy was performed. It showed hypercellularity (85%) of which 75% was due to atypical plasmocytes. A monoclonal Lambda multiple myeloma (IgD) was diagnosed. Plasma exchanges and intermittent hemodialysis were performed alternatively while awaiting the results of a kidney biopsy. Renal ultrasound showed a right kidney of 11.1 cm and a left kidney of 12.3 cm in diameter, with mild hyperechogenicity. The kidney biopsy revealed an altered tubulo-interstitium with the presence of tubular casts (Lambda+) associated with acute tubular necrosis lesions. The aspect of the glomeruli was normal with no evidence of amyloidosis. Chronic vascular lesions suggestive of hypertensive changes were also described. The final conclusion was compatible with Lambda cast nephropathy. Despite prompt chemotherapy, renal function did not improve, urine output decreased, and the patient remained dialysis-dependent. In early December 2009, the patient was readmitted for failure to thrive and a blastic transformation was found on the repeated bone marrow sampling. His prognosis is poor.

Classification of acute renal failure

Acute renal failure (ARF) is an important complication in oncologic patients that will negatively affect their outcome. Although ARF is frequent in hospitalized patients, epidemiologic data on its impact on morbidity and mortality of

---

* This chapter is an updated version of the original chapter written by Facundo Lugones and Martine Leblanc in the previous edition.

the oncologic population is scarce. However, it is clear that ARF has the potential to alter the outcome of cancer patients and sometimes prevent them from receiving optimal treatment. (1)

ARF is defined as a sustained and abrupt decline, within hours to days, of the glomerular filtration rate (GFR) (2–5). It usually alters extracellular volume status, electrolytes, and acid-base balance, and causes retention of nitrogen products released from protein catabolism (2, 5). Until recently, there was no consensus on the definition of ARF. The Acute Dialysis Quality Initiative group (ADQI) and more recently the Acute Kidney Injury Network (AKIN) proposed the broader term AKI for acute kidney injury as well as the RIFLE (Risk-Injury-Failure-Loss-ESRD) criteria for acute renal dysfunction, defining injury as a doubling of baseline serum creatinine or a GFR decrease >50% and failure as a tripling of serum creatinine or GFR decrease >75% (6). Several studies have shown that the RIFLE system is directly related to outcomes in critically ill patients with acute kidney injury (AKI) (7–9) (see Fig. 9.1 and Table 9.1).

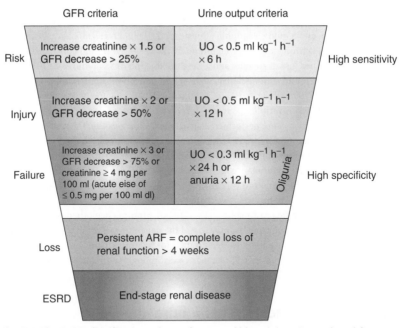

Fig. 9.1 The RIFLE classification scheme for acute kidney injury. Reproduced from Bellomo R, Ronco C, Kellum JA, et al; Acute Dialysis Quality Initiative workgroup: Acute renal failure–definition, outcome measures, animal models, fluid therapy and informations technology needs: The Second International Consensus Conference of the Acute Dialysis Quality Initiative (ADQI) Group. *CritCare* 2004;**8**:R204–R212. Copyright 2004 Bellomo et al; licensee BioMed Central Ltd.
* for serum creatinine, 4 mg/ dl = 350 μmol/L

Table 9.1 Classification/staging system for acute kidney injury (AKI)*

AKI stage	Serum creatinine criteria	Urine output criteria
1	Absolute increase ≥26.4 µmol/L (0.3 mg/dL) Or Value is 1.5–2X baseline value	<0.5 mL/kg/hr for >6 hr
2	Value is 2–3X baseline value	<0.5 mL/kg/hr for > 12 hr
3	Value ≥350 µmol/L (4.0 mg/dL) with absolute increase ≥44 µmol/L (0.5 mg/dL) Or Patient is receiving renal replacement therapy	<0.3 mL/kg/hr x 24 hr Or Anuria x 12 hr

* According to the 2005 AKIN (Acute Kidney Injury Network) Consensus Meeting modification of the RIFLE (risk, injury, failure, loss, end-stage renal disease) classification. Only one criterion (serum creatinine or urine output) has to be fulfilled for the case to qualify for a stage.

Renal failure in cancer patients is often multi-factorial; however, for diagnostic purposes and clinical management, the multiple causes of ARF are classified according to practical pathophysiology (2, 5, 10–16). Pre-renal causes represent the majority of cases of hospital-acquired ARF. The renal response to hypoperfusion is characterized by a fast and reversible rise in serum urea and creatinine. If the effective blood flow is rapidly restored, renal function returns to normal since the integrity of renal tissue is preserved. Intra-renal ARF occurs with pathologies affecting renal parenchyma. The spectrum of intrinsic renal diseases in the cancer population is broad and includes diseases of the renal vessels, glomeruli, and tubulo-intersitium. A frequent cause of intrinsic ARF is acute tubular necrosis secondary to renal hypoperfusion and/or toxins. Post-renal ARF is due to obstruction of the urinary tract usually distal to the bladder.

While the general approach to ARF in cancer patients is not different from that used in relation to other patients, there are some particularities that will be specified in this chapter.

Pre-renal ARF

Any reduction in renal perfusion can cause pre-renal ARF. It is a physiologic response to a decreased effective circulating volume. Renal parenchyma remains characteristically intact and renal function returns to normal when perfusion is restored.

Cancer patients appear particularly susceptible to pre-renal ARF for multiple reasons, including high comorbidity and exposure to multiple interventions. Pre-renal azotemia is commonly found in association with dehydration secondary to mucositis-related gastrointestinal losses, or bleeding due to thrombocytopenia or surgeries, or third spacing (17). Superior vena cava syndrome, pericardial effusion, and tamponade with or without myocardial dysfunction due to chemotherapy (e.g. doxorubicin) can reduce cardiac output and result in pre-renal ARF. Hepatorenal syndrome refers to ARF in the setting of advanced hepatic disease, such as liver metastases or veno-occlusive disease of the liver (VOD) after allogenic bone marrow transplant (BMT), and is associated with marked renal vasoconstriction (18).

Sepsis, a relatively common complication in cancer patients receiving chemotherapy or after BMT, may impair renal function through hemodynamic factors (ineffective circulation and altered local renal hemodynamics), but immunologic, toxic, and inflammatory mechanisms are also likely to be at work (19, 20). In addition, cancer patients often receive non-steroidal anti-inflammatory drugs (NSAIDs) that can precipitate pre-renal azotemia in a context of poor hydration or extra-renal fluid losses. Capillary leak syndrome associated with interleukin-2 administration may also induce pre-renal failure (21).

In pre-renal ARF, perfusion and glomerular filtration are maintained during moderate hypotension by autoregulation mechanisms that are effective until the mean arterial pressure falls below 60–70 mmHg (22). Autoregulation of renal blood flow is an attempt to maintain GFR constant at different levels of arterial pressure (4). This is achieved by afferent arteriolar vasodilatation (to decrease pre-glomerular resistance) as well as predominant efferent arteriolar vasoconstriction (23). When not corrected, persistent renal hypoperfusion will eventually lead to ischemic acute tubular necrosis.

Acute tubular necrosis (ATN)

Cancer patients are at high risk for pre-renal failure which frequently evolves towards ATN. Other causes of ATN include nephrotoxic compounds and intravascular hemolysis. In established ATN, there is evidence of renal vasoconstriction further reducing glomerular blood flow; this contrasts with the normal auto-regulatory renal vasodilatation that should occur in response to decreased perfusion pressure. Another important component is tubular cell injury and tubular obstruction (5). ATN is actually a misnomer since the presence of tubular necrosis upon histological examination of the kidney is only seen in occasional tubule cells, and much of the injury relevant to ARF remains sublethal (24). The most susceptible tubular segments are located in the outer medulla, a zone that is susceptible to ischemic injury.

Post-renal ARF

Serum creatinine can be maintained at normal levels by a single kidney. A lower urinary tract obstruction can produce azotemia if it occurs at the urethra or bladder neck. An upper obstruction is ureteral or intratubular (intra-renal). Rarely, an upper obstruction will cause renal failure if it involves

Table 9.2 Potential etiologies of postrenal ARF

Ureteral obstruction (bilateral or unilateral if single kidney)

Extra-ureteral
- Tumor: uterus, prostate
- Endometriosis
- Aneurysm of abdominal aorta
- Accidental surgical ligature
- Retroperitoneal hematoma

Intra-ureteral
- Lithiasis
- Uric acid crystals
- Clots
- Cellular debris (in papillary necrosis)
- Oedema
- Fungus ball

Vesical bladder obstruction
- Lithiasis
- Clots
- Tumor; uterus, prostate, bladder
- Functional: neurogenic bladder, medication

Urethral obstruction
- Congenital valve
- Stenosis

both ureteral lumens or the ureteral lumen of a single functioning kidney. Obstruction elevates the intratubular pressure which translates at the glomerular level by a reversal of the driving forces of glomerular filtration. Cancer patients are at risk for obstructive ARF (see Table 9.2).

Specific causes of acute renal failure in cancer patients

Hypercalcemia

Severe hypercalcemia is a specific cause of pre-renal ARF secondary to an associated nephrogenic diabetes insipidus. Cancer is one of the most common causes of hypercalcemia (25–26). Various cancers can cause hypercalcemia, including lung, breast, and kidney, as well as myeloma and prostate cancer.

Hypercalcemia of malignancy can be classified into different types or mechanisms: local osteolytic bone resorption, humoral hypercalcemia, and 1,25-vitamin-D overproduction (25–27). In patients with local osteolytic hypercalcemia secondary to extensive bone metastasis (typically breast cancer), the hypercalcemia results from the marked increase in osteoclastic bone resorption in areas surrounding the malignant cells secondary to resorptive cytokines (IL-1, IL-6, TGF-alpha, TNF-alpha). Multiple myeloma produces destructive bone lesions but unlike metastases of solid tumors, resorption is accompanied by an increased bone formation secondary to osteoblastic activity. In humoral hypercalcemia of malignancy (HHM), bone resorption is caused by secretion of parathyroid related protein (PTHrP) by malignant tumors with or without direct bone involvement such as squamous cell cancers of various organs, renal cancer, ovarian cancer and others. This hormone has paracrine and systemic effects similar to PTH on bone and kidney; thus PTHrP enhances bone resorption and renal reabsorption of calcium and phosphate. A less frequent mechanism is overproduction of 1,25-dihydroxyvitamin D3 in certain hematologic malignancies (Hodgkin's and non Hodgkin's lymphomas), resulting in intestinal absorption of calcium.

Clinical manifestations of hypercalcemia relate to its degree and rapidity of development. Symptoms can be general (anorexia, pruritus, polydipsia, polyuria, dehydration), neuromuscular (lethargy, muscle weakness, hyporeflexia, seizure, psychosis, obtundation, coma), gastrointestinal (vomiting, constipation, ileus), and/or cardiac (bradycardia, prolonged PR and shortened QT intervals, atrial or ventricular arrhythmias) (28). Nephrolithiasis and nephrocalcinosis, as consequences of interstitial deposition of calcium-phosphate complexes, can occur.

Treatment of cancer-related hypercalcemia is directed at the underlying disease. However, acute severe hypercalemia (>3.5 mmol/L) requires immediate treatment. Large volumes of normal saline given intravenously to enable volume repletion and enhanced urine calcium elimination (26, 29). Loop diuretics may be used although the efficacy of this historical practice was challenged by a recent systematic review (30). If diuretics are used, it should be only after normovolemia has been reached, otherwise they could worsen dehydration. Inhibition of bone resorption with bisphosphonates, e.g. by a single intravenous dose of pamidronate 30–90 mg, is effective for many weeks. Calcitonin given subcutaneously (4–8 IU/kg) has a rapid onset and minimal toxicity but a transient effect. Corticosteroids are effective in hematologic malignancies (myeloma, lymphoma, leukemia), exerting a cytostatic effect. Renal replacement therapy with low calcium dialysate may be needed for patients with renal failure. In general, dialysis should be considered in the treatment of cancer-related hypercalcemia when the GFR is below 20 mL per minute, or when the presence of congestive heart failure contraindicates the administration of saline (26).

Tumor lysis syndrome

Tumor lysis syndrome (TLS) is a critical condition resulting from massive cell death leading to severe hyperuricemia, hyperphosphatemia, hyperkalemia, hypocalcemia, and ARF in patients with high cell turnover tumors. It can be observed with high-grade lymphomas (particularly Burkitt's lymphoma), high leukocyte count leukemias, and less commonly with solid tumors, during rapid cellular destruction induced by chemotherapy. Although spontaneous TLS may rarely occur prior to any cancer treatment, hyperphosphatemia in such cases may not be as severe as after cytoreductive treatment. The clinical profile of patients at risk of TLS includes age < 25 years, male sex, lymphoproliferative disease with extensive abdominal burden, high serum LDH concentrations, volume depletion, acid and concentrated urine (31–33) (see Table 9.3).

During massive cellular lysis, released metabolites rapidly enter the circulation; enhanced renal elimination soon becomes insufficient, in part because of dehydration or underlying kidney impairment. In the pathophysiology of ARF in TLS, extracellular volume depletion and overload of uric acid and phosphate both play a role (31). A decrease in intravascular volume leads to a pre-renal state as well as to an increase in tubular uric acid concentration. Cellular breakdown of nucleic acids leads to purine release, and catabolism of hypoxanthine and xanthine by xanthine oxidase forms uric acid. At a

Table 9.3 Cairo–Bishop grading classification of tumor lysis syndrome

	Grade 0*	Grade I	Grade III	Grade IV	Grade V
LTLS	-	+	+	+	+
Creatinine	≤1.5XULN	1.5XULN	>3–6XULN	>6XULN	Death
Cardiac arrhythmia	None	Intervention not indicated	Symptomatic and incompletely controlled medically or controlled with device (e.g. defibrillator)	Life-threatening (e.g. arrhythmia associated with CHF, hypotension, syncope, shock)	Death
Seizure	None	One brief generalized seizure; seizure(s) well controlled by anticonvulsants or infrequent focal motor seizures not interfering with ADL	Seizure in which consciousness is altered; poorly controlled seizure disorder; with breakthrough generalized seizures despite medical intervention	Seizure of any kind which are prolonged, repetitive or difficult to control (e.g. status epilepticus, intractable epilepsy)	Death

LTLS = No laboratory tumor lysis syndrome
ULN = Upper limit of normal
Clinical tumor lysis syndrome requires one or more clinical manifestations along with criteria for LTLS
Reproduced with permission from Cairo MS, Bishop M (October 2004). Tumor lysis syndrome: new therapeutic strategies and classification. *Br. J. Haematol.* **127** (1): 3–11.

physiological pH, it is totally ionized; however, in the renal tubules, it becomes less ionized and insoluble. In the distal collecting system, urine is satured in uric acid and crystals may form, especially in an acid urine, leading to luminal obstruction and decreased GFR (34). Hyperphosphatemia may cause ARF by precipitation of calcium phosphate complexes in the renal interstitium and tubular system resulting in acute nephrocalcinosis (32, 35).

Aggressive intravenous hydration and diuresis are needed for the prevention of TLS and to enhance the excretion of uric acid. Urine alkalinization with sodium bicarbonate, has historically been recommended to enhance uric acid elimination, but its use is controversial and not recommended in recently published guidelines by the American Society of Oncology (ASO) (33). Two medications are available to reduce uric acid. Allopurinol decreases uric acid formation by inhibiting xanthine oxidase. Allopurinol may rarely lead to enhanced urinary xanthine and hypoxanthine; it has therefore been implicated in xanthine nephropathy (36). Urate oxidase is an enzyme that catalyzes the enzymatic oxidation of uric acid into allantoin, which is five times more soluble than uric acid. Rasburicase, a recombinant form of the urate oxidase enzyme, has been shown in children and adults as a safe and very effective alternative to allopurinol, allowing more rapid control and lower levels of plasma uric acid. The recently published guidelines by the ASO recommend the use of rasburicase for adults and children with TLS prone cancers for prevention and management of TLS (33)

With oliguric ARF, renal replacement may be required. Although the dialysis requirement in TLS has been reduced since the introduction of rasburicase, as many as 5% of adult patients still require renal replacement (37). Peritoneal dialysis is insufficient since achieved clearances for uric acid and phosphorus are low. Multiple modalities may be used in the management of TLS including conventional intermittent hemodialysis and continuous renal replacement therapies (CRRTs) (38). In adult TLS, phosphorus influx into the extracellular milieu can exceed 6 g/d. Such a solute burden has been effectively managed using CRRT with dialysate and replacement flow rates of 4L/h or more. These continuous methods were found almost equivalent to two 4-hour hemodialysis sessions/day (39–40).

Myeloma

Renal failure (RF) is a common complication of multiple myeloma. At the time of diagnosis, up to 40% of patients have evidence of renal impairment (41). Renal failure may shorten survival, but in some series, reversal of myeloma nephropathy occurs in 50% of patients and is associated with better long-term survival (42–43).

Plasma cells synthesize light chains independently from heavy chains and combine them in their endoplasmic reticulum, thus forming immunoglobulins. When a plasma cell clone exists, over-production of homogeneous, free light chains are released and can appear as Bence–Jones in urine. Monoclonal light chains cause renal damage by different mechanisms and in various segments of the nephron. Renal failure is caused mainly by the toxic effects of monoclonal light chains to renal tubules.

Light chain cast nephropathy represents the main cause of acute reversible renal impairment during myeloma (41, 44). Light chains (15 to 45 kDa) filter the glomeruli and are absorbed in the proximal tubules by endocytosis. There, they are degraded by lysosomal enzymes. In cast nephropathy, excess light chain production overcomes the capacity of the tubular cells to catabolize the free light chains. These then accumulate in the tubular fluid of distal nephron segments where they form tubular casts (Fig. 9.2). Casts contain Bence–Jones proteins coaggregated with the glycopeptide portion of Tamm–Horsfall protein. The histology shows intratubular protein casts located in the distal nephron surrounded by macrophages (Fig. 9.3).

While other factors often contribute to ARF in the myeloma patient, such as dehydration, hypercalcemia, nephrotoxic drugs (antibiotics, non-steroidal

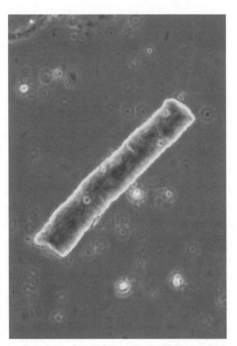

Fig. 9.2 Waxy cast in the urine of a patient with multiple myeloma.

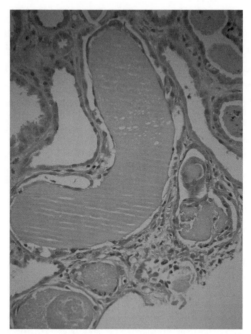

Fig. 9.3 Casts in a biopsy from a kidney of a patient with multiple myeloma.

anti-inflammatory drugs) and the use of contrast agents, these factors are rarely the primary reason for renal failure. Nonetheless, the finding of renal insufficiency with light chains in the urine is not necessarily diagnostic of light chain cast nephropathy. Serum dosing of free light chains is a useful diagnostic tool and serum levels above 500 mg/L are expected if renal failure is related to cast nephropathy. Other clinicopathological renal conditions associated with multiple myeloma include amyloidosis, light chain deposition disease, and interstitial nephritis (41, 45). To distinguish among these, a renal biopsy may be needed (45).

Therapy for cast nephropathy is directed at avoiding intratubular precipitation of light chains and reducing their production (41). Fluid intake resulting in a 2–3L daily alkaline diuresis is indicated. Loop diuretics should be used with caution to treat hypercalcemia owing to the adverse impact in the formation of casts in the renal tubule (46). Potential nephrotoxics (aminoglycosides, NSAIDs, and contrast media) should be avoided as much as possible. Hypercalcemia must be corrected by hydration and prompt intitiation of antimyeloma therapy, which includes steroids. Although urine alkalinization by itself has not been shown clearly benefical in humans, data from animal models suggest that alkalinization and low sodium chloride concentration in the distal nephron help prevent cast formation (46). The usefulness of plasmapheresis to rapidly reduce paraprotein levels while awaiting chemotherapy effect is controversial. In a recent trial, the routine addition of plasma exchange to conventional treatment did not improve either recovery from renal failure or patient survival (47). Dialysis should be started early to avoid uremia complications and to compensate the hypercatabolic state induced by high-dose steroids. If dialysis is required, recovery of renal function may be delayed by several months, but chronic dialysis is often needed. Newer approaches with highly permeable dialyzers to remove light chains before permanent renal damage has occurred appear promising (48).

Lymphoma-leukemia and kidney infiltration

Renal infiltration is not unusual in patients with lymphoma or leukemia. Approximately 30% and 50% of patients with lymphoma and leukemia, respectively, have kidney involvement at autopsy (49, 50). The infiltration is typically diffuse, bilateral. and symmetrical. However, this only rarely leads to significant renal dysfunction, and ARF is rarely the initial manifestation of lymphoma (51). Clinical manifestations of kidney lymphomatous infiltration are rather nonspecific, including flank pain, hematuria, abdominal distension, or palpable mass. Extra-renal symptoms (fever, weight loss, general malaise) may be present in such cases. Urinalysis can reveal microscopic hematuria and mild proteinuria. Imaging shows enlarged kidneys (51). Rapid renal function improvement and parallel decrease of kidney size have both been documented after chemotherapy/radiotherapy (50). Renal metastases from solid tumors occur infrequently, and only few case reports have been published (52).

ARF after bone marrow transplantation

Acute renal failure is one of the most frequent complications of bone marrow transplantation (BMT). The development of ARF seems to carry a negative impact on overall outcome in BMT patients, especially if severe enough to require dialysis. There are three types of hematopoeietic cell transplantation: (a) *myeloablative autologous* which involves high-dose myeloablative therapy for cancer followed by infusion of the patient's own stem cells; (b) *myeloablative allogeneic transplantation*, in which the infused stem cells derive from a donor who is another person; (c) *nonmyeloablative allogeneic transplantation* (mini-allo) which uses a lower dose of radiation and/or chemotherapy with subsequent infusion of non-self hematopoietic stem cells. It may exerts his curative effect via a graft-vs.-tumor effect mediated by the non-self donor cells (53).

The incidence of ARF after bone marrow transplantation is higher in myeloablative compared to non-myeloablative BMT. In one study, severe ARF occurred in 73% of patients undergoing myeloablative conditioning, vs. 47% in those undergoing non-myeloablative regimens (54). With autologous BMT, the incidence of ARF is much lower (22%) because graft vs. host disease (GVHD) does not occur and immunosuppressive agents, potentially nephrotoxic, are not used (53).

The pathogenesis of ARF after BMT is complex and is often multi-factorial including volume depletion, ATN, nephrotoxic drugs, TLS, and/or sepsis. Several distinct syndromes have been categorized according to time of onset (55). Within the first few days after autologous BMT, AKI may develop from TLS or toxicity from the infused marrow. Because most patients are in remission at the time of transplantation and thanks to appropriate prophylaxis, the incidence of TLS in this population is uncommon. The most common period for ARF after BMT is between 10 and 20 days after the transplant. It is during this period that patients with BMT are most at high risk for sepsis due to profound neutropenia. Medication used for treating infections (e.g. aminoglycoside, amphotericin B) may cause renal damage in kidneys already suffering from hypoperfusion. Sinusoidal obstruction syndrome, also known as venoocclusive disease (VOD) of the liver, is one of the most common causes of severe ARF after myeloablative BMT (55–57). It is caused by chemotherapy-induced hepatic venular thrombosis resulting in portal hypertension. The incidence of VOD varies between 5% and 70%, of which about 50% develop ARF, with similarities with hepato-renal syndrome. At least two of the following criteria are usually required to diagnose VOD: serum total bilirubin >34 μmol/L, hepatomegaly or right upper quadrant pain of liver origin, and rapid weight gain (>2 kg). Thrombotic microangiopathy may also occur within the first few months after BMT (58).

The mortality of ARF in the setting of BMT reaches 35% to 45%; it increases to more than 60% if ICU admission is required, increasing to above 80% if dialysis is needed, and it is nearly fatal if mechanical ventilation is needed (59–61). In a recent metanalysis in patients undergoing myeloablative allogeneic transplantation, the risk of death was independently related to the incidence of ARF, with a relative risk of death after ARF of 2.2 (p <0.001) (62). Mechanical ventilation is recognized as a predictor of poor outcome, suggesting a prognosis dismal enough to restrict its use in BMT patients (60–61, 63–67). In our center, ARF was present in 74% of BMT cases admitted to ICU for respiratory distress and hypotension (68). ARF occurred significantly more frequently with allogenic than autologous BMT. The prevalence of sepsis (83% versus 60%) and hepatic failure (69% versus 40%) were significantly higher in

ARF patients compared to those without ARF. ARF was usually considered multi-factorial by clinicians, being associated with extensive co-morbidity and multi-organ failure. ARF in this series occurred on average 27 days after BMT. Short-term mortality rates were higher in ARF vs. non-ARF BMT patients (88% versus 60%).

Nephrotoxic drugs

Many drugs and their metabolites are eliminated through the kidneys, sometimes causing potential toxic insults. Mechanisms of nephrotoxic drugs are very broad, including renal hemodynamic alterations, direct tubular injury, interstitial nephritis, and intratubular obstructions. The list of all the nephrotoxic drugs is very extensive but certain agents are particularly involved in the cancer population (1, 69).

Certain chemotherapeutics agents are commonly associated with nephrotoxicity but most of these cause subacute or chronic renal failure. Two agents are frequently associated with ARF: cisplatinum and methotrexate. Cisplatinum causes a nonoliguric renal impairment associated with relatively extensive tubular injury resulting in various electrolyte abnormalities. Cisplatinum-induced ARF is dose-dependent and can be minimized by means of hydration/forced diuresis. With current prototols, cisplatin is now associated with only mild renal failure and patients usually recover their renal function (1, 70).

Methotrexate (MTX) is an antimetabolite widely used in cancer treatment. In standard dose, either oral or intravenous, MTX is not nephrotoxic despite its 90% renal elimination. At high dose (>50 mg/kg), precipitation of the parent drug and the main metabolite (7-hydroxymethotrexate) occurs in renal tubules leading to ARF with rapid rise in serum creatinine (71). By appropriate hydration and urine alkalinization, one can prevent and/or greatly reduce tubular drug precipitation and renal injury (72). MTX-induced acute renal failure is reversible in almost all cases but when renal elimination of MTX is diminished, levels can rise progressively and accumulate to life-threatening levels. MTX-induced toxicity can be managed with a high dose of folinic acid (leucovorin) (73), hydration, and urine alkalinization. Peritoneal dialysis, hemodialysis, and plasma exchange do not increase MTX clearance because it is very much protein-bound.

Other chemotherapeutic agents, including cisplatin, bleomycin, mitomycin C, gemcitabine, and tamoxifen, may cause a thrombotic microangiopathy that resembles hemolytic uremic syndrome (74). This acute complication can be life-threatening. Discontinuing the offending drug is essential but efficacy of plasma therapy varies. Mitomycin-C (MMC) is an anti-tumor antibiotic that participates in alkylation reactions of DNA. The risk of developing hemolytic uremic syndrome (HUS) after therapy with MMC is between 4% and 15%, increasing when the cumulative dose exceeds 60 mg/m². Mortality rates above 50% have been observed after this complication (75).

Other agents commonly given to cancer patients can be nephrotoxic. They include some antibiotics, especially aminoglycosides, amphotericin B, and acyclovir. Aminoglycosides are excreted by glomerular filtration and toxicity may occur if the dose is not adjusted to renal clearance. Gentamicin serum levels should always be monitored to avoid toxicity (76). Single doses as compared to multiple daily doses of aminoglycosides have been suggested as less nephrotoxic but this has not been widely validated for neutropenic patients, and multiple daily doses may still be favored in such circumstances (77). The macrolide vancomycin, when used alone in recommended doses, is rarely toxic by itself. However, data suggests that concomitant use of an aminoglycoside is associated with an increased risk of renal toxicity (78). Amphotericin B is another potential cause of ARF but this is usually reversible when discontinuing treatment. The administration of amphotericin B in lipid emulsion as compared to standard dextrose solution has been found significantly less nephrotoxic (79). Intravenous acyclovir can crystallize in renal collecting tubules causing intratubular obstruction with reversible renal dysfunction.

NSAIDs and immunosupressants used in bone marrow transplant (e.g. cyclosporine/tacrolimus) can also be nephrotoxic. Cancer patients frequently receive more than one of these drugs during the course of their disease, leading them to higher risk of nephrotoxicity.

Cancer patients with pre-existing renal disease are particularly at risk of contrast-induced nephropathy. It is one of the most common causes of renal failure in hospitalized patients (80). Main risk factors include underlying chronic renal failure and diabetes. It is typically reversible and resolves within a few weeks, most often without dialysis. Unfortunately, sometimes the damage can be irreversible and lead to long-term need for dialysis. Use of intravenous crystalloid for volume expansion may prevent this complication (81).

Clinical and laboratory diagnosis of acute renal failure

When facing AKI in a cancer patient, it is always important to exclude a prerenal or a post-renal component. In addition, causes alternative to ATN should be considered in parenchymal ARF; indeed, the diagnosis of ATN becomes a diagnosis of exclusion. A complete clinical and drug history is essential since renal failure in hospitalized patients is often multi-factorial. If the duration of renal failure is uncertain, a few indices help distinguish an acute from a more chronic process. Small renal size/cortical hyperechogenicity, osteodystrophy, neuropathy, and anemia may all suggest chronicity of renal failure, although anemia is difficult to interpret in cancer patients.

Diuresis by itself does not indicate the etiology of AKI. However, anuria (<50 mL/d) suggests obstruction, rapidly progressive glomerulonephritis, or myeloma with tubular casts. Oliguria (<400 mL/d) is found in 50% to 60% of ATN cases.

Several indicators help differentiate pre-renal from renal failure (Table 9.4). Recently, a scoring system based on number on granular casts and renal tubular epithelial cells has been proposed to differentiate ATN from pre-renal AKI (Table 9.5) (82). With pre-renal ARF, the capacity to concentrate urine is preserved and high-urine osmolality is found, whereas in ATN, isosthenuria is expected. The two most reliable parameters for such a distinction are the fractional sodium excretion and the urinary/plasma creatinine ratio. Urine microscopy provides useful clues. Acute tubular necrosis is present when there are dirty brown casts, which are made of tubular cell debris and Tamm–Horsfall protein.

Management of acute renal failure

Prevention of AKI begins with avoidance of risk factors such as nephrotoxic drugs or constrast agents when possible and discontinuing certain drugs in high-risk situations (e.g. NSAIDs, angiotensin-conversion-enzyme inhibitors, or angiotensin receptor blockers).

Intravascular fluid expansion is clearly nephroprotective and is the mainstay for prevention of kidney injury (either from hypoperfusion or nephrotoxic agents such as contrast media) (83–85). However, the level of intravascular filling for optimal renal protection is not clearly established. Fluid resuscitation is

Table 9.4 Biochemical indices used to distinguish pre-renal and intrinsic ARF

	Pre-renal	Intrinsic
Osm (urine, mOsm/kg)	>500	<400
Na (urine, mmol/L)	<20	>40
Urea/creatinine (serum, mmol/μmol)	>0.1	<0.05
U/S creatinine (urine/serum)	>40	<20
U/S osmolality (urine/serum)	>1.5	>1
FE_{Na} (%)	<1	>2
FE_{urea} (%)	<35	>35

Fractional excretion (FE) is calculated as :
FE_{Na} = ([Na u/Na s]/ [creatinine u/creatinine s]) X 100
FE_{urea} = ([urea u/ urea s]/[creatinine u/creatinine s]) X 100

Table 9.5 Scoring system based on number of granular casts and renal tubular epithelial cells seen per high-power field for differentiating acute tubular necrosis from pre-renal acute kidney injury

Score description
1. RTE cells 0 and granular casts 0
2. RTE cells 0 and granular casts 1 to 5 or RTE cells 1 to 5 and granular casts 0
3. RTE cells 1 to 5 and granular casts 1 to 5 or RTE cells 0 and granular casts 6 to 10 or RTE cells 6 to 20 and granular casts 0

RTEC= renal tubular epithelial cells
From Perazella MA et al. Diagnostic value of urine microscopy for differential diagnosis of acute kidney injury in hospitalized patients. *Clin J Am Soc Nephrol*, **3**: 1615–1619, 2008.

based on clinical evaluation and can sometimes be assisted by invasive monitoring in the ICU. From a clinical perspective, maintenance of renal blood flow is highly desirable to prevent ARF given the vulnerability of the kidney to hypoxia. Therefore, besides restoring an adequate cardiac output and refilling intravascular volume, attempts should be made to maintain adequate arterial blood pressure. When volume expansion does not suffice, vasopressors are required, and may improve renal perfusion in hypotensive patients (83).

Many drugs have been tried in the primary prevention of AKI. Unfortunately, none conclusively demonstrated protection against ARF. Loop diuretics inhibit solute reabsorption at Henle's loop, and may facilitate the management of ARF by converting oliguria to non-oliguria. However, there is no evidence that loop diuretics prevent renal injury, improve mortality, or accelerate renal recovery in such a setting and, at high dose, they may be associated with ototoxicity (86). There is also strong evidence against the use of low-dose dopamine for prevention of ARF (87).

There is a lack of non-dialytic treatments so far and there is no clear guideline as to when renal replacement therapy (RRT) should be initiated in AKI (88). Oliguric ARF may require renal replacement earlier than non-oliguric ARF because of more difficult fluid management. Besides fluid overload, electrolyte abnormalities (hyperkalemia, hyperphosphatemia, hyponatremia) and metabolic acidosis associated with ARF are often the main indications for initiating dialysis. The degree of azotemia per se is not always easy to assess in ARF; in cancer patients, serum urea concentration may be particularly high because of a pre-renal component and enhanced catabolism due to corticosteroids, fever, or infections. Conversely, the serum urea concentrations usually considered alarming and indicating true need for dialysis, e.g.35 mmol/L, may not always indicate a severe ARF or need for renal replacement in cancer patients. When the GFR falls below 10 mL/min, dialytic support should be strongly considered to avoid uremic complications. Unfortunately, GFR is difficult to assess precisely.

Daily urinary collections are time-consuming and are not accurate in rapidly evolving situations. Equations to estimate GFR are also invalid when patients are not in a steady state. Finally, GFR measurements by nuclear markers are relatively expensive and unpractical. Therefore, one is left with clinical judgment to decide on the appropriate timing to initiate dialysis. Newer biomarkers potentially indicating AKI earlier than traditional parameters are of growing interest and should become extremely useful tools in the near future (89). As discussed in previous sections, besides traditional indications for initiating extracorporeal therapy in ARF, cancer patients may present particular indications such as hyperuricemia, hypercalcemia, TLS, or drug removal.

Renal replacement for ARF may include intermittent hemodialysis or CRRTs. It is generally accepted that CRRT confers an advantage over intermittent conventional hemodialysis in regard to hemodynamic stability. The available evidence, however, demonstrates no clear difference, in terms of clinically relevant outcomes, between continuous vs. intermittent modalities, even among the sickest patients with multi-organ failure (88, 90). In most patients, three to four intermittent dialysis sessions per week of four or more hours using blood flows of 300 mL/min or greater are usually sufficient. Some clinicians may still prefer CRRT in critically ill patients with ARF and severe hemodynamic instability. If using CRRT, since the target dose of 35 mL/kg per hour recommended following the Ronco study was challenged by the recent ATN and RENAL studies, no firm recommendation can be made at this point (88, 91–3).

Adequate protein and caloric intake is essential to ARF patients. Protein catabolism can be substantial in ARF, oftentimes above 250 g/day (94). Cancer, sepsis, and steroids have the potential to further increase catabolism. Such an increased protein degradation may accelerate the elevations in potassium, acid, and phosphate concentrations. Since a negative nitrogen balance accelerates endogenous proteolysis and muscle wasting and further impairs immune functions, efforts should be directed at obtaining a neutral or slightly positive nitrogen balance. The recommended protein intake should reach at least 1.2–1.8 g/kg/d in ARF, depending on the coexisting risk factors such as severe malnutrition, magnitude of hypermetabolic state, and whether the patient is receiving dialysis (95–6). Amino acid amounts lost through renal replacement should be accounted for (e.g. with CRRT, an additional 15g can easily be lost daily and should be replaced) (97). Feeding via the enteral route is by far preferable to parenteral alimentation when possible, since it keeps intestinal mucosa active and reduces bacterial translocation (98).

The approach to anemia management in the ICU has changed since the TRICC (transfusion requirements in critical care) trial, which showed no benefit of transfusing above a hemoglobin threshold of 70 g/L in patients without coronary disease (99–101). Erythropoietin (EPO) has not been formally evaluated in ARF patients even though animal studies suggest that erythropoietin administration could accelerate renal recovery (102). The use of erythropoietin supplementation has shown several benefits in chronic renal failure but may be associated with an increase of stroke in high doses (103) and there are some data suggesting an increase in mortality in cancer patients (104). Its use for critical illness is also controversial and may be associated with an increase in thromboembolic events (105). Available data suggests that EPO should thus not be used in cancer patients with ARF.

Advanced care planning (or advanced directives in health care) may be extremely useful in cancer patients and helps to ensure that consent will be respected should the patient become unable to participate in treatment decisions. Vague terms such as 'heroic or extraordinary' measures and 'unlikely recovery' may however make decisions difficult. Even severe ARF is potentially reversible; thus, ARF should not be the sole element in the decision process. In cancer patients, the decision to continue aggressive care may depend on the type and prognosis of the tumor, as well as the degree of co-morbidity. Age alone is not an acceptable predictor of mortality and quality of life after critical illness (106). On the other hand, there are limits to the physician's obligation. Indeed, according to ethical principles, physicians are not ethically required to provide unreasonable or futile care to patients who are considered critically or terminally ill with almost no chance of recovery (107). In some cases, a therapeutic trial may be the better option, whereas in others, improved palliative and comfort care will reduce prolonged suffering and improve the quality of death. At this point, it becomes a case-by-case story …

References

1 Lameire N, Flombaum C, Moreau D, Ronco C (2005). Acute renal failure in cancer patients. *Ann Med* **37**: 13–25.

2 Brady H, Singer G (1995). Acute renal failure. *Lancet* **346**: 1533–40.

3 Mindell J, Chertow G (1997). A practical approach to acute renal failure. *Med Clin North Am* **81**: 731–748.

4 Ratcliffe P (1998). The pathophysiology of acute renal failure. In: *Oxford Textbook of Clinical Nephrology* (ed. A Davison, JP Grünfeld, D Kerr et al.), pp. 1531–56. Oxford University Press, Oxford.

5 Lameire N, Van Biesen W and Vanholder R (2005). Acute renal failure. *Lancet* **365**: 417–30.

6 Bellomo R, Ronco C, Kellum JA, Mehta RL, Palevsky P. Acute Dialysis Quality Initiative (2004). Acute renal failure-definition, outcome measures, animal models, fluid therapy and information technology needs: the Second International Consensus Conference of the Acute Dialysis Quality Initiative (ADQI) Group. *Crit Care* **8**: R204–12.

7 Abosaif N, Tolba Y, Heap M, Russell J, El Nahas A (2005). The outcome of acute renal failure in the intensive care unit according to RIFLE: model application, sensitivity, and predictability. *Am J Kidney Dis* **46**: 1038–48.

8 Kuitunen A, Vento A, Suojaranta-Ylinen R and Pettilä V (2006). Acute renal failure after cardiac surgery: evaluation of the RIFLE classification. *Ann Thorac Surg* **81**: 542–6.

9 Bell M, Liljestam E, Granath F, Fryckstedt J, Ekbom A and Martling C (2005). Optimal follow-up time after continuous renal replacement therapy in actual renal failure patients stratified with the RIFLE criteria. *Nephrol Dial Transplant* **20**: 354–60.

10 Humphreys B, Soiffer R and Magee C (2005). Renal failure associated with cancer and its treatment: an update. *J Am Soc Nephrol* **16**: 151–61.

11 Anderson R (2001). Clinical and laboratory diagnosis of acute renal failure. In: *Acute renal failure: a companion to Brenner & Rector's the Kidney* (ed. B Molitoris), pp. 157–68. Saunders Company, Philadelphia.

12 Givens M, Wethern J (2009). Renal complications in oncologic patients. *Emerg Med Clin North Am* **27**: 283–91.

13 Darmon M, Ciroldi M, Thiery G, Schlemmer B, Azoulay E (2006). Clinical review: specific aspects of acute renal failure in cancer patients. *Crit Care* **10**: 211.

14 Lameire N, Van Biesen W, Vanholder R (2008). Acute renal problems in the critically ill cancer patient. *Curr Opin Crit Care* **14**: 635–46.

15 Kapoor M, Chan G (2001). Malignancy and renal disease. *Crit Care Clin* **17**: 571–98, viii.

16 Lameire N (2007). The kidney in oncology. *Acta Clin Belg* **62**: 141–54.

17 Da Silva JJ, Mesler D (2001). Acute renal failure as a result of malignancy.In: *Acute renal failure: a companion to Brenner & Rector's the Kidney* (ed. B Molitoris), pp. 312–21. Saunders Company, Philadelphia.

18 Munoz S (2008). The hepatorenal syndrome. *Med Clin North Am* **92**: 813–37, viii–ix.

19 Wan L, Bellomo R, Di Giantomasso D, Ronco C (2003). The pathogenesis of septic acute renal failure. *Curr Opin Crit Care* **9**: 496–502.

20 Bellomo R, Wan L, Langenberg C, May C (2008). Septic acute kidney injury: new concepts. *Nephron Exp Nephrol* **109**: e95–100.

21 Guleria A, Yang J, Topalian S, et al. (1994). Renal dysfunction associated with the administration of high-dose interleukin-2 in 199 consecutive patients with metastatic melanoma or renal carcinoma. *J Clin Oncol* **12**: 2714–22.

22 Badr K, Ichikawa I (1988). Pre-renal failure: a deleterious shift from renal compensation to decompensation. *N Engl J Med* **319**: 623–9.

23 Johnson P (1986). Autoregulation of blood flow. *Circ Res* **59**: 483–95.

24 Schrier RW, Wang W, Poole B, Mitra A (2004). Acute renal failure: definitions, diagnosis, pathogenesis, and therapy. *J Clin Invest* **114**: 5–14.

25 Lumachi F, Brunello A, Roma A, Basso U (2009). Cancer-induced Hypercalcemia. *Anticancer Res* **29**: 1551–5.

26 Stewart A (2005). Clinical practice. Hypercalcemia associated with cancer. *N Engl J Med* **352**: 373–9.

27 Clines G, Guise T (2005). Hypercalcaemia of malignancy and basic research on mechanisms responsible for osteolytic and osteoblastic metastasis to bone. *Endocr Relat Cancer* **12**: 549–83.

28 Bushinsky D, Monk R (1998). Electrolyte quintet: Calcium. *Lancet* **352**: 306–11.

29 Lumachi F, Brunello A, Roma A, Basso U (2008). Medical treatment of malignancy-associated hypercalcemia. *Curr Med Chem* **15**: 415–21.

30 LeGrand S, Leskuski D, Zama I (2008). Narrative review: furosemide for hypercalcemia: an unproven yet common practice. *Ann Intern Med* **149**: 259–63.

31 Davidson M, Thakkar S, Hix J, Bhandarkar N, Wong A, Schreiber M (2004). Pathophysiology, clinical consequences, and treatment of tumor lysis syndrome. *Am J Med* **116**: 546–54.

32 Haas M, Ohler L, Watzke H, Böhmig G, Prokesch R, Druml W (1999). The spectrum of acute renal failure in tumour lysis syndrome. *Nephrol Dial Transplant* **14**: 776–9.

33 Coiffier B, Altman A, Pui C, Younes A, Cairo M (2008). Guidelines for the management of pediatric and adult tumor lysis syndrome: an evidence-based review. *J Clin Oncol* **26**: 2767–78.

34 Klinenberg J, Kippen I, Bluestone R (1975). Hyperuricemic nephropathy: pathologic features and factors influencing urate deposition. *Nephron* **14**: 88–98.

35 Boles J, Dutel J, Briere J, Mialon P, Robasckiewicz M, Garre M (1984). Acute renal failure caused by extreme hyperphosphatemia after chemotherapy of an acute lymphoblastic leukemia. *Cancer* **53**: 2425–9.

36 LaRosa C, McMullen L, Bakdash S, et al. (2007). Acute renal failure from xanthine nephropathy during management of acute leukemia. *Pediatr Nephrol* **22**: 132–5.

37 Jeha S, Kantarjian H, Irwin D, et al. (2005). Efficacy and safety of rasburicase, a recombinant urate oxidase (Elitek), in the management of malignancy-associated hyperuricemia in pediatric and adult patients: final results of a multicenter compassionate use trial. *Leukemia* **19**: 34–8.

38 Tosi P, Barosi G, Lazzaro C, et al. (2008). Consensus conference on the management of tumor lysis syndrome. *Haematologica* **93**: 1877–85.

39 Agha-Razii M, Amyot S, Pichette V, Cardinal J, Ouimet D, Leblanc M (2000). Continuous veno-venous hemodiafiltration for the treatment of spontaneous tumor lysis syndrome complicated by acute renal failure and severe hyperuricemia. *Clin Nephrol* **54**: 59–63.

40 Pichette V, Leblanc M, Bonnardeaux A, Ouimet D, Geadah D, Cardinal J (1994). High dialysate flow rate continuous arteriovenous hemodialysis: a new approach for the treatment of acute renal failure and tumor lysis syndrome. *Am J Kidney Dis* **23**: 591–6.

41 Dimopoulos M, Kastritis E, Rosinol L, Bladé J. Ludwig H (2008). Pathogenesis and treatment of renal failure in multiple myeloma. *Leukemia* **22**: 1485–93.

42 Bladé J, Fernández-Llama P, Bosch F, et al. (1998). Renal failure in multiple myeloma: presenting features and predictors of outcome in 94 patients from a single institution. *Arch Intern Med* **158**: 1889–93.

43 Knudsen L, Hjorth M, Hippe E (2000). Renal failure in multiple myeloma: reversibility and impact on the prognosis. Nordic Myeloma Study Group. *Eur J Haematol* **65**: 175–81.

44 Winearls C (1995). Acute myeloma kidney. *Kidney Int* **48**: 1347–61.

45 Pillon L, Sweeting R, Arora A, et al. (2008). Approach to acute renal failure in biopsy proven myeloma cast nephropathy: is there still a role for plasmapheresis? *Kidney Int* **74**: 956–61.

46 Sanders P, Booker B (1992). Pathobiology of cast nephropathy from human Bence Jones proteins. *J Clin Invest* **89**: 630–9.

47 Clark W, Stewart A, Rock G, et al. (2005). Plasma exchange when myeloma presents as acute renal failure: a randomized, controlled trial. *Ann Intern Med* **143**: 777–784.

48 Hutchison C, Bradwell A, Cook M, et al. (2009). Treatment of acute renal failure secondary to multiple myeloma with chemotherapy and extended high cut-off hemodialysis. *Clin J Am Soc Nephrol* **4**: 745–54.

49 Richmond J, Sherman R, Diamond H, Craver L (1962). Renal lesions associated with malignant lymphomas. *Am J Med* **32**: 184–207.

50 Obrador G, Price B, O'Meara Y, Salant D (1997). Acute renal failure due to lymphomatous infiltration of the kidneys. *J Am Soc Nephrol* **8**: 1348–54.

51 Törnroth T, Heiro M, Marcussen N, Franssila K (2003). Lymphomas diagnosed by percutaneous kidney biopsy. *Am J Kidney Dis* **42**: 960–71.

52 Manning E, Belenko M, Frauenhoffer E, Ahsan N (1996). Acute renal failure secondary to solid tumor renal metastases: case report and review of the literature. *Am J Kidney Dis* **27**: 284–91.

53 Parikh C, Coca S (2006). Acute renal failure in hematopoietic cell transplantation. *Kidney Int* **69**: 430–5.

54 Parikh C, Schrier R, Storer B, et al. (2005). Comparison of ARF after myeloablative and nonmyeloablative hematopoietic cell transplantation. *Am J Kidney Dis* **45**: 502–509.

55 Zager R (1994). Acute renal failure in the setting of bone marrow transplantation. *Kidney Int* **46**: 1443–58.

56 Bearman S (1995). The syndrome of hepatic veno-occlusive disease after marrow transplantation. *Blood* **85**: 3005–20.

57 Carreras E (2000). Veno-occlusive disease of the liver after hemopoietic cell transplantation. *Eur J Haematol* **64**: 281–91.

58 Roy V, Rizvi M, Vesely S, George J (2001). Thrombotic thrombocytopenic purpura-like syndromes following bone marrow transplantation: an analysis of associated conditions and clinical outcomes. *Bone Marrow Transplant* **27**: 641–6.

59 Gruss E, Bernis C, Tomas J, et al. (1995). Acute renal failure in patients following bone marrow transplantation: prevalence, risk factors and outcome. *Am J Nephrol* **15**: 473–9.

60 Price K, Thall P, Kish S, Shannon V, Andersson B (1998). Prognostic indicators for blood and marrow transplant patients admitted to an intensive care unit. *Am J Respir Crit Care Med* **158**: 876–84.

61 Rubenfeld G, Crawford S (1996). Withdrawing life support from mechanically ventilated recipients of bone marrow transplants: a case for evidence-based guidelines. *Ann Intern Med* **125**: 625–33.

62 Parikh C, McSweeney P, Schrier R (2005). Acute renal failure independently predicts mortality after myeloablative allogeneic hematopoietic cell transplant. *Kidney Int* **67**: 1999–2005.

63 Faber-Langendoen K, Caplan A, McGlave P (1993). Survival of adult bone marrow transplant patients receiving mechanical ventilation: a case for restricted use. *Bone Marrow Transplant* **12**: 501–7.

64 Paz H, Garland A, Weinar M, Crilley P, Brodsky I (1998). Effect of clinical outcomes data on intensive care unit utilization by bone marrow transplant patients. *Crit Care Med* **26**: 66–70.

65 Torrecilla C, Cortés J, Chamorro C, Rubio J, Galdos P, Dominguez de Villota E (1988). Prognostic assessment of the acute complications of bone marrow transplantation requiring intensive therapy. *Intensive Care Med* **14**: 393–8.

66 Hennessy B, White M, Crotty G (1997). Predicting death in mechanically ventilated recipients of bone marrow transplants. *Ann Intern Med* **127**: 88.

67 Abraham B, Hardan I, Segal E, Stemmer S, Perel A (1996). Respiratory failure and intensive care treatment in bone marrow-transplanted patients. *Intensive Care Med* **22**: 269–70.

68 Létourneau I, Dorval M, Bélanger R, Légaré M, Fortier L, Leblanc M (2002). Acute renal failure in bone marrow transplant patients admitted to the intensive care unit. *Nephron* **90**: 408–12.

69 de Jonge M, Verweij J (2006). Renal toxicities of chemotherapy. *Semin Oncol* **33**: 68–73.

70 Arany I, Safirstein R (2003). Cisplatin nephrotoxicity. *Semin Nephrol* **23**: 460–4.

71 Abelson H, Fosburg M, Beardsley G, et al. (1983). Methotrexate-induced renal impairment: clinical studies and rescue from systemic toxicity with high-dose leucovorin and thymidine. *J Clin Oncol* **1**: 208–16.

72 Widemann B, Adamson P (2006). Understanding and managing methotrexate nephrotoxicity. *Oncologist* **11**: 694–703.

73 Flombaum C, Meyers P (1999). High-dose leucovorin as sole therapy for methotrexate toxicity. *J Clin Oncol* **17**: 1589–94.

74 Zakarija A, Bennett C (2005). Drug-induced thrombotic microangiopathy. *Semin Thromb Hemost* **31**: 681–90.

75 Montes A, Powles T, O'Brien M, Ashley S, Luckit J, Treleaven J (1993). A toxic interaction between mitomycin C and tamoxifen causing the haemolytic uraemic syndrome. *Eur J Cancer* **29A**: 1854–7.

76 Rougier F, Claude D, Maurin M, Maire P (2004). Aminoglycoside nephrotoxicity. *Curr Drug Targets Infect Disord* **4**: 153–62.

77 Warkentin D, Ippoliti C, Bruton J, Van Besien K, Champlin R (1999). Toxicity of single daily dose gentamicin in stem cell transplantation. *Bone Marrow Transplant* **24**: 57–61.

78 Somberg J (1994). Clinical Therapeutic Conference: vancomycin nephrotoxicity. *Am J Ther* **1**: 245–51.

79 Sorkine P, Nagar H, Weinbroum A, et al. (1996). Administration of amphotericin B in lipid emulsion decreases nephrotoxicity: results of a prospective, randomized, controlled study in critically ill patients. *Crit Care Med* **24**: 1311–15.

80 Nash K, Hafeez A, Hou S (2002). Hospital-acquired renal insufficiency. *Am J Kidney Dis* **39**: 930–6.

81 Barrett B, Parfrey P (2006). Clinical practice. Preventing nephropathy induced by contrast medium. *N Engl J Med* **354**: 379–86.

82 Perazella MA, Coca SG, Kanby M, Brewster UC, Parikh CR (2008). Diagnostic value of urine microscopy for differential diagnosis of acute kidney injury in hospitalized patients. *Clin J Am Soc Nephrol* **3**: 1615–19.

83 Venkataraman R (2008). Can we prevent acute kidney injury? *Crit Care Med* **36**: S166–71.

84 Venkataraman R, Kellum J (2007). Prevention of acute renal failure. *Chest* **131**: 300–8.

85 Kellum J, Leblanc M, Gibney R, Tumlin J, Lieberthal W, Ronco C (2005). Primary prevention of acute renal failure in the critically ill. *Curr Opin Crit Care* **11**: 537–41.

86 Ho K, Sheridan D (2006). Meta-analysis of frusemide to prevent or treat acute renal failure. *BMJ* **333**: 420.

87 Kellum J, M Decker (2001). Use of dopamine in acute renal failure: a meta-analysis. *Crit Care Med* **29**: 1526–31.

88 Pannu N, Klarenbach S, Wiebe N, Manns B, Tonelli M (2008). Renal replacement therapy in patients with acute renal failure: a systematic review. *JAMA* **299**: 793–805.

89 Naud J, Leblanc M (2008). Biomarkers in acute kidney injury. *Biomark Insights* **3**: 115–25.

90 Vinsonneau C, Camus C, Combes A, et al. (2006). Continuous venovenous haemodiafiltration versus intermittent haemodialysis for acute renal failure in patients with multiple-organ dysfunction syndrome: a multicentre randomised trial. *Lancet* **368**: 379–85.

91 Ronco C, Bellomo R, Homel P, et al. (2000). Effects of different doses in continuous veno-venous haemofiltration on outcomes of acute renal failure: a prospective randomised trial. *Lancet* **356**: 26–30.

92 Palevsky P, Zhang J, O'Connor T, et al. (2008). Intensity of renal support in critically ill patients with acute kidney injury. *N Engl J Med* **359**: 7–20.

93 Bellomo R, Cass A, Cole L, et al. (2009). Intensity of continuous renal-replacement therapy in critically ill patients. *N Engl J Med* **361**: 1627–38.

94 Leblanc M, Garred L, Cardinal J, et al. (1998). Catabolism in critical illness: estimation from urea nitrogen appearance and creatinine production during continuous renal replacement therapy. *Am J Kidney Dis* **32**: 444–53.

95 Chan L (2004). Nutritional support in acute renal failure. *Curr Opin Clin Nutr Metab Care* **7**: 207–12.

96 Kopple J (2001). National kidney foundation K/DOQI clinical practice guidelines for nutrition in chronic renal failure. *Am J Kidney Dis* **37**: S66–70.

97 Mokrzycki M, Kaplan A (1996). Protein losses in continuous renal replacement therapies. *J Am Soc Nephrol* **7**: 2259–63.

98 Baumgart D, Dignass A (2002). Intestinal barrier function. *Curr Opin Clin Nutr Metab Care* **5**: 685–94.

99 Hébert P, McDonald B, Tinmouth A (2004). Clinical consequences of anemia and red cell transfusion in the critically ill. *Crit Care Clin* **20**: 225–35.

100 Carson J, Hill S, Carless P, Hébert P, Henry D (2002). Transfusion triggers: a systematic review of the literature. *Transfus Med Rev* **16**: 187–99.

101 Hébert P, Wells G, Blajchman M, et al. (1999). A multicenter, randomized, controlled clinical trial of transfusion requirements in critical care. Transfusion Requirements in Critical Care Investigators, Canadian Critical Care Trials Group. *N Engl J Med* **340**: 409–17.

102 Bernhardt W, Eckardt K (2008). Physiological basis for the use of erythropoietin in critically ill patients at risk for acute kidney injury. *Curr Opin Crit Care* **14**: 621–6.

103 Pfeffer M, Burdmann E, Chen C, et al. (2009). A trial of darbepoetin alfa in type 2 diabetes and chronic kidney disease. *N Engl J Med* **361**: 2019–32.

104 Leyland-Jones B, Semiglazov V, Pawlicki M, et al. (2005). Maintaining normal hemoglobin levels with epoetin alfa in mainly nonanemic patients with metastatic breast cancer receiving first-line chemotherapy: a survival study. *J Clin Oncol* **23**: 5960–72.

105 Corwin H, Gettinger A, Fabian T, et al. (2007). Efficacy and safety of epoetin alfa in critically ill patients. *N Engl J Med* **357**: 965–76.

106 Chelluri L, Grenvik A, Silverman M (1995). Intensive care for critically ill elderly: mortality, costs, and quality of life. Review of the literature. *Arch Intern Med* **155**: 1013–22.

107 Luce J (1995). Physicians do not have a responsibility to provide futile or unreasonable care if a patient or family insists. *Crit Care Med* **23**: 760–6.

Chapter 10

Urinary tract obstruction in cancer patients

Marie Philipneri and Bahar Bastani

Introduction

Malignant upper or lower urinary tract obstruction is an ominous sign in cancer patients. It may be due to direct tumor invasion, retroperitoneal lymphadenopathy, or external tumor compression. The obstruction usually develops slowly, and therefore may produce only a few signs and symptoms or changes in the urinalysis. Every attempt should be made to avoid extensive surgical intervention or the placement of the chronic indwelling catheter in these often debilitated patients. The endourologic procedures of ureteral stenting, percutaneous nephrostomy, and intermittent bladder catheterization are effective palliative means.

Case report

A 47-year-old male was found to be confused without focal neurological signs. His vital signs were: blood pressure, 180/105 mmHg; heart rate, 87 beats per minute; respiratory rate, 16 per minute and very deep; and temperature, 94.2° F. He had pale conjunctiva and a few bibasilar crackles. His physical examination was otherwise unremarkable.

On initial laboratory evaluation, he was found to have serum sodium 138 mmol/L, potassium 9.5 mmol/L, chloride 110 mmol/L, bicarbonate 8 mmol/L, BUN 64 mmol/L (179 mg/dL), creatinine 1900 μmol/L (21.5 mg/dL), glucose 7.9 mmol/L (142 mg/dL), calcium 1.8 mmol/L (7.3 mg/dL), phosphorus 3.1 nmol/L (9.6 mg/dL), magnesium 1.1 mmol/L (2.6 mg/dL), albumin 32 g/L (3.2 g/dL), hemoglobin 1.3 mmol/L (8.4 g/dL), hematocrit 25%, platelets 268×10^9/L (268,000/mm3), white blood cell count 10×10^9 cells/L (10,000/mm3) with 80% neutrophils. His arterial blood gas revealed pH 7.14, pCO2 29 mmHg, and pO2 104 mmHg on 2 L nasal oxygen. EKG revealed prolonged PR and QRS intervals with peaked T-waves. Chest X-ray showed a mild pulmonary vascular congestion.

Because of the problems of uremic encephalopathy, severe metabolic acidosis, life-threatening hyperkalemia, and hypothermia, the patient was managed with emergency hemodialysis. A renal ultrasound revealed 11 cm kidneys with increased cortical echogenicity, significant bilateral hydronephrosis, hydroureter, and a mildly distended bladder with trabeculated wall (Fig. 10.1 (A–C)). A non-contrast CT scan of the abdomen and the pelvis confirmed bilateral hydronephrosis and hydroureter and suggested the presence of a mass

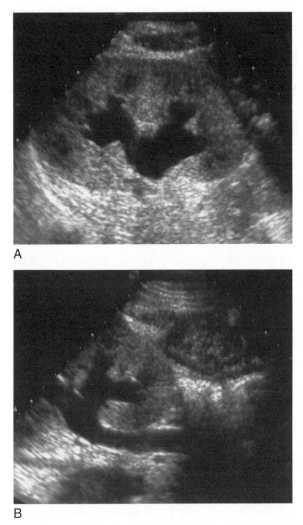

Fig. 10.1 Renal ultrasound showed significant bilateral hydronephrosis (A) with increased echogenicity and separation of the central echoic complexes bilaterally, bilateral hydroureter (B).

within the posterior aspect of the bladder wall. After infusion of 50 mLs of water-soluble contrast into the urinary bladder, via a Foley catheter, the prostate gland was found to be enlarged, impressing upon the base of the bladder (Fig. 10.1(D)). The serum prostatic cancer antigen (PSA) was 2000 units.

An ultrasound-guided prostate biopsy revealed adenocarcinoma of the prostate gland with a Gleason score of 7. A bone scan revealed multiple metastatic lesions.

With the impression of an advanced metastatic prostate cancer, causing bilateral ureteral and bladder outlet obstruction, the patient underwent bilateral nephrostomy tubes as well as the insertion of a Foley catheter in his bladder. He maintained a total urine output in the

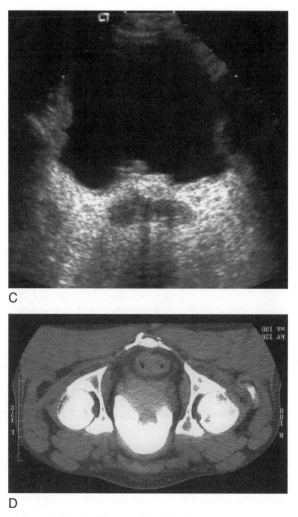

Fig. 10.1 (*continued*) and a significantly dilated bladder with trabeculated wall (C). CT scan of pelvis after infusion of 50 mL of water soluble contrast into the urinary bladder revealed an enlarged prostate gland, measuring 5.5 x 6.5 cm in greatest axial dimensions, which was impressing upon the base of the bladder (D). The bladder wall was diffusely thick and irregular suggesting chronic bladder outlet obstruction.

range of 2–3 L per day; however, he required maintenance hemodialysis. The patient refused any further management for his metastatic prostatic cancer.

Anatomy of the urinary tract

Obstruction can occur anywhere along the urinary tract, from the kidneys to the urethral meatus (Fig. 10.2). However, some areas are more susceptible to

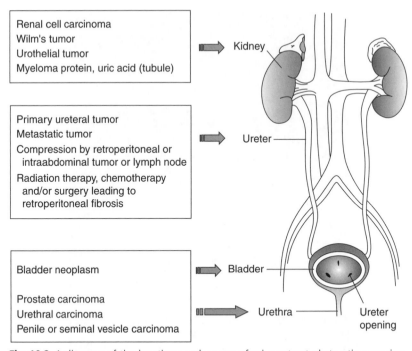

Fig. 10.2 A diagram of the locations and causes of urinary tract obstruction causing renal failure in cancer patients.

obstruction due to physiological narrowing. Three such areas along the ureter include the uretero-pelvic junction (UPJ), the crossing of the ureter over the common iliac vessels at the pelvic brim, and the ureterovesical junction (UVJ).

At the UPJ, the diameter of the ureter is only 2–3 mm. Distally, the ureter widens to a diameter of 10 mm, until it reaches the pelvic brim. Then, it narrows again to approximately 4–6 mm, as it crosses over the common iliac vessels. At the UVJ, the ureter is at its narrowest diameter at 1–5 mm, as it enters the bladder.

Moreover, in women, a fourth area of the ureteral narrowing can be noted as the distal ureter crosses posterior to the pelvic blood vessels and the broad ligament in the posterior pelvis. Urethral obstruction in men is frequently due to compression from an enlarged prostate.

Tumors associated with urinary tract obstruction

The most frequent malignancies causing urinary tract obstruction are prostate cancer in men and cervical cancer in women. Prostate, cervical, and bladder tumors account for nearly three-fourths of the tumors causing urinary tract obstruction. Breast, gastrointestinal malignancies, and lymphomas are responsible for the majority of the remaining one-fourth of the patients. Rarely, remote metastatic tumors, such as insular thyroid carcinoma (1), adenocarcinoma of the lung (2), gastric cancer with peritoneal metastasis (3), and small-cell cervical carcinoma (4) may cause urinary tract obstruction.

Prostate cancer is second only to lung cancer as a cause of cancer mortality in men worldwide, and urinary tract obstruction is its frequent presentation. Neheman et al. screened 300 men for prostate cancer using the serum levels of PSA and a digital rectal examination (DRE). Those men diagnosed with prostate cancer had at least one symptom of urinary tract obstruction, and the symptoms correlated well with the high serum PSA levels (5).

Urethral cancer is a relatively uncommon neoplasm. It has a predilection for women with a female to male ratio of 4:1, yet it accounts for only 0.02% of all cancers found in women. Tiguert et al. reported a case of primary clear cell cancer of the urethra in a woman who presented with acute urinary retention (6). Primary ureteral tumors are even more uncommon (less than 5% of all urothelial tumors) and they are at times difficult to diagnose (7).

Genital tumors are common causes of urinary tract obstruction in women. Semczuk et al. reported a patient who presented with bilateral hydronephrosis due to giant uterine leiomyoma that coexisted with endometrial cancer (8). The uterus measured 35 x 29 x 18 cm and weighed 15.2 kg. Advanced ovarian cancer (stages III/IV) may also lead to urinary tract obstruction in women (9).

Lymphomas can rarely present with, or develop during their course, a renal failure secondary to either bilateral ureteral obstruction from external compression by the enlarged retroperitoneal lymph nodes, or from a lymphomatous infiltration of the kidneys. Obrador et al. reported a patient with non Hodgkin's lymphoma who developed severe acute renal failure with enlarged kidneys (24–25 cm in length) due to massive lymphomatous infiltration of the kidneys. Following chemotherapy, the renal function of the patient improved markedly, with a significant reduction in his kidney size to 16–19 cm within one week of a pulse steroid therapy (10). Similarly, patients with multiple myeloma may present with acute renal failure and enlarged kidneys due to intratubular obstruction with cast nephropathy, diffuse light chain disease, or plasma cell infiltration of the kidneys. Hence, prompt initiation of therapy is warranted for patients presenting with acute renal failure due to infiltrative disorders, such as lymphoma or multiple myeloma.

Causes of urinary tract obstruction in cancer patients

The causes of urinary tract obstruction in cancer patients can be classified by their locations (i.e. renal, ureteral, and infravesical) (Table 10.1 and Fig. 10.2).

Table 10.1 Causes of urinary tract obstruction in cancer patients according to the location of the obstruction

Location	Cause
Renal	Myeloma protein, uric acid (tubule) Renal cell carcinoma Wilm's tumor Urothelial tumor
Ureteral	Primary renal, ureteral or bladder carcinoma Metastatic carcinoma Compression by retroperitoneal or intraabdominal tumor or lymph node Retroperitoneal fibrosis secondary to radiation therapy, chemotherapy &/ or surgery
Infravesical	Prostate carcinoma Urethral carcinoma Penile or seminal vesicle carcinoma

Alternatively, one may classify cases of obstruction according to the mechanisms of urinary tract obstruction as follows:

- Obstructive uropathy as a direct consequence of the malignancy, such as direct invasion or compression of the urinary tract. Obstructive uropathy due to an encasement of the urinary tract, often due to retroperitoneal metastasis, may be difficult to recognize. There may be little or no dilatation of the collecting system and the patients may be non-oliguric. Harrison et al. reported a 57-year-old male with anuric renal failure due to encasement of the ureters by poorly differentiated lymphocytic lymphoma. The excretory urogram revealed only minimal dilatation of the collecting systems, a delayed pyelogram and a dense nephrogram (11). Spector et al. described a patient with acquired immunodeficiency syndrome, who developed acute renal failure due to encasement of the renal pelvis and ureters by histiocytic lymphoma. Ultrasonography and computerized tomography did not show any urinary tract dilatation. Obstructive uropathy was only revealed by retrograde pyelography (12).

Rarely, tumors involving the central nervous system can interfere with the neurophysiology of micturition, thus resulting in urinary retention. Spinal cord compression due to metastasis may present acute urinary retention. Helweg-Larsen (13) followed 153 consecutive patients with known cancers and myelographically verified spinal cord compression. The primary cancers were breast (37%), prostate (28%), lung (18%), or kidney (4%). At the time of diagnosis, 57 patients (37%) presented with bladder dysfunction requiring urinary catheterization. During follow-up visits, 10 of these

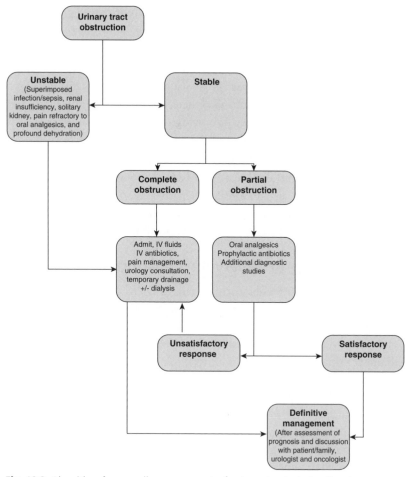

Fig. 10.3 Algorithm for overall management of urinary tract obstruction in cancer patients.

57 patients required urinary catheter. Acute urinary retention due to spinal cord compression may also be the first manifestation of malignancy (14). A prompt diagnosis is of utmost importance to prevent any permanent neurological dysfunction, especially hypotonic/atonic bladder, thereby resulting in renal failure. Corticosteroids are often administered immediately and are followed by radiation therapy and/or surgical decompression, based on the type and the extent of the tumor.

◆ Obstructive uropathy as a consequence of treatment of a malignancy, e.g. following radical cystectomy and urinary diversion for bladder cancer (15), interstitial radiation (brachytherapy) for localized prostate cancer (16), urinary retention due to a combination of narcotics and anti-emetics during chemotherapy, tumor lysis syndrome (17), or retroperitoneal fibrosis following radiation therapy (18–19).

Lee et al. reviewed 91 consecutive patients with prostate cancer, who underwent permanent radioactive seed implantation of whom 11 (12%) developed urinary retention, thus requiring catheterization. The significant factors predicting urinary retention following the above procedure were the number of needles required, and the pre-treatment prostate volume as measured by the ultrasound (20).

- Obstructive uropathy as a consequence of pre-existing conditions, such as urethral stricture or benign prostatic hypertrophy. A combination of treatment-related injury and pre-existing conditions can account for any obstruction occurring in the treatment of prostrate cancer.

Pathophysiology of urinary tract obstruction

Long-term bladder outlet obstruction leads to trabeculation in the bladder wall secondary to hypertrophied muscles, mucosal diverticula, and ultimately detrusor muscle decompensation. Urinary stasis secondary to incomplete bladder emptying increases the risk of urinary tract infection, stone formation, and upper urinary tract injury.

Hydroureter and hydronephrosis result from progressive back pressure on the ureter and kidney calyces. Increased ureteral peristaltic activity, in an attempt to propel urine forward, leads to hypertrophy of the ureteral musculature and ultimately, elongation and tortuosity of the ureter. The ureter may eventually resemble a loop of bowel.

Under normal circumstances, urine production is brought about by a combination of the following: pressure gradient from the glomerulus to the Bowman's capsule, peristalsis of the renal pelvis and the ureter, and the effect of gravity. When the urinary tract is obstructed, intraluminal pressure proximal to the site of obstruction rises, since the glomerular filtration is maintained initially. As the intraluminal pressure continues to rise, ureteral peristalsis is eventually overcome and results in the dilatation of the collecting systems, and hydroureter and hydronephrosis follow. Increased intraluminal hydrostatic pressure is also transmitted directly back to the proximal tubule to the extent that the pressure gradient from the glomerulus to the Bowman's space falls, thereby lowering the glomerular filtration rate (GFR). Moreover, the elevated intratubular pressure augments the reduction in the GFR by the release of vasoactive substances, mainly angiotensin II and thromboxanes, both of which reduce the renal blood flow (21– 24). This may be considered an appropriate physiological response where the blood flow is shunted away from the obstructed nephrons to the non-obstructed functioning nephrons in an effort to maintain the overall kidney function. Chronic reduction in the GFR is felt to be mainly secondary to this vasoconstrictive action and decreased renal perfusion.

In addition to renal vasoconstriction and ischemia, inflammation is also known to contribute to the tubulointerstitial injury of obstructive uropathy. Oxidative stress and higher levels of angiotensin II from the obstructed kidney can up-regulate several growth factors and cytokines, such as transforming growth factor-beta (TGF-β), tumor necrosis factor (TNF), platelet-derived growth factor (PDGF), insulin-like growth factor (IGF), osteopontin, vascular cell adhesion molecule-1 (VCAM-1), nuclear factor-kB (NF-kB), monocyte chemoattractant peptide, intracellular adhesion molecule-1 (ICAM-1) and CD 14 (25). TGF-β is a potent stimulus for glomerulosclerosis and fibrogenesis (26–27). TNF is up-regulated mainly in the tubules of the obstructed kidney. It contributes to the inflammatory injury of the kidney, via various mechanisms including the recruitment of monocytes and macrophages, which in turn release oxygen-free radicals and proteases, myofibroblast differentiation, and NF-kB activation (28). Longstanding urinary tract obstruction can also lead to apoptosis of the tubular epithelial cells (29). Several genes and factors involved in apoptosis have been described. Fibrosis and renal epithelial cell loss would explain long-term, permanent reductions in the renal function after an episode of urinary tract obstruction.

Clinical presentation

The clinical presentation depends on the nature, location and mode of onset of an obstruction.

The frequent presentation of an acute upper urinary tract obstruction is with flank pain, often radiating down to the ipsilateral groin, along the course of the ureter. On the other hand, a chronic unilateral obstruction may be silent and detected only incidentally as hydronephrosis, with or without the loss of corticomedullary differentiation, on abdominal imaging studies performed for other reasons. Hematuria is also common with malignancies involving the urinary tract. Severe renal failure and uremia can be associated with nausea, vomiting, and poor appetite. Fever, chills, dysuria, and cloudy urine suggest a concomitant urinary tract infection. Bilateral obstruction or obstruction of a solitary kidney can result in decreased or even absent urine output, and uremic symptoms including weakness, pallor, weight loss, peripheral edema, and change in mental status. On physical examination, palpation or percussion may reveal an enlarged kidney, secondary to significant hydronephrosis.

Similarly, large retroperitoneal or pelvic masses causing extrinsic compression of the urinary tract may also be palpable. Costovertebral angle tenderness is often present. Rarely, ascites might be noted due to urinary extravasation from bladder rupture.

Partial obstruction of the lower urinary tract is commonly associated with urinary frequency, hesitancy, straining to void, decreased force of the urinary stream, sensation of inadequate emptying, and/or post-void dribbling. Significant long-term obstruction may lead to urinary retention and stress incontinence. Suprapubic fullness or pain could suggest urinary retention. Hematuria is common in malignancies of the lower urinary tract, whereas dysuria and cloudy urine suggest an infectious process. On examination, an enlarged bladder with or without tenderness on palpation or percussion indicates urinary retention. Digital rectal examination must be performed to look for prostate enlargement, lower gastrointestinal tumors and peritoneal metastasis into the rectovesical or rectouterine pouch (Blumer's shelf). Meatal stenosis is usually readily apparent on examination. In women, a large lower genitourinary tract mass can be easily visualized on pelvic examination, especially with the aid of a half-speculum device.

A commonly held misconception is that patients with bilateral ureteral or bladder neck obstruction should be oliguric or even anuric. However, anuria only occurs with complete obstruction. Patients with a partial obstruction generally show a normal urine output or even polyuria, secondary to an acquired concentration defect in the distal nephron. Thus, a normal urine output does not exclude obstruction as the cause of renal failure.

Diagnosis

Laboratory studies

- ◆ Urinalysis. The presence of pyuria (>3 white blood cells (WBCs) per high-power field) suggests inflammation and/or infection. Positive nitrites and/or leukocyte esterase tests, as well as the presence of bacteriuria on microscopic examination, further indicate an infectious process. When an infection is suspected, the urine culture should be sent for microbial identification and specific antibiotic susceptibility. Urine cytology should be obtained when hematuria is otherwise unexplained.

- ◆ Serum electrolytes. Bilateral renal obstruction can lead to renal insufficiency. Typical metabolic abnormalities, which are associated with renal insufficiency, include hyperkalemia and metabolic acidosis. In an elegant study by Batlle et al. of the 13 patients who had developed renal insufficiency with hyperkalemic metabolic acidosis secondary to obstructive uropathy, five of them had impaired potassium excretion associated with decreased ammonium excretion, a urinary pH <5.5, and renin and aldosterone deficiency (hyporenin, hypoaldosteronism). In the remaining eight patients, the urinary pH did not fall below 5.5 despite systemic acidosis, and they failed to lower their urinary pH and did not increase fractional potassium excretion after the administration of mineralocorticoids and sodium sulfate infusion, indicating a voltage-defect hyperkalemic distal RTA (30). Hyperkalemia could be life-threatening and urgent treatment including dialysis might be warranted when potassium levels are above 6 mmol/L and refractory to medical management or immediate relief of obstruction (31).

- Complete blood count. Leukocytosis (especially neutrophilia with shift to the left) could suggest systemic or local infection. Anemia is a frequent complication associated with malignancy and/or chronic renal insufficiency. It is often due to erythropoietin deficiency and/or resistant state. Anemia may also be acute, due to blood loss.

Imaging studies

- Ultrasonography is a valuable screening test because it is non-invasive and does not carry the risk of radiation or contrast exposure. It is relatively inexpensive and useful even in patients with advanced renal insufficiency. It is especially useful in differentiating solid versus cystic lesions of kidneys. Moreover, hydronephrosis, hydroureter, and/or distended bladder can be readily delineated with ultrasound. However, subtle anatomical details could be missed, particularly if the ultrasonographer is inexperienced. Huang et al. used vaginal ultrasonography with three-dimensional scanning and Doppler flow techniques to demonstrate a distal urethral obstruction by an infiltrating tumor and avoided more invasive diagnostic procedures. They concluded that this diagnostic technique may be used as a screening tool for women who present with voiding dysfunction (32).

- Computed tomography (CT) is an extremely valuable tool to detect the source of an extrinsic compression, along the course of the urinary tract. Retro-peritoneal, pelvic, and intra-abdominal tumors are readily visible on the CT scan.

- Magnetic resonance imaging (MRI) has the advantage over CT scan in its ability to delineate specific tissue planes for surgical intervention. Moreover, diffusion-weighted MRI might have a role in detecting urinary epithelial cancer non-invasively (33). It is particularly useful in patients with a high clinical suspicion for upper urinary tract malignancies but whose hydronephrosis cannot be explained by conventional imaging or endoscopic techniques (34). However, MRI is costly and time-consuming. MRI with gadolinium-containing contrast agents has been associated with nephrogenic systemic fibrosis in patients with advanced renal insufficiency (35–36). Nonetheless, Okayama et al. recently reported a patient with hydronephrosis secondary to testicular cancer and concluded that MRI without contrast could provide valuable information (37).

• Intravenous pyelogram (IVP) is the study of choice for visualization of the entire course of the urinary tract in patients with normal renal function (serum creatinine <1.5 mg/dL (<133 µmol/L)). It provides both anatomical and functional information. Urinary tract obstruction is characterized by a prolonged nephrogram phase, delayed excretion of the contrast material, delayed calyceal filling, and dilation proximal to the point of obstruction. Initial non-visualization of the collecting system often indicates severe obstruction. Hence, following the administration of contrast, additional delayed films up to several hours should be obtained to assess for the delayed excretion. Moreover, IVP has an advantage over the CT scan in detecting small urothelial upper tract lesions. Since the urothelial tumors of the urinary tract have a tendency for multifocal growth, the excretory urography has been widely used in the follow-up of multicentric bladder neoplasms. However, Goessl et al. (38) have suggested that a routine IVP is not necessary at the first diagnosis of uncomplicated cases of primary bladder cancer.

• Retrograde urethrogram is a useful test to visualize the entire length of the urethra and especially useful to delineate the urethral valves and strictures.

• Retrograde pyelogram is especially useful in patients with severely impaired renal function. By injecting contrast material directly into each ureteric orifice, it visualizes the entire upper collecting system. However, this test is performed in the operating room under anesthesia.

• Radionuclide study is a useful test in assessing the differential functional contribution of each kidney. Moreover, in patients who present with dilatation of the upper urinary tract, it is a useful test to distinguish a true anatomical obstruction from functional dilatation. A delayed excretion following the administration of furosemide suggests an obstructive process, whereas prompt excretion of the radionuclide after furosemide, indicates functional dilatation.

Diagnostic procedures

• Cystoscopy allows direct visualization of the entire urethra and the bladder. A simple flexible or rigid cystoscopy is a well-tolerated outpatient office procedure for the urologist, but when additional invasive procedures are required it is best performed in the operating room, under anesthesia.

Management

Medical therapy

Urologic consultation should be obtained in the event of any newly diagnosed hydronephrosis or urinary retention.

In the absence of infection, partial obstruction can be initially managed with analgesics and prophylactic antibiotics, until complete evaluation and a definitive management can be executed.

Pain due to obstruction is managed with non-steroidal anti-inflammatory drugs (NSAIDs) and/or opioid analgesics. The former should be avoided if renal dysfunction or hyperkalemia already exists, or if there is a risk of renal insufficiency, such as coexisting intravascular volume depletion or the concomitant use of other nephrotoxic agents. If NSAIDs are used, renal function should be followed closely and these agents promptly discontinued if renal dysfunction or severe hyperkalemia is detected. Prophylactic antibiotics should be used to cover common urinary tract infection micro-organisms.

Chye et al. (39) and Hamdy et al. (40) have shown that a short-term use of corticosteroids reduces edema around obstructing tumors and/or has an anti-tumor effect, thereby possibly avoiding the need for invasive decompression procedures. However, the use of high-dose corticosteroids may be dangerous, resulting in life-threatening gastrointestinal hemorrhage or perforation in patients with advanced malignancies and urinary tract obstruction. Hence, in the current era, when highly effective and relatively safe endourologic procedures are available, the use of corticosteroids by themselves is seldom recommended for the treatment of a urinary tract obstruction.

Expeditious intervention and/or hospitalization is indicated for patients with complete obstruction, a solitary kidney, obstruction associated with superimposed infection (fever, leukocytosis, bacteriuria), renal insufficiency, pain refractory to oral analgesics, or nausea, vomiting, and dehydration too severe to be managed on an outpatient basis.

Surgical therapy

Complete urinary tract obstruction is a urological emergency, and a relief of obstruction should be achieved without delay. Success in the recovery of renal function is dependent on the duration and the degree of obstruction. Hence, temporary drainage procedures, such as insertion of a Foley catheter, ureteral stent, and/or percutaneous nephrostomy tube should be implemented immediately to decompress the urinary system, until complete evaluation and planning for a definitive correction can be accomplished.

In dog experiments, renal impairment became evident only after 18 hours of complete obstruction. Moreover, ureteral ligation in dogs resulted in considerable renal cortical loss, 'with often nothing left … but a shell' by the fourth week (41), and relief of a complete obstruction of longer than 42 days' duration was followed by almost no return of kidney function (42–43). However, limited clinical data in human subjects suggests that even with severe renal failure requiring dialysis support, and after a bilateral ureteral obstruction of greater than six weeks, a relief of obstruction may lead to gradual recovery (over days to months) of enough renal function to alleviate the need for further dialysis (44). A recent single-center study of 104 patients revealed relatively stable renal function for up to three years after relief of obstruction. Specifically, 45 (43%) patients who were left with moderate to severe renal impairment (mean GFR 25.3 mL/min) three months after relief of obstruction did not demonstrate progression of their renal disease at three years (45). Bad prognostic signs which could indicate severe and often irreversible renal failure are a total non-visualization of the kidney on the renal nuclear scan, and the marked thinning of the renal cortex on ultrasound examination. However, these signs do not absolutely preclude a substantial return of the renal function in some individual cases (46–47). While most of the recovery of the renal function occurs within the first 7–10 days of the relief of obstruction (45, 47), some patients with severe renal failure, after a prolonged period of urinary tract obstruction, may require dialysis for a period of weeks after relief of obstruction, until sufficient recovery of the renal function occurs (44).

Obstruction coexisting with infection is a more serious urological emergency, as irreversible renal parenchymal damage can occur within a few days, as well as a serious risk of urosepsis. It requires prompt relief from the obstruction and appropriate broad-spectrum parenteral antibiotics to avoid the potentially life-threatening urosepsis (48).

Decompression of the lower urinary tract (i.e. urethra, bladder) is accomplished by the following:

◆ Placement of a urethral catheter. Nursing staff can usually place this catheter under local anesthesia. However, the urologist should place the catheter in difficult cases with prostatic enlargement or urethral stricture. Sterile intermittent catheterization is a preferred alternative to a long-term indwelling catheter in the setting of chronic urinary retention secondary to bladder dysfunction.

◆ Percutaneous placement of a suprapubic catheter through the lower anterior abdominal wall, immediately superior to the pubis, and directly into the bladder under local anesthesia. Alternatively, it may be placed during an open surgical procedure in the operating room by the urologist under general anesthesia.

Decompression of the upper urinary tract (i.e. renal pelvis and ureter) is accomplished by either of the following:

♦ Percutaneous nephrostomy. This is the first line of urinary diversion, which provides a rapid and reliable ureteral and renal decompression. A small tube is placed directly into the renal pelvis through the flank. It is placed percutaneously in the radiology suite by the interventional radiologist, under local anesthesia. In patients with bilateral hydronephrosis due to advanced malignancies, the value of unilateral versus bilateral nephrostomy tubes is being debated. Nariculum et al. conducted a retrospective study involving 25 men with advanced prostate cancer and bilateral ureteral obstruction. They found that nadir serum creatinine did not differ between bilateral and unilateral nephrostomies insertion (49).

♦ Ureteral stent. In the operating room, a small caliber tube running the length of the ureter from the renal pelvis to the bladder is placed endoscopically by the urologist. The procedure is performed with significant intravenous sedation and/or general anesthesia. During extensive pelvic debulking surgeries, ureteral stents may also be successfully placed transureterically, through a longitudinal incision in the ureter near the pelvic brim (9). In a retrospective study involving 17 patients with hydronephrosis due to bladder cancer involving ureteral orifice, 10 patients underwent resection of bladder including ureteral orifice without stent placement, and only one patient had successful resolution of hydronephrosis. The authors recommended ureteric stenting at the time of cystectomy in patients with muscle invasive bladder cancer and hydronephrosis (50).

More definitive intervention is dependent upon the type, location, cause, and duration of the obstruction.

For many years, an open surgical diversion has been the treatment of choice for extrinsic ureteral obstruction due to urologic malignancies. However, the rate of major complications was as high as 45% (51). Moreover, a quarter of the patients undergoing open nephrostomy procedures died within a month and the average survival following the procedure was only about six months. Over the past decade, there have been significant improvements in the endoscopic and the percutaneous diversion techniques used to relieve a malignant urinary tract obstruction. The contemporary endourologic techniques have allowed less invasive therapeutic measures in the management of the urinary tract obstruction. The ultimate goal is to sustain a long-lasting ureteral patency, preserve renal function, and maintain the quality of life of these patients. There are many reports supporting that application of one or more of these techniques, even for palliation in the advanced malignancies, helps to improve the quality of life of the patients, primarily by improving their renal function and avoiding the complications of uremia (52–54).

Patients with ureteral obstruction due to pelvic malignancy typically undergo urinary diversion with a percutaneous nephrostomy tube or an insertion of a Double-J ureteral stent made of flexible synthetic materials (e.g. polyurethane). The former is especially useful for immediate relief of life-threatening consequences of obstructive uropathy (55–56) but carries many complications, such as infection, bleeding, obstruction, and tube displacement (57). More importantly, percutaneous nephrostomies are uncomfortable. Therefore, percutaneous nephrostomy for patients with advanced malignancies should be individualized and the patients or their families should be informed of the expected outcome of this procedure (58).

A survey of over 400 urologists and oncologists revealed significant differences in practice patterns in regards to use of percutaneous nephrostomy and stent insertion. Oncologists were mostly concerned about infection while urologists worried about potential mechanical complications and quality of life (59). Chitale et al. reviewed their management of upper tract obstruction secondary to malignant pelvic disease in 65 patients treated over a period of two years. Fifty-eight patients had urological malignancies and the rest had non-urological malignancies. Forty-one patients had percutaneous nephrostomy followed by antegrade ureteric stenting, while a cystoscopic retrograde ureteric stenting was performed in 24 patients as a primary method of decompression. The two-stage antegrade stenting had a success rate of 98%, whereas endoscopic retrograde stenting was successful in only 21% of the patients. Moreover, the antegrade approach was associated with minimal morbidity (60). Table 10.2 compares the indications, advantages, and disadvantages of retrograde and antegrade approaches to ureteral stent placements for malignant ureteric obstruction (61).

The Double-J ureteral stent is superior to the regular ureteral stent and the nephrostomy tube. It has the 'double-J' stent configuration with one end coiled in the bladder and the other in the renal pelvis, which minimizes the risk of stent migration. However, the insertion of this stent may not always be successful and/or may prove to be ineffective, after its placement (62). Hence, there may be a need for frequent stent replacements (63), which is often proved to be technically challenging due to the advanced malignant ureteral obstruction, and is a great inconvenience for the debilitated patients. Recently, a group of urologists demonstrated that simultaneous placement of two ipsilateral

Table 10.2 Comparison of retrograde and antegrade approaches to ureteral stent placements for malignant ureteric obstruction

	Retrograde approach	Antegrade approach
Indications	◆ No evidence of ureteral orifice involvement of tumor per imaging studies ◆ Technically difficult nephrostomy due to body habitus or other reasons ◆ Solitary functioning kidney and risk of nephrostomy-related bleeding	◆ Significant tumor involvement of the bladder ◆ Gross bladder hemorrhage
Advantages	◆ Single-stage procedure ◆ Low risk of bleeding ◆ Length of stent left in bladder may be adjusted to minimize irritation	◆ High technical success rate of placement
Disadvantages	◆ Modest technical success rate of placement	◆ Multi-stage procedure-Higher risk of bleeding ◆ Ideal stent length in bladder is challenging

double-J ureteral stents are feasible and safe (64). Moreover, Barbalias et al. (65) demonstrated that intraureteral metallic stents, both balloon and self-expandable, were safe and effective for palliative management of ureteral obstruction due to pelvic malignancies. Similar results were reported in eight patients with ureteral strictures, secondary to metastatic prostate cancer (66), and by other urologists, who have used the metallic stents successfully (67–72). In a retrospective analysis of 78 patients with ureteral obstruction due to non-urological malignancies and ureteral stents, systemic chemotherapy did not increase the risk of acute pyelonephritis (73).

Others have tried various subcutaneous urinary diversion techniques, such as anterior nephrostomy with subcutaneous pyelovesical bypass stenting, to improve the quality of life of the patients with pelvic malignancies (74). This technique requires a functional bladder. In ten cases Nissenkorn et al. presented their successful experience with nephrovesical subcutaneous stent as an alternative to the permanent nephrostomy tube (75).

In a series involving 58 patients with bladder cancer and obstructive nephropathy (mean serum creatinine 1.85 mg/dL), radical cystectomy, bilateral pelvic lymphadenectomy and urinary diversion were performed in 36 suitable patients. Fifteen (26%) patients were disease-free after 34 months of follow-up. The authors concluded that radical cystectomy is not associated with additional morbidity in patients with renal insufficiency whose renal function was optimized pre-operatively, compared to those with relatively preserved renal function (76). For patients with muscle-invasive cancer of the bladder, undergoing radical cystectomy, orthotopic ileal neobladder may be the preferred diversion procedure. Kaouk et al. (77) successfully performed this procedure laparoscopically, in a porcine model. In patients who have had previous pelvic irradiation, urinary diversion can be challenging. The use of irradiated bowel as a neo-bladder can be followed by complications in the irradiated bowel segment. Thus, the use of non-irradiated bowel segments is now the preferred technique in these patients (78). In a study of 17 patients with advanced cervical cancer, the authors concluded that for patients with bilateral hydronephrosis and impaired renal function (creatinine clearance less than 50 mL/min) urinary diversion should be considered prior to radiation (79). Laparoscopic ureterolysis is an alternate treatment option for patients with persistent hydronephrosis due to external compression despite successful tumor management by surgery, chemotherapy, and/or radiation. Laparoscopic ureterolysis provides a shorter recovery period and lower mortality compared with the open procedure (80).

Finally, major reconstructive surgical procedures, such as formal urinary diversion, via an ileal orthotopic neobladder, as a modification of the method described by Hauptman (81), revision of ileal ureteral anastomosis, ureteral reimplantation, and ileal ureter interposition should be considered for patients with complete remission from their malignancies and good prognosis. Castellan and Gosalbez reported good long-term results in two patients following ureteral replacement with refigured tubes of small or large bowel using the Yang–Monti principle (82).

Post-operative management

The polyuric phase, following the relief of a long-standing urinary tract obstruction, is due to a physiologic diuresis, known as post-obstructive diuresis. This is usually a self-limiting process and can be managed conservatively with fluid and electrolyte replacement. The urine output may initially exceed 500–1000 mL/h, and is often an appropriate attempt to excrete the fluid and salt retained during the period of obstruction.

There are three types of post-obstructive diuresis. Urea diuresis is the most common, and is due to the excretion of the retained urea and other osmotic agents (high osmotic load) after relief of obstruction. It is often self-limiting and usually resolves when blood urea nitrogen (BUN) normalizes within 24–48 hours. Fluid balance and electrolytes must be monitored closely and replaced accordingly when indicated, during this phase.

The second most common post-obstructive diuresis is sodium diuresis. This is due to the excretion of the retained salt and water after relief of obstruction, and continues until a euvolemic state is achieved. It is usually self-limiting, but may last longer than 72 hours. Fluid balance and electrolytes (i.e. intake and output (I/O), central venous pressure (CVP), urine and serum electrolytes) should be monitored more aggressively during this phase. Replacement of fluids, often with isotonic sodium chloride solution at 0.5 mL per 1 mL urine, becomes especially important, if the diuresis is prolonged after normalization of volume status (pathological diuresis), in order to avoid dehydration and hyponatremia.

The last form of post-obstructive diuresis, is water diuresis, which is a temporary nephrogenic diabetes insipidus, secondary to an impaired renal tubular response to anti-diuretic hormone (ADH). Often, it resolves with recovery of the renal tubular function over a period of several months.

There is a common misunderstanding regarding the rate at which an enlarged bladder can be decompressed. Two complications that can occur after sudden drainage of large urine volumes from a completely obstructed bladder are: (a) gross hematuria (from sudden expansion of the stretched, compressed, ischemic bladder wall veins) and, on rare occasions, (b) reflex hypotension. It has been suggested that after an initial drainage of 500 mL, the catheter be clamped with subsequent slow drainage over several hours. However, the pressure inside a tensely enlarged, obstructed bladder is very sensitive to small changes in volume. The intravesical pressure is reduced by 50% after removal of 100 mL, and by 75% after removal of 250 mL of urine (83–84). Thus, an intermittent or partial clamping after 500 mL urinary drainage is not likely to protect against hematuria, especially in the setting of chronic obstruction. Hence, we do not recommend routine clamping of the catheter. However, one should closely monitor the volume status, and replace in time the fluid and electrolytes in order to avoid volume depletion. If gross hematuria occurs, the following should be performed: serial hematocrit measurements, transfusion of blood products as indicated, correction of coagulopathy, if present, and urology consultation if not already obtained.

A temporary detrusor muscle dysfunction may result due to prolonged bladder distention. Therefore, following the relief of obstruction, the urinary catheter may need to remain in place for several days to allow for recovery of detrusor function before attempting a voiding trial. It is also recommended that post-void residual be checked several hours after the removal of the urinary catheter, in order to ensure regained bladder function.

Follow-up care

After successful placement of a ureteral stent or nephrostomy tube, periodic monitoring of renal function, frequent urine cultures, and timely stent or tube replacements (typically every 4–6 months) are recommended. An imaging study of the renal collecting system, i.e. IVP, renal ultrasound, or a CT scan, should be obtained four to six weeks after the complete relief of obstruction to ensure normalization of hydronephrosis and the absence of any untoward sequel.

Serious complications from urinary tract obstruction include the following:

◆ Renal insufficiency due to renal parenchymal loss following long-term urinary tract obstruction

◆ Infectious complications, such as pyelonephritis, pyonephrosis (i.e. gross pus within the obstructed renal pelvis of a functionless kidney), abscess formation, and urosepsis

◆ Urinary extravasation into the renal sinus with perinephric urinoma formation

◆ Urinary fistula formation

◆ Atonic bladder due to bladder decompensation

◆ Rarely, intraperitoneal rupture of hydronephrosis (85)

Complications following endourologic procedures include the following:

◆ Bleeding manifested as gross hematuria and/or perinephric hematoma

◆ Injury to nearby organs, such as the spleen, intestine, and rarely pleural space

◆ Ureteral stent obstruction with proteinaceous material

◆ Stent migration and rarely erosion through the urinary tract

◆ Bladder spasm due to irritation of the trigone

◆ Vesicoureteral reflux

◆ Urinary tract infection.

Prognosis

Prognosis depends on several factors, including the etiology, location, degree (tumor volume), and duration of the obstructive process, as well as the presence of a concomitant infection. A favorable prognosis is generally expected, if the renal function is preserved, obstruction is alleviated, and infection is eradicated. In a series of 54 patients with bladder cancer, incidence of hydronephrosis was 2.7-fold higher with bulky tumors compared to less bulky or flat tumors (86). In another series of 788 patients with transitional cell carcinoma of the bladder who underwent radical cystectomy, 108 (13.7%) patients had unilateral and 25 (3.2%) patients had bilateral hydronephrosis. The presence of hydronephrosis at the time of diagnosis of bladder cancer was associated with a higher likelihood of advanced tumor stage, and it was an independent risk factor for bladder cancer recurrence-free survival (87). Hydronephrosis reduces the likelihood of successful complete surgical resection of recurrent tumor in patients with pelvic recurrence from colon and rectal cancers (88).

Overall, ureteral obstruction due to malignancy is an ominous sign in patients with cancer. Median survival for patients with malignant ureteral obstruction is less than seven months, regardless of the tumor origin (89–90). Donat et al. reported their experience on the outcome of 78 patients with advanced malignancies referred for ureteral decompression at the Memorial Sloan-Kettering Cancer Center. The overall median survival following the first decompression procedure was 6.8 months. Only 55% and 30% of the patients were alive at one and three years, respectively. The prognosis of patients with gastric or pancreatic malignancies were particularly poor, with only 12.5% surviving at one year and none at three years, and a median survival of only 1.4 months (91). Median survival after the diagnosis of cancerous spinal cord compression is also poor, being 3.6 months (13). Hence, the decision to intervene in a patient with an untreatable malignancy and urinary tract obstruction should be carefully considered in close consultation with the oncologist. It is reasonable to perform the palliative procedures to relieve the urinary tract obstruction, if undesirable symptoms can be alleviated or an improvement in the renal function would facilitate the use of palliative chemotherapy.

Hydronephrosis is an independent prognostic factor in bladder cancer patients (92). However, whether both unilateral and bilateral hydronephrosis have a similar impact on the outcome is controversial. The presence of hydronephrosis (unilateral or bilateral) in patients with recurrent rectal adenocarcinoma portends a very poor prognosis and curative surgery is not recommended (93–94).

Brown et al. reviewed 75 patients in whom hydronephrosis developed after resection of colorectal cancer. A focal plaque-like mass centered on the peritoneum, was the most common (49%) cause of hydronephrosis. Patients with residual tumor (microscopic or macroscopic) developed hydronephrosis at a median time of 13 months compared with 22 months for those having curative resection. Furthermore, they concluded that hydronephrosis is an important early indicator of colorectal cancer recurrence, even in the absence of a demonstrable mass. Of the 26 patients without an obvious cause of hydronephrosis on the initial CT examination, a follow-up CT scan demonstrated a definite mass lesion in 50% of the cases. The median survival after the onset of hydronephrosis was six months (range, 1–34 months) with a one-year mortality rate of 62% (95).

Recently, a group of investigators from Japan examined 140 patients with ureteral obstruction secondary to advanced incurable malignant disease and developed a prognostic model for predicting survival after palliative urinary diversion. On multivariate analysis the number of events related to malignant dissemination (three or more), degree of hydronephrosis (grade 1 or 2), and serum albumin before nephrostomy (3 gm/dl or less) were significantly associated with a short survival time. The patients were divided into three risk groups of favorable—zero risk factors (34 patients)—intermediate—one risk factor (60 patients)—and poor—two or three risk factors (46 patients). The six-month survival rates for the favorable, intermediate, and poor risk groups were 69%, 24%, and 2%, respectively (96).

Future trends

Successful percutaneous and endoscopic urinary tract procedures based on new advances in imaging techniques, equipments, and devices will make less invasive measures a high priority in the management of these challenging patients.

References

1 Meyer-Rochow GY, McMullen TP, and Gill AJ, Sywak MS, Robinson BG, (2009). Intra-abdominal insular thyroid carcinoma metastasis. *Thyroid* **19**: 527–-30.

2 Hiraki A, Ueoka H, Gemba K, et al. (2003). Hydronephrosis as a complication of adenocarcinoma of the lung. *Anti-cancer Research* **23**: 2915–16.

3 Tamura S, Miki H, Nakata K, et al. (2007). Intraperitoneal administration of paclitaxel and oral S-1 for a patient with peritoneal dissemination and hydronephrosis due to advanced gastric cancer. *Gastric Cancer* **10**: 251–5.

4 Boyle E, Nzewi E, Khan I, et al. (2009). Small cell cervical cancer: an unusual finding at cholecystectomy. *Arch Gynecol Obstet* **279**: 251–4.

5 Neheman A, Shotland Y, Metz Y, Stein A. (2001). Screening for early detection of prostate cancer (first experience in Israel). *Harefuah* **140**: 4–10.

6 Tiguert R, Ravery V, Madjar S, Gousse AE (2001). Acute urinary retention secondary to clear cell adenocarcinoma of the urethra. *Prog Urol* **11**: 70–2.

7 Goel A, Singh D, and Goel A. (2008). Transitional cell cancer of ureter misdiagnosed as pelviureteric junction obstruction: pitfalls of standard diagnostic tools. *Indian Journal of Cancer* **45**: 184–5.

8 Semczuk A, Skorupski P, Olcha P, et al. (2009). Giant uterine leiomyomas causing bilateral hydronephrosis coexisting with endometrial cancer in polyp: a case study. *Eur J Gynaecol Oncol* **30**: 344–6.

9 Ang C, Naik R (2009). The value of ureteric stents in debulking surgery for disseminated ovarian cancer. *Int J Gynecol Cancer* **19**: 978–80.

10 Obrador GT, Price B, O'Meara Y, and Salant DJ (1997). Acute renal failure due to lymphomatous infiltration of the kidneys. *J Am Soc Nephrol* **8**: 1348–54.

11 Harrison RB, Widner LA, Johnstone WH, Wyker Jr AW (1979). Subtle obstructive uropathy from encasement of the ureters by tumor. *J Urol* **122**: 835–6.

12 Spector DA, Katz RS, Fuller H, Cristiano LM, Vitalis S, Jarrow, J (1989). Acute non-dilating obstructive renal failure in a patient with AIDS. *Am J Nephrol* **9**: 129–30.

13 Helweg-Larsen, S. (1996). Clinical outcome in metastatic spinal cord compression. A prospec-tive study of 153 patients. *Acta Neuro Scand* **94**: 269–75.

14 Tintinalli JE (1986). Acute urinary retention as a presenting sign of spinal cord compression. *Ann Emerg Med* **15**: 1235–57.

15 Tal R, Sivan B, Kedar D, Baniel J. (2007). Management of benign ureteral strictures following radical cystectomy and urinary diversion for bladder cancer. *J Urol* **178**: 538–42.

16 Blaivas JG, Weiss JP, Jones M. (2006). The pathophysiology of lower urinary tract symptoms after brachytherapy for prostate cancer. *BJU International* **98**: 1233–7.

17 Wright JL, Lin DW, Dewan P, Montgomery RB (2005). Tumor lysis syndrome in a patient with metastatic, androgen independent prostate cancer. *Int J Urol* **12**: 1012–13.

18 Fujikawa,K, Miyamoto T, Ihara Y, Matsui Y, Takeuchi H. (2001). High incidence of severe urologic complications following radiotherapy for cervical cancer in Japanese women. *Gynecol Oncol* **80**: 21–3.

19 McIntyre JF, Eifel PJ, Levenback C, Oswald MJ (1995). Ureteral stricture as a late complication of radiotherapy for stage IB carcinoma of the uterine cervix. *Cancer* **75**: 836–43.

20 Lee N, Wuu CS, Brody R, Laguna JL, Katz AE, Bagiella E, and Ennis RD (2000). Factors predicting for postimplantation urinary retention after permanent prostate brachytherapy. *Int J Rad Oncol, Biol, Phys* **48**: 1457–60.

21 Klahr S (1991). New insights into the consequences and mechanisms of renal impairment in obstructive nephropathy (editoral). *Am J Kidney Dis* **18**: 689–99.

22 Hwang SJ, Haas M, Harris Jr HW (1993). Transport defects of rabbit medullary thick ascending limb cells in obstructive nephropathy. *J Clin Invest* **91**: 21–8.

23 Tanner GA, Knopp LC (1986). Glomerular blood flow after single nephrom obstruction in the rat kidney. *Am J Physiol* **250**: F77–85.

24 Klotman P, Smith S, Volpp B, et al. (1986). Thromboxane inhibition improves func-tion of hydronephrotic rat kidneys. *Am J Physiol* **250**: F282.

25 Klahr S (2001). Urinary tract obstruction. *Semin Nephrol* **21**: 133–45.

26 Schnermann JB, Zhy XL, Shu X, et al. (1996). Regulation of endothelin production and secretion in cultured collecting duct cells by endogenous transforming growth factor-beta. *Endocrinology* **137**: 5000–8.

27 Hocher B, Thone-Reineke C, Rohmeiss P, et al. (1997). Endothelin-1 transgenic mice develop glomerulosclerosis, interstitial fibrosis, and renal cysts but not hypertension. *J Clin Invest* **99**: 1380–9.

28 Guo G, Morrissey JJ, McCracken R, et al. (1999). The role of TNFR1 and TNFR2 receptors in the interstitial fibrosis of obstructive nephropathy. *Am J Physiol* **277**: F766–F72.

29 Troung LD, Petrusevska G, Yang G, et al. (1996). Cell apoptosis and proliferation in experimental chronic obstructive uropathy. *Kidney Int* **50**: 200–7.

30 Batlle DC, Arruda JA, Kurtzman NA (1981). Hyperkalemic distal renal tubular acidosis associated with obstructive uropathy. *N Eng J Med* **304**: 373–80.

31 Ali Y, Gupta RK, Kehinde EO, Johnny KV (2006). Extreme hyperkalaemia secondary to malignant ureteric obstruction: case report. *East African Medical Journal* **83**: 637–40.

32 Huang WC, Yang SH, Yang JM. (2007). Two- and 3-dimensional ultrasonography in acute urinary retention due to distal urethral obstruction by infiltrating metastatic colon cancer. *J Ultras Med* **26**: 255–9.

33 Takeuchi M, Matsuzaki K, Kubo H, Nishitani H (2008). Diffusion-weighted magnetic resonance imaging of urinary epithelial cancer with upper urinary tract obstruction: preliminary results. *Acta Radiologica* **49**: 1195–9.

34 Chahal R, Taylor K, Eardley I, Lloyd SN, and Spencer JA. (2005). Patients at high risk for upper tract urothelial cancer: evaluation of hydronephrosis using high resolution magnetic resonance urography. *J Urol* **174**(2): 478–82.

35 Bhave G, Lewis JB, and Chang SS. (2008). Association of gadolinium based magnetic resonance imaging contrast agents and nephrogenic systemic fibrosis. *J Urol* **180**(3): 830–5.

36 Idee JM, Port M, Dencausse A, Lancelot E, Corot C. (2009). Involvement of gadolinium chelates in the mechanism of nephrogenic systemic fibrosis: an update. *J Am Acad Dermatol* **61**: 868–74.

37 Okayama S, Matsui M, Somekawa S, Iwano M, Saito Y (2009). Non-contrast MRI for the evaluation of hydronephrotic and dysfunctioning kidney secondary to testicular cancer. *Renal Failure* **31**: 153–8.

38 Goessl C, Knispel HH, Miller K, Klan R (1997). Is routine excretory urography necessary at first diagnosis of bladder cancer? *J Urol* **157**: 480–1.

39 Chye R, Lickiss N (1994). The use of corticosteroids in the management of bilateral malignant ureteric obstruction. *J Pain Symp Manage* **9**: 537–40.

40 Hamdy FC, Williams JL (1995). Use of dexamethasone for ureteric obstruction in advanced prostate cancer: Percutaneous nephrostomies can be avoided. *Br J Urol* **75**: 782–5.

41 Chaulk JR, Fisher RF (1920). An experimental study of ureteral ligation: demonstration of late results to ureter and kidney. *Surg Gynecol Obstet* **30**: 343–9.

42 Vaughn Jr ED, Gillenwater JY (1971). Recovery following complete chronic unilateral occlusion: functional, radiographic and pathologic alterations. *J Urol* **106**: 27–36.

43 Vaughan Jr ED, Sweet RE, Gillenwater JY (1973). Unilateral ureteral occlusion: pattern of nephron repair and compensatory response. *J Urol* **109**: 979–82.

44 Cohen E, Sobrero M, Roxe DM, Levin ML (1992). Reversibility of long-standing urinary tract obstruction requiring long-term dialysis. *Arch Intern Med* **152**: 177–9.

45 Ravanan R and Tomson CRV (2007). Natural history of postobstructive nephropathy: a single-center retrospective study. *Nephron Clin Pract* **105**: c165–c170.

46 McAfee JG, Singh A, O'Callaghan JP (1980). Nuclear imaging supplementary to the urography in obstructive uropathy. *Radiology* **137**: 487–96.

47 Green J, Vardy Y, Munichor M, Better OS (1986). Extreme unilateral hydronephrosis with normal GFR: Physiologic studies in a case of obstructive uropathy. *J Urol* **136**: 361–5.

48 Conrad S, Busch R, Huland H (1991). Complicated urinary tract infections. *Eur Urol* **19**: 16–22.

49 Nariculam J, Murphy DG, Jenner C, et al (2009). Nephrostomy insertion for patients with bilateral ureteric obstruction caused by prostate cancer. *Brit J Radiol* **82**: 571–6.

50 Thiruchelvam N, Ubhayakar G, Mostafid H (2006). The management of hydronephrosis in patients undergoing TURBT. *International Urology & Nephrology* **38**: 483–6.

51 Holden S, McPhee M, Grabstald H (1979). The rationale of urinary diversion in the cancer patient. *J Urol* **121**: 19–21.

52 Feng, M.I, Bellman, G.C, and Shapiro, C.E (1999). Management of ureteral obstruction secondary to pelvic malignancies. *J Endourol* **13**: 521–4.

53 Harrington KJ, Pandha HS, Kelly SA, Lambert HE, Jackson JE, Waxman J (1995). Palliation of obstructive nephropathy due to malignancy. *Br J Urol* **76**: 101–7.

54 Barton DP, Morse SS, Fiorica JV, Hoffman MS, Roberts WS, Cavanagh D (1992). Percutaneous nephrostomy and ureteral stenting in gynecologic malignancies. *Obstetr Gynecol* **80**: 805–11.

55 Rotariu P, Yohannes P, Alexianu M, Puppo P, Perachino M, Ricciotti G, Bozzo W (1994). Laparoscopic cutaneous ureterostmy for palliation of ureteral obstruc-tion caused by advanced pelvic cancer. *J Endourol* **8**: 425–8.

56 Ekici S, Sahin A, Ozen H (2001). Percutaneous nephrostomy in the management of malignant ureteral obstruction secondary to bladder cancer. *J Endourol* **15**: 827–9.

57 Cardona AF, Garzon JR, Burgos E, et al. (2006). Mortality and complications associated with percutaneous nephrostomy in patients with ureteral obstruction related to advanced cervical cancer. *Journal of Palliative Care* **22**: 315.

58 Chang HL, Lim HW, Su FH, Tsai ST, Wang YW (2006). Win or lose? Percutaneous nephrostomy for a terminal-stage cervical-cancer patient featuring obstructive uropathy. *Journal of Palliative Care* **22**: 57–60.

59 Hyams ES, Shah O (2008). Malignant extrinsic ureteral obstruction: a survey of urologists and medical oncologists regarding treatment patterns and preferences. *Urology* **72**: 51–6.

60 Chitale SV, Scott-Barrett S, Ho ETS, Burgess NA (2002). The management of ureteric obstruction secondary to malignant pelvic disease. *Clin Radiol* **57**: 1118–21.

61 Uthappa MC, Cowan NC (2005). Retrograde or antegrade double-pigtail stent placement for malignant ureteric obstruction? *Clin Radiol* **60**: 608–12.

62 Ganatra AM, Loughlin KR (2005). The management of malignant ureteral obstruction treated with ureteral stents. *J Urol* **174**: 2125–8.

63 Alsikafi NF, O'Connor RC, Kuznetsov DD, Dachman AH, Bales GT, Gerber GS (2002). Prospective evaluation of ureteral stent durability in patients with chronic ureteral obstruction. *Urology* **59**: 847–50.

64 Rotariu P, Yohannes P, Alexianu M (2001). Management of malignant extrinsic compression of the ureter by simultaneous placement of two ipsilateral ureteral stents. *J Endourol* **15**: 979–83.

65 Barbalias G, Siablis D, Liatsikos E, et al. (1997). Metal stents: A new treatment of malignant ureteral obstruction. *J Urol* **158**: 54–8.

66 Lopez-Martinez R, Singireddy, S, and Lang, E.K (1997). The use of metallic stents to bypass ureteral strictures secondary to metastatic prostate cancer: Experience with 8 patients. *J Urol* **158**: 50–3.

67 Daskalopoulos G, Hatzidakis A, and Triantafyllou T (2001). Intraureteral metallic endoprosthesis in the treatment of ureteral strictures. *Eur J Rad* **39**: 194–200.

68 Barbalias GA, Liatsikos EN, Kalogeropoulou C, Karnabatidis D, Siablis D (2000). Metallic stents in gynecologic cancer: an approach to treat extrinsic ureteral obstruction. *Eur Urol* **38**: 35–40.

69 Wakui M, Takeuchi S, Isioka J, Iwabuchi K, Morimoto S (2000). Metallic stents for malignant and benign ureteric obstruction. *BJC Int* **85**: 227–32.

70 Tekin MI, Aytekin C, Aygun C, PeSkircioglu L, Boyvatn F, Ozkardes H (2001). Covered metallic ureteral stent in the management of malignant ureteral obstruc-tion: preliminary results. *Urol* **58**: 919–23.

71 Nagele U, Kuczyk MA, Horstmann M et al. (2008). Initial clinical experience with full-length metal ureteral stents for obstructive ureteral stenosis. *World J Urol* **26**: 257–62.

72 Borin JF, Melamud O, Clayman RV (2006). Initial experience with full-length metal stent to relieve malignant ureteral obstruction. *J Endourol* **20**: 300–4.

73 Oh SJ, Ku JH, Byun SS, et al. (2005). Systemic chemotherapy in patients with indwelling ureteral stenting. *Int J Urol* **12**: 548–51.

74 Desgrandchamps F, Cussenot O, Meria P, Cortesse A, Teillac P, Le Duc A (1995). Subcutaneous urinary diversions for palliative treatment of pelvic malignancies. *J Urol* **154**: 367–70.

75 Nissenkorn I, Gdor Y (2000). Nephrovesical subcutaneous stent: An alternative to permanent nephrostomy. *J Urol* **163**: 528–30.

76 Gupta NP, Kolla SB, Seth A, et al (2007). Oncological and functional outcome of radical cystectomy in patients with bladder cancer and obstructive uropathy. *J Urol* **178**(4 Pt 1): 1206–11.

77 Kaouk JH, Gill IS, Desai MM (2001). Laparoscopic orthotopic ileal neobladder. *J Endourol* **15**: 131–42.

78 Leissner J, Black P, Fisch M, Hockel M, Hohenfellner R (2000). Colon pouch (Mainz pouch III) for continent urinary diversion after pelvic irradiation. *Urol* **56**: 798–802.

79 Horan G, McArdle O, Martin J, Collins CD, Faul C (2006). Pelvic radiotherapy in patients with hydronephrosis in stage IIIB cancer of the cervix: renal effects and the optimal timing for urinary diversion? *Gynecologic Oncology* **101**: 441–4.

80 Wen CC, Wang DS (2005). Laparoscopic ureterolysis for benign and malignant conditions. *J Endourol* **19**: 710–14.

81 Sevin G, Soyupek S, Armagan A, Hoscan MB, Oksay T (2004). Ileal orthotopic neobladder (modified Hautmann) via a shorter detubularized ileal segment: experience and results. *BJU International* **94**: 355–9.

82 Castellan M, Gosalbez R (2006). Ureteral replacement using the Yang-Monti principle: long-term follow-up. *Urol* **67**: 476–9.

83 Foster, MC, Upsdell SM, O'Reilly PH (1990). Urological myths. *Br Med J* **301**: 1421.

84 Osius TG, Hynman Jr F (1963). Dynamics of acute urinary retention: A manomet-ric, radiographic and clinical study. *J Urol* **90**: 702.

85 Fukasawa M, Kobayashi H, Matsushita K, Araki I, Takeda M (2002). Intraperitoneal rupture of giant hydronephrosis due to ureteral cancer accompanied by renal cell carcinoma. *J Urol* **167**: 1393–4.

86 Yuh B, Padalino J, Butt ZM (2008). Impact of tumour volume on surgical and patho-logical outcomes after robot-assisted radical cystectomy. *BJU International* **102**: 840–3.

87 Bartsch GC, Kuefer R, Gschwend JE (2007). Hydronephrosis as a prognostic marker in bladder cancer in a cystectomy-only series. *Eur Urol* **51**: 690–7.

88 Larsen SG, Wiig JN, Giercksky KE (2005). Hydronephrosis as a prognostic factor in pelvic recurrence from rectal and colon carcinomas. *Am J Surg* **190**: 55–60.

89 Russo P (2000). Urologic emergencies in the cancer patient. *Semin Oncol* **27**: 284–98.

90 Wong LM, Cleeve LK, Milner AD, Pitman AG (2007). Malignant ureteral obstruction: outcomes after intervention. Have things changed? *J Urol* **178**: 178–83.

91 Donat SM, Russo P (1996). Ureteral decompression in advanced non-urologic malignancies. *Ann Syrg Oncol* **3**: 393–9.

92 Canter D, Guzzo TJ, Resnick MJ (2008). Hydronephrosis is an independent predictor of poor clinical outcome in patients treated for muscle-invasive transitional cell carcinoma with radical cystectomy. *Urol* **72**: 379–83.

93 Lev-Chelouche D, Keidar A, Rub R, Matzkin H, Gutman M (2001). Hydronephrosis associated with colorectal carcinoma: treatment and outcome. *Eur J Surg Oncol* **27**: 482–6.

94 Cheng C, Rodriguez-Bigas MA, Petrelli N (2001). Is there a role for curative surgery for pelvic recurrence from rectal carcinoma in the presence of hydronephrosis? *Am J Surg* **182**: 274–7.

95 Brown G, Grury AE, Cunningham D, Husband JE (2003). Clinical CT detection of hydronephrosis in resected colorectal cancer: a predictor of recurrent disease. *Clin Radiol* **58**: 137–42.

96 Ishioka J, Kageyama Y, Inoue M, Higashi Y, Kihara K (2008). Prognostic model for predicting survival after palliative urinary diversion for ureteral obstruction: analysis of 140 cases. *J Urol* **180**: 618–21.

Chapter 11

Acquired cysts and cancer of failing kidneys

Isao Ishikawa

Case report

A 59-year-old male had begun chronic hemodialysis treatment at 35 years of age (1984) because of chronic renal failure due to IgA nephropathy (bilateral kidney volume: 162 mL). Periodic plain computed tomography (CT) scan was carried out once a year and the kidneys showed the greatest contraction three years after starting of hemodialysis (99 mL); thereafter, the kidneys became enlarged due to acquired renal cysts. Although gross hematuria was noted in May 2005 and renal cell carcinoma (RCC) was suspected, imaging study showed only acquired renal cysts in the kidneys (423 mL). A tumor at the middle part of the right kidney was suspected in June 2007. However, the suspected mass was not enhanced by dynamic CT and pre-operative diagnosis of RCC could not be established. Therefore, follow-up was continued. The top of Fig. 11.1 demonstrates the dynamic CT scan obtained 23.4 years after the start of hemodialysis (2007/6), which did not show any contrast enhancement (471 mL). Six months afterward (2007/12) the dynamic CT was re-examined. As shown at the bottom of Fig. 11.1, the size of the tumor in the right kidney had increased from 3 cm to 4 cm in diameter and the tumor was slightly enhanced by dynamic CT, indicating a hypovascular tumor. A contrast-enhanced ultrasonographic image obtained with perflubutane microbubble (Sonazoid ®) is demonstrated in Fig. 11.2(a). The tumor is indicated by arrows, and tumor enhancement by contrast media was obtained. The time-intensity curve showed clear tumor enhancement. The PET/CT scan shown in Fig. 11.2(b) demonstrates uptake of F-18 FDG into the tumor as indicated by an arrow in the right lower panel. In the fusion images of PET and CT, the uptake of F-18 FDG is observed in accordance with the part of a tumor in each tomographic section of CT. When right nephrectomy was performed in February 2008, the tumor measured 3.7 x 3.4 x 4.8cm. Figs. 2(c) and (d) demonstrate the histology of the tumor, which showed papillary RCC (2(c)), containing the deposition of many Ca oxalate crystals (2(d)). The tumor was diagnosed as pT1b, Nx, M0, INFα, and G2, Stage I, and met the criteria for an acquired cystic disease (ACD)-associated RCC (1) (Fig. 11.3).

In summary, gross hematuria had occasionally developed during the previous two-and-a-half years in this patient with a 24-year history of hemodialysis. Since the tumor was hypovascular, surrounded by many acquired renal cysts and did not bulge beyond the kidney outline, a pre-operative diagnosis of RCC was difficult to establish. The pre-operative diagnosis was finally made based on repeated dynamic CT scans, contrast-enhanced ultrasonography, and PET/CT. This patient has not shown any sign of metastasis as of August 2010.

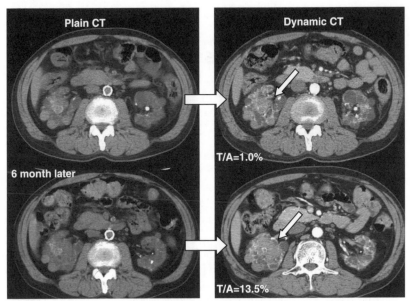

Fig. 11.1 Dynamic CT in June and December 2007. In his case: CT in December 2007 demonstrated an enlarged mass, compared with June 2007, and slight enhancement of the tumor on dynamic CT. RCC in this patient with long-term hemodialysis was surrounded by many cysts and showed poor contrast enhancement, resulting in difficulty in establishing a pre-operative diagnosis of RCC. T/A = Ratio of contrast enhancement of tumor to aorta. (Left panel: plain CT; right panel: contrast-enhanced dynamic CT).

Introduction

Dunnill et al. (2) first reported renal cell carcinoma (RCC) occurring in the diseased kidneys with acquired renal cysts in dialysis patients based on an autopsy study. The first clinical case (a 24-year-old male on hemodialysis for seven years due to chronic glomerulonephritis) of RCC complicated by acquired cystic disease of the kidney (ACDK) was reported by Ishikawa et al. (3) in 1980. This patient developed bladder cancer eight years ago; however, he is being treated by hemodialysis as of August 2010.

Acquired cysts of failing kidneys

Definition of acquired cystic disease of the kidney (ACDK)

ACDK is defined as acquired renal cysts developing in bilateral contracted kidneys regardless of the original renal disease (2–3). When three or more cysts in a kidney are clinically observed on imaging, or 25% or more of the

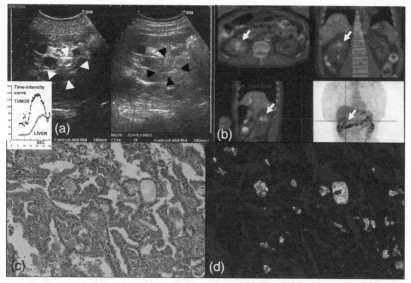

Fig. 11.2 Contrast-enhanced ultrasonography, PET/CT and histology of this case.
(a) Contrast-enhanced ultrasonography demonstrated clear enhancement by
perflubutane microbubble, as shown by a time-intensity curve. (Left panel: contrast
harmonic image; right panel: tissue harmonic image.) (b) As shown by PET/CT, there
was FDG uptake by this tumor. (c) ACD-associated RCC (H and E stain, x100). (d)
Polarized microscopy demonstrated abundant deposition of Ca oxalate crystals on (c).
Reproduced with permission from Ishikawa, I (2008). Present status of acquired cystic disease of the kidney, *J Jpn Ass Dial Physicians*, **23**: 179–187.

cut surface of a kidney is occupied by cysts on pathology, a diagnosis of ACDK
is made, although the numbers of cysts and area occupied by cysts are arbitrary.
However, when a renal cyst is demonstrated on imaging study, the fact that 20
or more cysts were demonstrated by pathology should be made known (3).

Factors related to development and enlargement of ACDK

1 The most important factor related to the development and enlargement of
  ACDK is the duration of chronic renal failure and dialysis (3). The longer
  the duration of dialysis becomes, the greater is the incidence and severity of
  acquired renal cysts. When renal function decreases to low normal (creatinine clearance: 52–71 mL/min), microscopic acquired renal cysts begin to
  develop (4). Acquired renal cysts have been observed in 12% of patients
  before the start of dialysis. Thereafter, acquired renal cysts develop in 44% of
  patients within less than three years after starting hemodialysis and develop

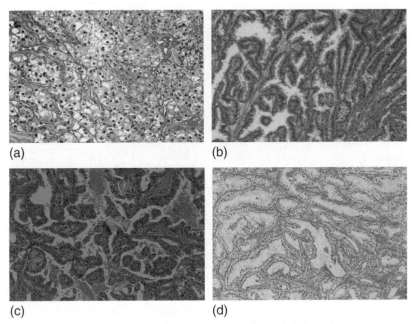

Fig. 11.3 Main histological subtypes in RCC seen in hemodialysis patients.
(a) Conventional clear cell RCC. (b) Papillary RCC. (c) ACD-associated RCC. (d) Clear cell papillary RCC.

in 79% of patients after more than three years (5). Acquired renal cysts are observed in 90% of patients after more than ten years of hemodialysis (3) or 90% between five and ten years (6). We performed a cross-sectional study of the present status of ACDK in our dialysis center in 2007 (7). The volume of diseased kidneys in 178 dialysis patients was investigated by CT scan. As a result, there were 90 glomerulonephritic patients; the male to female ratio was 55:35 and the mean age was 60.8 ± 10.9 years old, showing an increase of 20.5 years compared with data from 1979 (5), and the mean duration of hemodialysis was 15.5 ± 9.4 years with an increase of 12.2 years compared with the data of 1979 (5). Mean volume of the bilateral kidneys was 196.8 ± 263.0 mL and increased by 2.3 times compared to 1979 (5); the bilateral kidney volume exceeded 400 mL in 13 of 90 chronic glomerulonephritic patients (14.4%) and the maximum bilateral kidney volume was 1655 mL. ACDK sometimes becomes enlarged, mimicking autosomal dominant polycystic kidney disease. The maximal weight of a single kidney with ACDK was reported to be 1094g (8) and 1250g (9) (including RCC).

A twenty-year follow-up (10) of the bilateral kidney volume in 96 dialysis patients with chronic glomerulonephritis starting in 1979 demonstrated that the bilateral kidney volume increased from 57.8 (1.51) mL (geometric mean (geometric standard deviation)) to 185.3 (2.03) mL in males and from 57.3 (1.64) mL to 99.7 (2.36) mL in females. Therefore, ACDK and ACDK-related RCC are important issues especially for chronic glomerulonephritic patients in whom long-term survival is feasible.

2 There is a gender difference in ACDK. ACDK demonstrates a male preponderance (11). The incidence and severity of acquired renal cysts are higher and more severe in males than in females. The extent of increased kidney volume from 1979 to 1999 was 3.2(2.06)-fold in males and 1.7(2.57)-fold in females, showing a larger value in males than in females (10).

3 ACDK (acquired renal cysts) regresses after successful renal transplantation (12). If renal graft function is good and the acquired cysts are small, regression of acquired cysts occurs more rapidly (3). This is an important observation when considering the pathogenesis of ACDK.

4 ACDK develops regardless of the underlying renal disease. However, the incidence and development of acquired renal cysts in patients with diabetic nephropathy and hypoplastic kidneys are low and slow (13). Fifty-six age-, gender-, and duration-of-dialysis- matched patients with diabetic nephropathy and chronic glomerulonephritis were compared with regard to kidney size on CT scan for an average of 59 months (13). From the start of hemodialysis until seven years after the start of dialysis, kidney volume was larger in patients with diabetic nephropathy than in those with chronic glomerulonephritis. Furthermore, renal atrophy was delayed and the development of acquired renal cysts was retarded in patients with diabetic nephropathy.

5 Although ACDK develops regardless of age, the incidence and severity of acquired renal cysts are comparatively higher in younger patients (3). ACDK also develops in pediatric patients with chronic renal failure. Our patients whose kidney volume increased 3.2 or more-fold during the 20-year follow-up were younger than 40 years old at the start of observation.

6 ACDK develops regardless of dialysis modality and develops both hemodialysis patients and peritoneal dialysis patients (14). ACDK development shows greater severity in black patients than in white patients (6).

7 There are no differences in the severity of ACDK between hemodialysis patients using cuprophan membrane and those using synthetic membrane.

8 Histologically, ACDK contains precursor lesions for malignant growth, such as hyperplastic epithelial cells of atypical cysts and renal adenoma (2). Ca oxalate crystals are often present in the cyst wall and cyst cavity, as well as the renal parenchyma (2).

Two major complications of ACDK

Retroperitoneal bleeding due to rupture of acquired renal cysts

Bleeding from rupture of acquired renal cysts, such as bleeding into the renal parenchyma and renal pelvis, peri-renal bleeding and retroperitoneal bleeding, are known. We consider that the prevalence of retroperitoneal bleeding is about 0.5% or one-third of that of RCC (3). Seventy percent of retroperitoneal bleeding is caused by minor trauma and the action of heparin. Thirty percent of retroperitoneal bleeding may be due to bleeding from RCC (9).

RCC as a complication of ACDK

RCC is the most important complication of ACDK and is described in the following section.

Cancer of failing kidneys

Incidence and epidemiology of RCC

In 81 % of RCC in patients with end-stage renal failure receiving dialysis, RCC develops in relation to acquired renal cysts (15). The incidence of RCC in failing kidneys with acquired renal cysts is related to the duration of chronic renal failure and hemodialysis. However, in patients with end-stage renal disease (ESRD), the incidence of RCC was high within one year before the start of hemodialysis. Distribution of the incidence of RCC in hemodialysis patients shows two peaks; the first peak is within one year after the start of dialysis (RCC unrelated to ACDK) and the second peak occurs after long-term dialysis (RCC related to ACDK). The reason many RCCs are detected within one year before and after the start of hemodialysis currently remains unknown.

The prevalence of RCC is 1.5% in whole hemodialysis patients and it is 4.0% in hemodialysis patients with ACDK (3). Denton et al. (16) reported that the prevalence of RCC before renal transplantation in 260 patients with short duration of hemodialysis (median duration of dialysis of one year) was 4.2%. Annual incidence of RCC per 100,000 dialysis patients was 191 patients overall, but decreased to 112 patients among those with less than ten years of dialysis and increased to 438 patients among those with more than ten years of dialysis (17). The incidence of RCC in male dialysis patients was four times greater than in female patients, similarly to the incidence of ACDK.

In our 20-year follow-up of ACDK and RCC in 96 dialysis patients (10), six RCCs developed during this period and there was no new development of RCC between 15- and 20-year follow-up except for a recurrence of RCC in one patient. Although 44 patients died over a 20-year period and malignant tumors were the cause of death in seven patients, there were no deaths due to RCC.

As a death related to ACDK, one patient died of retroperitoneal bleeding due to the rupture of ACDK. In addition, RCC newly developed in a patient between 20 and 28 years of follow-up, and finally eight RCCs developed in seven of 96 dialysis patients during a 28-year follow-up.

The age-adjusted standardized incidence ratio (SIR) of RCC in dialysis patients was 14.3–17.1 according to Ishikawa (17), and it was 3.6 according to Maisonneuve et al. (18). Ishikawa reported that RCC in dialysis patients aged 30 to 40 years was 54 to 143 times higher in male patients and 284 to 412 times higher in female patients than in the general population. Maisonneuve et al. reported from analysis of 1,303 US dialysis patients that younger patients demonstrated a high SIR of RCC, i.e. SIR was 41.5 in patients aged 0–34 years, 5.2 in patients aged 35–64 years and 2.3 in patients aged more than 65 years. The incidence of ACDK in peritoneal dialysis patients did not differ from that in hemodialysis patients (14). Therefore, the incidence of RCC in peritoneal dialysis patients is the same as that in hemodialysis patients. According to Savaj et al. (19), the annual incidence of RCC was estimated to be 130 per 100,000 peritoneal dialysis patients. In subjects with a kidney transplant, Doublet et al. (20) found five cases of RCC (3.9%) among 129 recipients, up to 106 months after transplantation, with a pre-transplant duration of dialysis of 30 months. He reported that the incidence of RCC is 100 times higher than that in the general population. Neuzillet et al. (21) reported that 12 RCCs were observed in 11 of 933 allograft recipients (1.2%, compared to 0.12% in the general population), within an average of 70.9 months (8–156 months) after transplantation. Besarani et al. (22) reported that 87 RCCs among 10,847 allograft recipients were found (0.8%). Schwartz et al. showed that the prevalence of patients with RCC in native kidneys after renal transplantation is 5% (23). Although we detected four RCCs in 269 renal transplantation recipients, RCCs in three of four patients appeared to have developed before renal transplantation according to our detailed examination. RCC diagnosed after renal transplantation should be investigated to determine whether it is a carry-over of the tumor that developed during hemodialysis or a de novo development after transplantation.

Results of nationwide questionnaire surveys in Japan

Nationwide questionnaire surveys of RCC arising in dialysis patients in Japan have been performed 12 times in total, once every two years between 1982 and 2004 (17). During this period, 2873 RCCs were collected. The male to female ratio was 4:1 and the mean age was 55.5 ± 11.5 (2004 survey: 58.9 ± 10.9) years old, which was younger than in the general population. Mean duration of dialysis was 126.9 ± 84.9 (2004 survey: 145.7 ± 95.0) months. The relation between the incidence of RCC and the age of patients with RCC has already been described. The SIR of RCC was higher in patients with chronic glomerulonephritis than in patients with nephrosclerosis or diabetic nephropathy. Diagnostic modalities for RCC were mainly ultrasonography and CT scan, and symptoms such as gross hematuria only appeared in 8%. Metastases were observed in 15.4%, and the 73% of these were detected at the diagnosis of RCC. Some patients with RCC died from cancer (6.3%) during the two-year observation period. RCC in dialysis patients develops in both kidneys (14.5%). There are two types of RCC in dialysis patients. One is RCC unrelated to ACDK (older patients with short duration of dialysis) and the other is RCC related to ACDK in 81%. The latter is seen in relatively younger male patients with a longer duration of dialysis. Histologic classification of RCC (7) according to the duration of dialysis demonstrated that clear cell RCC comprised the majority of tumors arising 0–10 years after the start of dialysis, but thereafter non-clear cell RCC comprised the majority of tumors arising more than ten years after the start of dialysis and clear cell RCC comprised only 20% of those arising after more than 25 years of hemodialysis (Fig. 11.4). Numbers of RCC in each year after the start of dialysis were studied in patients with chronic glomerulonephritis and diabetic nephropathy (Fig. 11.5). RCC in patients

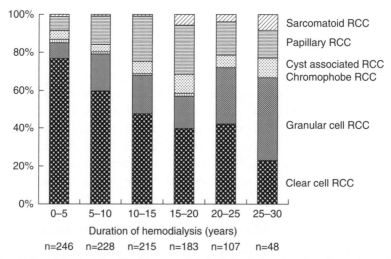

Fig. 11.4 Histological classification of RCC (*General rule for clinical and pathological studies on RCC*, 1999) collected by a nationwide Japanese questionnaire survey, depending on the duration of hemodialysis: It is shown that the incidence of granular cell RCC increases in patients with long-term hemodialysis while that of clear cell RCC decreases in patients with long-term hemodialysis.
Reproduced with permission from Ishikawa, I (2008). Present status of acquired cystic disease of the kidney, *J Jpn Ass Dial Physicians*, **23**: 179–187.

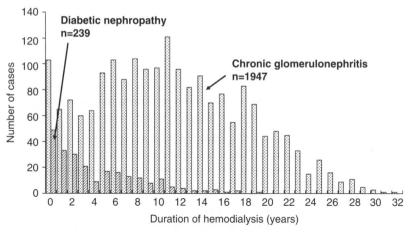

Fig. 11.5 RCC in patients with chronic glomerulonephritis and diabetic nephropathy, classified by the duration of hemodialysis: RCC in diabetic nephropathy develops during short-term hemodialysis and RCC in chronic glomerulonephritis increases in long-term hemodialysis.

Reproduced with permission from Ishikawa, I (2008). Present status of acquired cystic disease of the kidney, *J Jpn Ass Dial Physicians*, **23**: 179–187.

with chronic glomerulonephritis increased with long-term dialysis, while RCC in patients with diabetic nephropathy were higher at the introduction for dialysis.

When a comparison of patients with RCC was made between those with fewer than ten years of hemodialysis and those with more than 20 years of hemodialysis, patients with more than 20 years of hemodialysis were younger, predominantly males, more frequently complicated by ACDK, and had larger tumor sizes, higher ratios of papillary RCC, a higher metastatic rate, and a higher rate of renal cancer death (15). Risk factors for RCC developing in dialysis patients are being a young male, being a long-term dialysis patient, and having enlarged kidneys due to severe acquired renal cysts (3).

Diagnosis of RCC in dialysis patients

1 Although dynamic CT scan is currently the most useful modality for pre-operative diagnosis of RCC when a suspicious tumor is detected by ultra-sonography or plain CT scan, judging the presence of enhancement of a hypovascular tumor on dynamic CT is sometimes difficult. To diagnose RCC pre-operatively we have to confirm the presence of vascularity (blood flow) in a solid mass by any diagnostic modality, such as dynamic CT or contrast-enhanced ultrasonography, in order to differentiate between RCC and bleeding cysts (24).

Diagnosis of RCC in short-term dialysis patients is comparatively easy because RCC projects beyond the atrophic kidney contour and clear cell RCC, which often occurs in short-term dialysis patients, demonstrates hypervascularity on dynamic CT in many cases. The ratio of contrast enhancement of the tumor to aorta was 1:4 for these tumors. In contrast, diagnosis of RCC in long-term dialysis patients is remarkably difficult because RCC is surrounded by many acquired renal cysts, and RCC in long-term dialysis patients is hypovascular in many cases (3), as shown in the case report in this chapter. The ratio of contrast enhancement of the tumor to aorta was 1:11 for these hypovascular tumors. Furthermore, diagnosis is difficult when a papillary RCC exists in the wall of a cyst with hematoma. In subjects with a functioning kidney transplant, acquired renal cysts may regress in a few months, and the diagnosis of RCC becomes easier (25).

2 In the diagnostic procedure for hypovascular tumor surrounded by many acquired renal cysts in long-term hemodialysis a T2-weighted image of plain MRI is added to the conventional ultrasonography and CT scan. A diffusion-weighted image in MRI may also be performed. A hypovascular tumor by dynamic CT may be shown as a clearly enhanced mass by contrast-enhanced ultrasonography. Ultrasonographic contrast media forms an image by the vibration of perflubutane microbubble (26). The contrast-enhanced ultrasonography image can be observed in real time, facilitating the determination of blood flow in the renal mass. Because gadolinium-containing MR contrast media cause nephrogenic systemic fibrosis and are contraindicated for hemodialysis patients, contrast-enhanced ultrasonography by perflubutane microbubble or sulfurhexafluoride microbubble (SonoVue®) (27) may be useful, after dynamic CT. Because of anuria in long-term dialysis patients, F-18 FDG is not excreted into the urinary tract. Therefore, F-18 FDG PET/CT may be useful to make a diagnosis of RCC in dialysis patients (28–9) as shown in our case report. However, the false negative rate of RCC in dialysis patients by F-18 FDG PET/CT is currently unknown.

Screening of RCC in dialysis patients

Periodic screening for RCC is recommended for selected dialysis patients (3, 30), because the incidence of RCC in dialysis patients is high, patients usually do not show symptoms, and the post-operative prognosis of RCC detected on screening is good (31). Examination for RCC is necessary when a patient complains of symptoms of RCC, and even if there are no symptoms, periodic screening is required according to the risks of developing RCC described above. Screening is recommended from the start of hemodialysis. Screening is not recommended for all dialysis patients from the perspective of cost effectiveness

(32) because of the growing number of older patients with diabetic nephropathy and nephrosclerosis. However, it is necessary for renal allograft recipients to be screened for RCC before renal transplantation (16, 23, 33). Since the diagnosis of RCC becomes easier when the acquired renal cysts regress after transplantation in patients with severe cystic changes, screening may need to be repeated a few months after renal transplantation (3) for patients showing severe cystic changes of the kidneys before renal transplantation. Screening may be carried out in patients who can tolerate nephrectomy when RCC is discovered. When there is no contrast enhancement of the tumor on dynamic CT in male patients with a duration of dialysis of more than ten years who show severe ACDK, plain MRI and/or contrast-enhanced ultrasonography are carried out to detect RCC, and nephrectomy should be performed if RCC is suspected. Otherwise, follow-up one or two times a year should be continued (7).

New histologic classification of RCC in dialysis patients

Characteristics of RCC in failing kidneys are the development of multiple tumors in the kidney and a high incidence of bilateral RCCs. Conventionally, RCC in dialysis patients shows a high incidence of papillary RCCs (dialysis patients: 48.8%, general population: 4.8%) (34). However, Sule et al. (35), Tickoo et al. (1), Cossu-Rocca et al. (36) and Gobbo et al. (37) proposed a new classification by histological and histochemical studies, because RCC in dialysis patients showed histological findings that cannot be classified into the subtypes of RCC seen in the general population (see Fig. 11.3).

Tickoo et al. (1) described tumors occurring in kidneys with ESRD as follows: (a) those resembling sporadic renal tumors are clear cell RCC, papillary RCC type1 and type 2, and chromophobe RCC; (b) tumors distinct from sporadic renal tumors are ACD-associated RCC, and clear cell papillary RCC of end-stage kidneys; and (c) other tumor-like lesions are cysts, putative precursor lesions, clustered microcystic lesions, and papillary adenomas. According to Tickoo et al. (1), the usual RCC seen in the general population occurred in only 41% of RCCs in patients with ESRD and dialysis, and characteristic 'ACD-associated RCC' in dialysis patients was seen in 36%, and 'clear cell papillary RCC of end-stage kidneys' was seen in 23%.

In ACD-associated RCC, tumor cells are large, have eosinophilic (acidophilic) and granular cytoplasm, have a Fuhrman's grade 3 nucleus, and have conspicuous nucleoli. ACD-associated RCC shows the same structure as type 2 classic papillary RCC. The deposition of Ca oxalate crystals is observed in 80% of these tumors. Tumor cells demonstrate a unique cribriform appearance and the architecture of tumor cells is solid acinar, solid sheet-like, and microcystic or macrocystic. Immunohistological study shows positive α-methylacyl-CoA racemase (AMACR) and negative cytokeratin 7 (CK7). Differentiation between ACD-associated RCC and type 2 classic papillary RCC is necessary. Existence of intratumoral deposition of Ca oxalate crystals and the presence of intracellular and intercellular clear spaces facilitates histological differentiation (38). Sarcomatoid changes of ACD-associated RCC were also observed in progressive cases (1, 39–40).

However, clear cell papillary RCC of end-stage kidneys is also seen in ESRD patients without ACDK. Tumor cells have clear cytoplasm, the nucleus is Fuhrman's grade 1 or 2, and the main structural type is papillary. Immunohistological study demonstrates negative AMACR and positive CK7. Cytogenetically, the profile also differs from classic clear cell RCC or classic papillary RCC (37). Histological subtypes of RCC, according to the new histological classification proposed by Tickoo et al. (1), the classification of RCC in dialysis patients that we collected by questionnaire studies (17), are shown in Fig. 11.6. The compatibility of the new histological classification in patients with ESRD proposed by Tickoo et al. and the Japanese classification of RCC in dialysis patients collected from questionnaire studies based on the *General rule for clinical and pathological studies on renal cell carcinoma* (3 edn, 1999) (41), is an issue that should be further evaluated. Although the proportion of ACD-associated RCC was high in our long-term dialysis patients, this relationship was not clear in

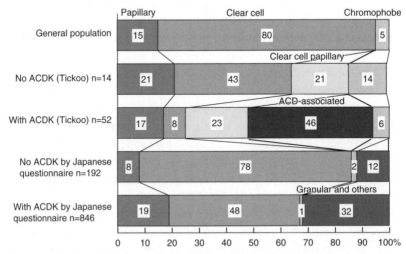

Fig. 11.6 Histological subtypes of RCC in ESRD, according to Tickoo et al. (1), and the histological types of RCC, based on the *General rule for clinical and pathological studies on RCC* of 1999 (41). Many granular and some of clear RCCs may be classified as ACD-associated RCC and many clear RCC may be classified as clear cell papillary RCC.

the patients reported by Tickoo et al. (1). Recently, Nouh et al. described the relationship between the new classification and the Japanese classification in 27 RCCs in dialysis patients and compared histological subtypes and duration of dialysis, and showed a higher incidence of classic clear cell RCC in short-term dialysis patients with fewer than ten years, and higher incidence of ACD-associated RCC in long-term dialysis patients with more than ten years (40).

Classic papillary RCC is divided into type 1 (small cell papillary RCC) and type 2 (large cell papillary RCC) (42). Papillary RCC in dialysis patients is classified as type 2 in the majority of cases.

Treatment of RCC in dialysis patients

The main treatment for RCC in dialysis patients is nephrectomy.

In nephrectomy, laparoscopic radical nephrectomy using a retroperitoneo-scope is being performed more frequently than open nephrectomy (43). When a tumor is large, a transperitoneal approach is used. Usually, nephrectomy ipsilateral to the RCC is performed, and then the contralateral kidney is followed closely. Cytokine therapies such as interferon or IL-2 are less frequently conducted as adjuvant therapy. Molecular target drugs, such as sorafenib or sunitinib, are tried when radical therapy or excision of the tumor is impossible, or RCC has metastasized in dialysis patients. Sorafenib may inhibit tumor growth by a dual mechanism, acting either directly on the tumor (through inhibition of Raf and Kit signaling) and/or on tumor angiogenesis (through inhibition of VEGFR and PDGFR signaling). The dose of sorafenib for dialysis patients is one-half to one-quarter of the dose prescribed for patients with normal renal function (44).

Prognosis of dialysis patients with RCC

The survival rate was assessed using the life table method in 848 patients with RCC collected by 9 previous nationwide questionnaire surveys (45). The actuarial five-year survival rate was 64.0%, and cancer-specific five-year survival rate was 81.5%. When based only on surgically treated cases, the actuarial five-year survival rate was 79.7% and the cancer-specific five-year survival rate was 91.7%. The prognosis of surgically treated cases is good and, in particular, patients detected by screening showed a better prognosis than patients demonstrating symptoms (31). Although the prognosis of RCC in dialysis patients is good on the whole, metastasis has already occurred by the time RCC is diagnosed in a few patients, and a small number of patients demonstrate rapidly growing cancer. Therefore, the death rate within two years after the discovery of RCC is high (45). How to detect a rapidly growing tumor is a very important issue. A method of screening or follow-up to recognize these cases is needed. When the grade and stage of RCC are matched between dialysis patients and the general population, the prognoses for RCC in dialysis patients and for RCC in the general population are the same (3, 6).

Pathogenesis of ACDK and RCC in dialysis patients

Genetic analysis in RCC in dialysis patients

Genetic analysis in RCC in dialysis patients is summarized in Table 11.1. Classic clear cell RCC in dialysis patients demonstrates deletion of 3p25 less frequently than in the general population (46). Classic papillary RCC in the general population demonstrated +7, −Y, and (+17), however, papillary RCC in dialysis patients demonstrated +7 and +17 in a minority of cases (47–48). In two of three patients with ACD-associated RCC, a gain of chromosomes 1, 2, 6, and 10 was observed (36). Gain of chromosomes 1, 2, 6, and 10 was demonstrated in only one or two of 25 patients in our collection of karyotype analyses for papillary RCCs (48). Chromosomal aberrations (clustering gains of chromosome 3, 7, 16, 17, and Y) in multifocal ACD-associated RCCs in the kidney or in the same patient were not identical on studies of comparative genomic hybridization and fluorescence in situ hybridization (49). This finding indicates the field effect of multiplicity of the tumors induced by multiple independent clones. Neither deletion of 3p25 nor +7, −Y, and (+17) were present in clear cell papillary RCC (37). Gain of chromosome 7 and 17 and loss of chromosome Y were demonstrated in non-tumorous lesions such as hyperplastic and dysplastic tubular epithelial cells on fluorescence in situ hybridization (50). We need

Table 11.1 Genetic changes in RCC in dialysis patients

Histology	Genetic changes	Frequency	Authors
Classic clear cell RCC	deletion of 3p25	3/7 tumors	Yoshida, et al[46]
Classic papillary RCC	Gain of chromosome 7 and 17	5/14 tumors, 5/25 tumors	Hughson, et al[47], Ishikawa[48]
Classic papillary RCC	Gain of chromosome 16	17/25 tumors	Ishikawa[48]
ACD-associated RCC	Gain of chromosome 1, 2, 6 and 10	2/3, 2/3, 2/3, 1/3 tumors, respectively	Cossu-Rocca, et al[36]
ACD-associated RCC	Gain of chromosome 3, 7, 16, 17 and Y	8/9, 6/9, 7/9, 4/9, 5/9 tumors, respectively	Pan, et al[49]
Clear cell papillary RCC	No deletion of 3p25, No gain of chromosome 7, 17 and loss of Y	in 7 tumors	Gobbo, et al[37]
Hyperplastic or dysplastic tubular epithelial cells	Gain of chromosome 7, 17 and loss of Y	6/11, 8/11, 2/11 patients, respectively	Hes, et al[50]

further accumulation of genetic data from pre-cancerous lesions to RCC under the new histological classification in dialysis patients.

Etiology of ACDK and RCC in dialysis patients

The relationship between the development of acquired renal cysts and RCC is considered from the histological observation of ACDK (2). Hypothetical mechanisms of developing acquired renal cysts and RCC are as follows (3, 51). First, by progression of renal disease, nephron loss occurs and a compensatory hypertrophic factor (uremic metabolite) begins to affect mainly the proximal tubules of residual nephrons. If the renal disease progresses further, mitogenic factors, such as further accumulation of uremic metabolites, electrolyte imbalance, acidosis, and renal ischemia, are an ongoing stimulus to the proximal tubules. Subsequently, epithelial cells of the proximal tubules proliferate, fluid accumulates into the tubular lumen, and acquired renal cysts develop. Uremic metabolites activate latent oncogenes of renal tubules by growth factors and oxidative stress. Renal adenoma and RCC develop in response to provoking factors, such as the reduction of active oxygen scavenger and apoptosis, disturbance of the DNA repair mechanism, and depressed immunosurveillance. Thus, a multi-step process of oncogenesis progresses (3, 51).

Some theories of the development of ACDK and RCC have already been summarized (52). Recent research has investigated Connexin32, which functions as a tumor suppressor gene and shows inactivation on histology of the cancerous and non-cancerous areas (53). Due to hypermethylation of P16INK4a, the inactivation of the tumor suppressor gene is observed (54). HGF and its receptor, c-met are stained strongly and upregulated in the epithelium of atypical renal cysts (55). Cytokine concentration, for example IL-6, IL-8, and VEGF, is high in the cystic fluid of ACDK (56). Phosphorylated c-Jun, the activated form of c-Jun, which constitutes activator protein-1 related to the signal transduction of these cytokines, is positive on staining of atypical cyst epithelium and in the early stage of RCC (57). This demonstrates that stimulation by cytokines may be related to the proliferation of cyst epithelium. Ca oxalate crystals are often found in the histology of ACDK and the blood concentration of Ca oxalate is high in dialysis patients. Dry et al. (58) and Sule et al. (35) considered the possibility of cystogenesis and tumorigenesis, based on the obstruction of renal tubules by Ca oxalate crystals, and the abnormal regulation of the tubular cell cycle. Since hemodialysis patients are under oxidative stress status, over expression of iNOS and COX2 and a high labeling index of 8-OHdG are seen in RCC in dialysis patients compared to that in sporadic RCC (54). Moreover, superoxide dismutase is low in dialysis patients. Hypoxia-inducible protein 2 due to the disorder of VHL gene or renal ischemia is highly expressed in atypical renal cysts or papillary RCC (59). Despite the research described above, uremic metabolites that cause ACDK and RCC have still not been identified and the pathogenesis of ACDK and RCC in dialysis patients has not yet been thoroughly elucidated.

Summary

1 Acquired renal cysts develop in the failing contracted kidney and RCC develops in some patients thereafter. The incidence and severity of acquired renal cysts are both high in relatively young males, and in patients on long-term hemodialysis. Most acquired renal cysts regress following successful renal transplantation. Histology of ACDK demonstrates pre-cancerous changes, such as atypical renal cysts and renal adenomas.

2 The incidence of RCC in dialysis patients is higher than that in the general population, and 81% of RCC in dialysis patients develop as a complication of ACDK.

3 RCC complicated with acquired renal cysts develops mainly by the mechanism of cyst-atypical cyst-adenoma-RCC sequences, although this is genetically unproven. RCC with acquired renal cysts is often seen in comparatively young males with long-term hemodialysis, is surrounded by many acquired renal cysts, and does not bulge from the kidney outline. The diagnosis of such RCC is difficult because there is little enhancement by dynamic helical CT.

4 New histologies, ACD-associated RCC, and clear cell papillary RCC of end-stage kidneys which do not fit the classification of classic RCCs have been proposed and account for about 60% of ESRD patients. Moreover, pathogenesis of these tumors may differ from that of classic sporadic RCC.

5 Since RCC in dialysis patients shows a high incidence, is asymptomatic, and has a good post-operative prognosis, screening for RCC is recommended for selected dialysis patients. In particular, screening for RCC is necessary before renal transplantation. Screening for RCC should be based on the risks of age and gender, and on the general condition of the patient. In 15.4% of dialysis patients with RCC, RCC had metastasized by the time of our surveys. Some hemodialysis patients develop rapidly progressive RCC. Laparoscopic radical nephrectomy is preferred. Sorafenib or sunitinib is also beginning to be used in patients with progressive RCC.

References

1 Tickoo SK, dePeralta-Venturina MN, Harik LR, et al. (2006). Spectrum of epithelial neoplasms in end-stage renal disease: an experience from 66 tumor-bearing kidneys with emphasis on histologic patterns distinct from those in sporadic adult renal neoplasia. *Am J Surg Pathol* **30**: 141–53.

2 Dunnill MS, Millard PR, Oliver D (1977). Acquired cystic disease of the kidneys: a hazard of long-term intermittent maintenance haemodialysis. *J Clin Pathol* **30**: 868–77.

3 Ishikawa I (2007). *Acquired cystic disease of the kidney and renal cell carcinoma-complication of long-term hemodialysis.* Springer, Tokyo, pp. 1–111.

4 Liu JS, Ishikawa I, Horiguchi T (2000). Incidence of acquired renal cysts in biopsy specimens. *Nephron* **84**: 142–7.

5 Ishikawa I, Saito Y, Onouchi Z, et al. (1980). Development of acquired cystic disease and adenocarcinoma of the kidney in glomerulonephritic chronic hemodialysis patients. *Clin Nephrol* **14**: 1–6.

6 Matson MA, Cohen EP (1990). Acquired cystic kidney disease: occurrence, prevalence, and renal cancers. *Medicine (Baltimore)* **69**: 217–26.

7 Ishikawa I (2008). Present status of acquired cystic disease of the kidney (in Japanese). *J Jpn Ass Dial Physician* **23**: 179–87.

8 Kessler M, Testevuide P, Aymard B, Huu TC (1991). Acquired renal cystic disease mimicking adult polycystic kidney disease in a patient undergoing long-term hemodialysis. *Am J Nephrol* **11**: 513–17.

9 Gehrig JJ, Gottheiner TI, Swenson RS (1985). Acquired cystic disease of the end-stage kidney. *Am J Med* **79**: 609–20.

10 Ishikawa I, Saito Y, Asaka M, et al. (2003). Twenty-year follow-up of acquired renal cystic disease. *Clin Nephrol* **59**: 153–9.

11 Ishikawa I, Onouchi Z, Saito Y, et al. (1985). Sex differences in acquired cystic disease of the kidney on long-term dialysis. *Nephron* **39**: 336–40.

12 Ishikawa I, Yuri T, Kitada H, Shinoda A (1983). Regression of acquired cystic disease of the kidney after successful renal transplantation. *Am J Nephrol* **3**: 310–14.

13 Watanabe M, Ishikawa I (2005). Kidney volume and development of acquired cystic disease of the kidney in diabetic nephropathy after the start of hemodialysis (in Japanese with English abstract). *J Kanazawa Med Univ* **30**: 191–7.

14 Ishikawa I, Shikura N, Nagahara M, Shinoda A, Saito Y (1991). Comparison of severity of acquired renal cysts between CAPD and hemodialysis. *Adv Perit Dial* **7**: 91–5.

15 Ishikawa I (2004). Present status of renal cell carcinoma in dialysis patients in Japan: questionnaire study in 2002. *Nephron Clin Pract* **97**: c11–16.

16 Denton MD, Magee CC, Ovuworie C, et al. (2002). Prevalence of renal cell carcinoma in patients with ESRD pre-transplantation: a pathologic analysis. *Kidney Int* **61**: 2201–9.

17 Ishikawa I (2005). Present status of renal cell carcinoma in dialysis patients: a questionnaire study in 2004 and review of past questionnaires since 1982 (in Japanese with English abstract). *J Jpn Soc Dial Ther* **38**: 1689–700.

18 Maisonneuve P, Agodoa L, Gellert R, et al. (1999). Cancer in patients on dialysis for end-stage renal disease: an international collaborative study. *Lancet* **354**: 93–9.

19 Savaj S, Liakopoulos V, Ghareeb S, et al. (2003). Renal cell carcinoma in peritoneal dialysis patients. *Int Urol Nephrol* **35**: 263–5.

20 Doublet JD, Peraldi MN, Gattegno B, Thibault P, Sraer JD (1997). Renal cell carcinoma of native kidneys: prospective study of 129 renal transplant patients. *J Urol* **158**: 42–4.

21 Neuzillet Y, Lay F, Luccioni A, et al. (2005). De novo renal cell carcinoma of native kidney in renal transplant recipients. *Cancer* **103**: 251–7.

22 Besarani D, Cranston D (2007). Urological malignancy after renal transplantation. *BJU Int* **100**: 502–5.

23 Schwarz A, Vatandaslar S, Merkel S, Haller H (2007). Renal cell carcinoma in transplant recipients with acquired cystic kidney disease. *Clin J Am Soc Nephrol* **2**: 750–6.

24 Ishikawa I (2000). Hemorrhage versus cancer in acquired cystic disease. *Semin Dial* **13**: 56.

25 Ishikawa I, Shikura N, Ozaki M (1993). Papillary renal cell carcinoma with numeric changes of chromosomes in a long-term hemodialysis patient: a karyotype analysis. *Am J Kidney Dis* **21**: 553–6.

26 Akiyama T, Onoue A (2007). Sonazoid-enhanced ultrasonography: a diagnosis of kidney and prostate disease (in Japanese). *Innervision* **22**: 41–5.

27 De Wilde K, Peeters P, Praet M, Petrovic M, Vanholder R (2008). Contrast-enhanced ultrasonography with microbubbles for successful screening of kidney tumours. *NDT Plus* **1**: 469.

28 Ak I, Can C (2005). F-18 FDG PET in detecting renal cell carcinoma. *Acta Radiol* **46**: 895–9.

29 Ozawa N, Okamura T, Koyama K, et al. (2007). Usefulness of F-18 FDG-PET in a long-term hemodialysis patient with renal cell carcinoma and pheochromocytoma. *Ann Nucl Med* **21**: 239–43.

30 Fujioka T, Obara W (2009). Evidence-based clinical practice guidelines for renal cell carcinoma (Summary-JUA 2007 Edition). *Int J Urol* **16**: 339–53.

31 Ishikawa I, Honda R, Yamada Y, Kakuma T (2004). Renal cell carcinoma detected by screening shows better patient survival than that detected following symptoms in dialysis patients. *Ther Apher Dial* **8**: 468–73.

32 Sarasin FP, Wong JB, Levey AS, Meyer KB (1995). Screening for acquired cystic kidney disease: a decision analytic perspective. *Kidney Int* **48**: 207–19.

33 Scandling JD (2007). Acquired cystic kidney disease and renal cell cancer after transplantation: time to rethink screening? *Clin J Am Soc Nephrol* **2**: 621–2.

34 Ishikawa I, Kovacs G (1993). High incidence of papillary renal cell tumours in patients on chronic haemodialysis. *Histopathology* **22**: 135–9.

35 Sule N, Yakupoglu U, Shen SS, et al. (2005). Calcium oxalate deposition in renal cell carcinoma associated with acquired cystic kidney disease: a comprehensive study. *Am J Surg Pathol* **29**: 443–51.

36 Cossu-Rocca P, Eble JN, Zhang S, Martignoni G, Brunelli M, Cheng L (2006). Acquired cystic disease-associated renal tumors: an immunohistochemical and fluorescence in situ hybridization study. *Mod Pathol* **19**: 780–7.

37 Gobbo S, Eble JN, Grignon DJ, et al. (2008). Clear cell papillary renal cell carcinoma: a distinct histopathologic and molecular genetic entity. *Am J Surg Pathol* **32**: 1239–45.

38 Rivera M, Tickoo SK, Saqi A, Lin O (2008). Cytologic findings of acquired cystic disease-associated renal cell carcinoma: a report of two cases. *Diagn Cytopathol* **36**: 344–7.

39 Kuroda N, Tamura M, Taguchi T, et al. (2008). Sarcomatoid acquired cystic disease-associated renal cell carcinoma. *Histol Histopathol* **23**: 1327–31.

40 Nouh MA, Kuroda N, Yamashita M, et al. (2010). Renal cell carcinoma in patients with end-stage renal disease: relationship between histological type and duration of dialysis. *BJU Int* **105**: 620–7.

41 Japanese Urological Association, Japanese Society of Pathology, Japan Radiological Society (1999). *General rule for clinical and pathological studies on renal cell carcinoma*. 3 ed. Kanehara Syuppan, Tokyo.

42 Delahunt B, Eble JN (1997). Papillary renal cell carcinoma: a clinicopathologic and immunohistochemical study of 105 tumors. *Mod Pathol* **10**: 537–44.

43 Iwamura M, Koh H, Soh S, et al. (2001). Retroperitoneoscopic radical nephrectomy by the posterior lumber approach for renal-cell carcinoma associated with chronic renal failure. *J Endourol* **15**: 729–34.

44 Ruppin S, Protzel C, Klebingat K, Hakenberg O (2009). Successful sorafenib treatment for metastatic renal cell carcinoma in a case with chronic renal failure. *Eur Urol* **55**: 986–8.

45 Ishikawa I (2002). Prognosis in dialysis patients complicated with renal cell carcinoma (in Japanese with English abstract). *J Jpn Ass Soc Dial Ther* **35**: 287–93.

46 Yoshida M, Yao M, Ishikawa I, et al. (2002). Somatic von Hippel-Lindau disease gene mutation in clear-cell renal carcinomas associated with end-stage renal disease/ acquired cystic disease of the kidney. *Genes Chromosomes Cancer* **35**: 359–64.

47 Hughson MD, Bigler S, Dickman K, Kovacs G (1999). Renal cell carcinoma of end-stage renal disease: an analysis of chromosome 3, 7, and 17 abnormalities by microsatellite amplification. *Mod Pathol* **12**: 301–9.

48 Ishikawa I (2005). Cancer in dialysis patients. In: *Cancer and the kidney* (ed. EP Cohen), pp. 227–47. Oxford University Press, Oxford.

49 Pan CC, Chen YJ, Chang LC, Chang YH, Ho DM (2009). Immunohistochemical and molecular genetic profiling of acquired cystic disease-associated renal cell carcinoma. *Histopathology* **55**: 145–53.

50 Hes O, Sima R, Nemcova J, et al. (2008). End-stage kidney disease: gains of chromosomes 7 and 17 and loss of Y chromosome in non-neoplastic tissue. *Virchows Arch* **453**: 313–19.

51 Grantham JJ (1991). Acquired cystic kidney disease. *Kidney Int* **40**: 143–52.

52 Ishikawa I (1991). Acquired cystic disease: mechanisms and manifestations. *Semin Nephrol* **11**: 671–84.

53 Yano T, Ito F, Kobayashi K, et al. (2004). Hypermethylation of the CpG island of connexin 32, a candiate tumor suppressor gene in renal cell carcinomas from hemodialysis patients. *Cancer Lett* **208**: 137–42.

54 Hori Y, Oda Y, Kiyoshima K, et al. (2007). Oxidative stress and DNA hypermethylation status in renal cell carcinoma arising in patients on dialysis. *J Pathol* **212**: 218–26.

55 Konda R, Sato H, Hatafuku F, Nozawa T, Ioritani N, Fujioka T (2004). Expression of hepatocyte growth factor and its receptor C-met in acquired renal cystic disease associated with renal cell carcinoma. *J Urol* **171**: 2166–70.

56 Ito F, Nakazawa H, Ryoji O, Okuda H, Toma H (2000). Cytokines accumulated in acquired renal cysts in long-term hemodialysis patients. *Urol Int* **65**: 21–7.

57 Oya M, Mikami S, Mizuno R, Marumo K, Mukai M, Murai M (2005). C-jun activation in acquired cystic kidney disease and renal cell carcinoma. *J Urol* **174**: 726–30.

58 Dry SM, Renshaw AA (1998). Extensive calcuim oxalate crystal deposition in papillary renal cell calcinoma:report of two cases. *Arch Pathol Lab Med* **122**: 260–1.

59 Konda R, Sugimura J, Sohma F, Katagiri T, Nakamura Y, Fujioka T (2008). Overexpression of hypoxia-inducible protein 2, hypoxia-inducible factor-1alpha and nuclear factor kappaB is putatively involved in acquired renal cyst formation and subsequent tumor transformation in patients with end stage renal failure. *J Urol* **180**: 481–5.

Chapter 12

Kidney cancer

Elizabeth R. Plimack and Roger B. Cohen

Case report

A 60-year-old male former smoker with no family history of cancer developed right flank pain and weight loss. CT scan demonstrated a large right renal mass as well as metastases to the lungs and contralateral adrenal gland. He underwent cytoreductive right radical nephrectomy and adrenalectomy. Pathology revealed a 17 cm clear cell renal cell carcinoma extending into the perinephric soft tissue and ipsilateral adrenal gland. Six weeks later, he was started on sunitinib as treatment for his metastatic disease. His disease remained stable for six months, at which time he progressed in the lungs and remaining adrenal gland. After a brief trial of sorafenib which was poorly tolerated due to hypertension, the patient was started on everolimus. After two months of treatment his disease again stabilized. After four months of treatment he developed symptomatic pneumonitis requiring steroid treatment. He is currently maintained on everolimus and steroids with periodic attempts at tapering the latter.

Introduction

Renal cell cancer is the most malignant urologic cancer, eventually killing more than 35% of affected patients. Renal cell cancer is actually a group of cancers with a common cellular origin, distinct genetic abnormalities and unique morphologic features. The clinical presentation and management of renal cell cancer are changing very rapidly, driven by advances in medical imaging, genetics, molecular pathology, surgery, and a new generation of targeted cancer therapeutics.

The incidence of renal cell cancer worldwide is upwards of 208,000 new cases per year, and continues to rise at approximately 2% per year with the highest rate seen in North America, Australia, New Zealand and Europe (1, 2). This increased incidence is felt to reflect more than detection of a greater number of incidental cases via modern imaging techniques and remains largely unexplained. Despite contemporary imaging technologies and earlier detection, kidney cancer presents in more than 30% of cases at an advanced stage with local and distant metastases (2). Up to 30% of patients treated by radical or partial nephrectomy for localized disease will eventually relapse. The five-year survival rate for all incident cases of renal cancer has doubled in the past forty years but the five-year survival for metastatic renal cell cancer prior to the advent of new targeted therapies was no better than 10% (3). New agents began to become available in 2006 and updated five-year survival rates will be forthcoming in the near future.

Insights into the genetics of sporadic and hereditary renal cancer, growing use of partial nephrectomy as an alternative to radical nephrectomy, and an increasing number of novel, often 'targeted', medical treatments have created new roles for internists, nephrologists, and urologists in the management of patients with this disease. Renal cancer is also in the vanguard of contemporary concepts about cancer staging, highlighted by recent advances that integrate traditional anatomic staging with genetic and biologic factors to provide vastly better prognostic information and guidance for patient selection for medical therapy, including clinical trials.

This chapter will present an overview of kidney cancer from the perspective of the medical oncologist, focusing on renal cell cancer and emphasizing those areas in which practice is rapidly evolving. This chapter will not discuss the less common malignancies of the kidney, including Wilms' tumor (nephroblastoma, nearly always a disease of childhood), cancer of the renal pelvis (usually transitional cell cancer, often related to tobacco exposure), or renal sarcomas.

Epidemiology and clinical presentation

Renal cell cancer accounts for approximately 4% of adult malignancies in the United States, and approximately 2% worldwide (1, 4). In 2009 there will be more than 58,000 new cases and 12,000 deaths from kidney cancer in the USA (4). The majority (>85%) of kidney cancers are adenocarcinomas (renal cell carcinoma). Over the past 20 years there has been a ~2% annual increase in the age-adjusted incidence for renal cell cancer (2). This increase reflects, in part, an increase in the number of asymptomatic cases detected incidentally during the course of CT, ultrasound, and MRI scans ordered for other purposes (5). These 'incidentalomas' now account for 25–60% of renal tumors (6–9). By contrast, approximately 10% of kidney cancers were discovered in this manner 30 years ago. Incidentally discovered cancers tend to be of lower grade and stage with improved patient survival. The median age at presentation of kidney cancer continues to be mid-60s, with a significantly lower age at presentation (mid-40s) in patients with inherited forms of kidney cancer. The male:female ratio is 2:1.

Classically, renal cell cancer presented as a triad of symptoms (hematuria, abdominal pain, and palpable mass), but this syndrome is uncommon today, occurring in fewer than 10% of patients. Less frequent symptoms at presentation include cough, bone pain, enlarged lymph nodes, fever, weight loss, anemia, and varicocele; these are symptoms of advanced, usually metastatic, disease. Paraneoplastic manifestations are present in up to 20% of patients with renal cell carcinoma, and include hypercalcemia, weight loss, fever, reversible hepatic dysfunction (Stauffer's syndrome), anemia or erythrocytosis, and amyloidosis (6). Many of these symptoms or findings are caused by cytokines produced by the cancer itself, including parathyroid hormone-related protein, interleukin-6, and erythropoietin. Renal cancer presents as bilateral disease in 2–6% of cases (7). Older autopsy series revealed bilateral disease in 12% of cases (8). Metachronous disease in the same or contralateral kidney will eventually occur in up to 13% of patients in long-term follow-up (9).

Exogenous risk factors

All USA and European cohort and case-control studies have shown that cigarette smoking is the key risk factor (14, 15), accounting for a 1.4-fold dose-dependent increase in risk for developing the disease. Stated another way, cigarette smoking is felt to account for one in four cases of renal cell cancer in men and one of ten cases in women. Long-term quitters (for more than 15 years) may reduce their risk 15–25% relative to current smokers (10). There is no established association with cigars, pipes, or smokeless tobacco.

A number of other risk factors have been described. There is an apparent increase in risk associated with elevated body mass index, especially in women; those women with BMI in the top 5% have a three-fold increase in risk compared with those in the lowest quartile (11). The mechanism for this association remains unclear; speculation surrounds the roles of elevated estrogen and insulin levels associated with obesity (18–19). There are no convincing associations with other reproductive factors such as number of births, age at menarche, use of oral contraceptives, or hormone replacement therapy (12).

There is a moderate elevation in risk among users of anti-hypertensive drugs (16, 21–22). This excess risk is not restricted to specific drugs (such as diuretics) and it has been difficult to distinguish etiologic factors related to hypertension itself from the effects of the drugs used in its treatment. The relative risk for hypertension alone appears to be ~ 1.4 (13–18). There are also links with high per capita protein and fat consumption that are independent of obesity, perhaps because high protein intake may produce renal tubular damage that, in turn, increases the cancer risk (19). Some of these associations may explain why renal cell cancer is more common in African Americans (20–22) who are more likely to smoke, be obese, and require anti-hypertensive therapy. The association with hypertension is intriguing and may be relevant to cancer etiology as a number of angiogenic/growth factors are elevated in hypertension (33–36). Interestingly, drugs such as captopril inhibit the growth of renal cell cancer cell lines (23), leading to speculation that improved blood pressure control might be a strategy for kidney cancer prevention (24).

Having one first-degree relative with kidney cancer is associated with a significantly increased risk of renal cell cancer (odds ratio 1.6–2.5, independent of von Hippel-Lindau syndrome) (25–27). Blacks with hemoglobin SS and SC disease are at a higher risk of renal medullary cancer (21), but medullary cancer is rare, accounting for less than 1% of incident cases. Patients with end-stage renal disease who develop acquired cystic kidney disease are also at an elevated risk of renal adenocarcinoma (28). Up to 30–50% of hemodialysis patients will develop cystic disease and between 5% and 9% of patients with acquired cystic disease will develop renal cancer (29). Most of these cancers are small, however, and discovered at autopsy. Whether renal cell cancer associated with acquired cystic disease after long-term hemodialysis is less proliferative and aggressive than sporadic renal cell cancer remains a matter of debate (30).

Other associations are more tenuous. Despite case reports and speculation that genetic anomalies leading to dysplasia might occur in unilateral renal agenesis or dysgenesis, there are no convincing data showing that kidney cancer is more common in congenital single or horseshoe kidneys (31). Among dietary factors, there is an inverse relationship between risk and consumption of vegetables and fruits (20). There is no relation, however, to coffee, alcohol, or any other beverage. There are also no consistent epidemiologic associations with any of a variety of environmental and occupational exposures, including trichloroethylene, petroleum products, asbestos, iron processing fumes, gasoline, lead, or cadmium (32–35).

Recommended diagnostic work-up

Imaging studies are critical in determining whether a renal mass is benign or malignant. Ultrasonography (Fig. 12.1), CT (Figs 12.2 and 12.3) and MRI scanning (Fig. 12.4) have largely replaced excretory urography (IVP) (Fig. 12.5) in the initial diagnostic evaluation. Most incidental renal masses discovered by ultrasound prove to be simple cysts that do not require further evaluation. On the other hand, solid lesions are highly suspicious for malignancy and should be evaluated further with CT and MRI; approximately half prove to be malignant. The differential diagnosis of a solid mass is renal cell cancer, oncocytoma (a well-differentiated renal tumor that behaves in a biologically

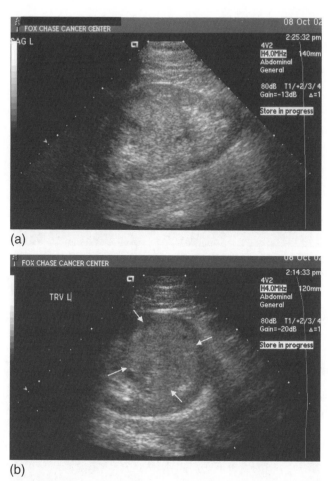

Fig. 12.1 Sagittal (a) and transverse (b) ultrasound of the left kidney. The left kidney measures 12.6 cm. There is a hypervascular solid mass (arrows) arising from the mid pole of the left kidney. This measures 6 cm x 4.9 cm x 4.9 cm. The mass occupies most of the central portion of the kidney and causes some compression of the collecting system. Photograph courtesy of Dr. Rosaleen Parsons.

indolent fashion, without metastasis), and angiomyolipoma. Most solid lesions should be removed surgically unless they are clearly an angiomyolipoma or a complex cyst. MRI (Fig. 12.4) is especially useful for evaluating the renal vein and inferior vena cava for tumor thrombus and has replaced inferior venacavography as the preferred imaging modality for this purpose.

The pathological diagnosis of renal cancer is usually made at the time of surgery (nephrectomy—radical or partial—for diagnosis and treatment

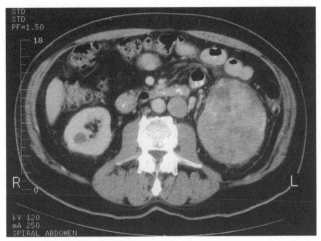

Fig. 12.2 Contrast enhanced axial CT showing a large left renal carcinoma. Photograph courtesy of Dr. Rosaleen Parsons.

of a solid mass). In some patients the diagnosis will be made via biopsy of an obvious distant metastatic lesion (node, lung, liver, or bone).

Pathology

Nearly all malignant kidney tumors arise from the tubular epithelium in the renal parenchymal cortex (renal cell cancer or adenocarcinoma), with the rest

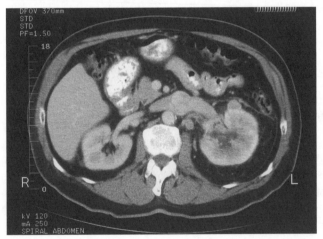

Fig. 12.3 Contrast enhanced axial CT showing tumor thrombus extending from the left kidney into the enlarged left renal vein. Photograph courtesy of Dr. Rosaleen Parsons.

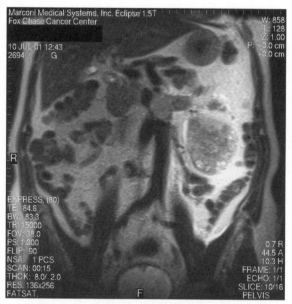

Fig. 12.4 Coronal T2-weighted MRI showing tumor thrombus (black arrow) extending from the left renal vein into the inferior vena cava. The open arrow shows the large partially necrotic tumor arising off the lower pole of the left kidney. The lesion measures 7 cm x 8 cm. Photograph courtesy of Dr. Rosaleen Parsons.

deriving from the renal pelvis (transitional cell cancers). The cell of origin of renal cell cancer is felt to be the proximal convoluted tubule (36). The majority (75–85%) of renal cell cancers are highly vascular and overexpress a number of growth factors, including vascular endothelial growth factor (VEGF), platelet-derived growth factor (PDGF), and fibroblast growth factor (FGF) (37). In addition, renal cell cancers frequently overexpress the receptors for these ligands, thereby creating autocrine loops for cancer establishment and maintenance. Abnormalities in the angiogenic pathway may be linked to renal cancer etiology through abnormal function of the VHL gene protein (see below).

The Heidelberg classification of renal cell tumors, presented in Table 12.1, represents a consensus pathologic classification that integrates traditional histopathological descriptions and emerging genetic knowledge about sporadic and hereditary renal cancer (38). A number of other molecular markers are also under evaluation in order to improve renal cancer staging and prognostication, including proliferation markers, DNA ploidy, cyclin dependent kinases, p27, bcl-2, p53, mdm2, carbonic anhydrase IX (G250 antigen), VHL mutations, and human telomerase (52–55). To date, however, none of these markers has achieved the status of an accepted part of the staging classification and

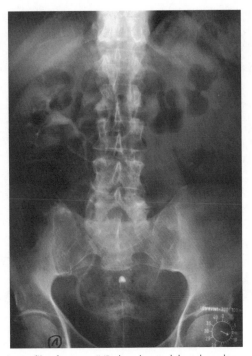

Fig. 12.5 Eight-minute film from an IVP showing a delayed nephrogram and an enlarged left kidney. The right kidney is normal. A radio-opaque Foley catheter is in the bladder. Other characteristic features of renal cell cancer on an IVP include mass effect, distortion of the renal contour and collecting system, central kidney calcification, absent visualization, and urethral notching (indicating thrombosis of the renal vein). Photograph courtesy of Dr. Rosaleen Parsons.

no molecular feature of renal cell carcinoma fulfills the College of American Pathologists' criteria for a marker that should be used to make patient treatment decisions.

There are four major histological subtypes of renal cell cancer—clear cell (Fig. 12.7), papillary (chromophilic) (Fig. 12.8), chromophobe, and collecting (Bellini) duct (39). As shown in Table 12.1, non-clear cell histologies account for fewer than 20% of patients with renal cell cancer. Most kidney cancers (75–80%) are clear cell adenocarcinomas (3), which appear histologically as clear lipid-rich cells (Fig. 12.7). Intratubular epithelial dysplasia is felt to be the precursor lesion for this disease (40) but there are no data on the epidemiology of this premalignant lesion.

Localized papillary and chromophobe renal cell cancers have a relatively favorable prognosis with >90% 5-year survival after nephrectomy (39, 41).

Table 12.1 Heidelberg classification of renal cell cancers

Cell type	Frequency	Most commonly documented genetic abnormalities
Common or conventional renal cell carcinoma (most are 'clear cell') (Fig. 12.7)	75–80%	VHL mutations (intragenic or aberrant hypermethylation) Duplication of 5q22 Deletion of arms 6q, 8p, 9p, 14q
Papillary (chromophilic) renal cell carcinoma (Fig. 12.8)	10%	Trisomy of 3q, 7,8,12,16,17,20 Loss of Y
Chromphobe	5%	LOH 1,2,6,10,13,17,21 Hypodiploidy
Collecting (Bellini) duct and medullary	1%	No consistent cytogenetic patterns
Unclassified	3–5%	N/A

Sarcomatoid change is not felt to be a sub-type of renal cell cancer but rather to reflect histological progression of any one of the four common subtypes to a more aggressive, less differentiated phenotype. Carcinoid tumors and small cell cancers occur rarely and their cell of origin within the kidney is uncertain. Metanephric adenoma, metanephric adenofibroma, papillary renal cell adenoma, and renal oncocytoma are considered benign parenchymal neoplasms. Wilms' tumor is also considered a separate category. This classification does not include tumors metastatic to the kidney or transitional cell cancer of the renal pelvis.

By contrast, collecting duct, unclassified, medullary, and sarcomatoid cancer are highly aggressive tumors (3). Medullary cancer occurs almost exclusively in African Americans and is associated with SS trait or hemoglobin-SC disease (42). Non-clear cell cancers have an especially dismal prognosis when metastatic, with resistance to systemic therapy and very poor survival when compared with the more common clear cell variant (43).

Genetics

Inherited types of kidney cancer account for only a small percentage of patients with the disease, but they are of critical importance in the leads they offer regarding kidney cancer pathogenesis (44). The most common inherited form of kidney cancer is associated with VHL disease in which there is a germline mutation of the VHL tumor-suppressor gene on chromosome 3p (at 3p25-26) (45–46). VHL disease is a rare familial monogenic cancer syndrome with autosomal dominant inheritance (47–48). Associated findings of the VHL syndrome include retinal hemangiomas, CNS hemangioblastomas, renal cysts, pheochromocytoma, endocrine pancreatic tumors, epididymal cystadenomas, and pancreatic cysts. VHL tumors follow the two-hit model of carcinogenesis with a germline mutation of the VHL gene (the 'first hit') as the central event in cancer development. In VHL disease tumors arise from cells in which the remaining wild-type copy of the VHL acquires a somatic inactivating mutation (the 'second hit') via mutation, loss of heterozygosity (LOH), or silencing of the VHL gene promoter by hypermethylation. Renal cell cancer will occur in at least two-thirds of VHL patients and is often bilateral and multicentric (48). Median age of onset of hereditary renal cell cancer is young (44 years) (49).

A second type of familial kidney cancer, much less common than VHL disease, involves a balanced translocation affecting chromosome 3 in the absence of the VHL mutation (t(3;8)(p14;q24), involving the fragile histidine triad (FHIT) gene) (50). Associated lesions of this familial cancer syndrome include thyroid, bladder, pancreatic, and gastric cancer, but the other characteristic tumors of the VHL syndrome do not occur.

The other forms of hereditary renal cancer (hereditary papillary and non-papillary RCC) are *not* associated with VHL mutation or 3p abnormality. Hereditary papillary RCC (HPRCC) is linked to germline mutations of the c-met proto-oncogene on chromosome 7q with lesions in 7q34. The c-met gene encodes the receptor for hepatocyte growth factor/scatter factor, a tyrosine kinase involved in tumor angiogenesis, motility, growth, and invasion. HPRCC is also a familial cancer syndrome; associated tumors include breast, pancreas, lung, skin, and stomach cancers. Of note, some sporadic cases of clear cell and papillary renal cancer also involve mutations of the c-met proto-oncogene (51). Children and adults with the tuberous sclerosis complex (TSC) are also at a higher risk of renal cancer. These tumors do not contain mutations in the VHL gene, implying that mutations of the TSC1 and TSC2 genes lead to renal cell cancers via alternative pathways (52).

A key observation is that acquired abnormalities of the VHL gene occur in the majority of sporadic clear cell renal cancers (53). Thus, clear cell renal cell carcinomas are characterized almost universally by loss of heterozygosity on chromosome 3p, which usually involves any combination of three regions: 3p25–p26 (harboring the VHL gene), 3p12–p14.2 (containing the FHIT gene), and 3p21–p22 (71–72). By contrast, 3p deletions are rare in papillary and chromophobe renal cell cancer. Inactivation of the VHL gene is felt to be an early if not the initiating event in most sporadic renal cancers (54). Intragenic VHL mutations are found in 40–60% and aberrant methylation of the VHL promoter region is seen in up to 20% of sporadic clear cell renal cancers, respectively (44, 54–55). As in VHL kindreds, this combination of allelic loss (loss of heterozygosity) and somatic mutation or hypermethylation leads to VHL gene inactivation and renal cancer via a classic two-hit mechanism. While most clear cell renal cancers have somatic VHL mutations or changes in the VHL promoter, 30–40% do not, which suggests that there must also be

VHL-independent tumorigenic pathways (72–4). More than 750 mutations of the VHL gene have been catalogued. The most common intragenic mutation is GC→ AT transition at CpG dinucleotides. The VHL protein has been cloned and its functions defined. The VHL gene product associates with the elongin B/C, Cul2, and Rbx-1 proteins to form a ubiquitin-ligase complex that is involved in the ubiquitination of hypoxia induced factor (HIF-1α). In the presence of O_2 the VHL protein normally targets HIF-1α for destruction. HIF-1α is a transcription factor that activates several genes, the products of which increase O_2 delivery (including erythropoietin and angiogenic growth factors). In VHL-associated renal cell cancer HIF-1α accumulates to high levels regardless of O_2 concentrations, which then leads to constitutive overexpression of HIF-1α target genes such as VEGF and other angiogenic factors. This process is believed to account for the hypervascular nature of tumors related to VHL (40, 75–7). VHL also negatively regulates TGF-α, a growth factor for primary renal proximal tubule epithelial cells. Overproduction of TGF-α might promote development and growth of RCC cells through an autocrine TGF-α/ epidermal growth factor receptor (EGFR) circuit (56).

Staging and prognosis

The goal of cancer staging (Fig. 12.6) is to determine the extent of regional and distant metastatic disease in order to assess operability and provide an accurate prognosis. Common metastatic sites are regional lymph nodes, lung, bone, liver, ipsilateral adrenal, and contralateral kidney. Most patients should undergo CT scanning of the chest through the kidneys and pelvis as part of the initial work-up before surgery or medical therapy. Asymptomatic patients do not need a bone scan or survey. Brain scan (CT or MRI) should be performed in the presence of symptoms that suggest CNS involvement. PET scanning is specific but not sensitive for detection of renal cell carcinoma metastases, and therefore is not used for routine staging in this disease (57).

In general, the extent of the tumor at diagnosis has the greatest impact on prognosis. Next to tumor size, grade is the most important prognostic pathologic factor (58–61). The four-point scheme proposed by Fuhrman et al. (59) is the most commonly used system in the USA although inter-observer variability will compromise the value of any tumor grading system. High nuclear grade correlates with mitotic activity and poor clinical outcome; for example, five-year cancer specific survival ranges from ~90% for grade I tumors to ~45% for grades III and IV (59, 62–63).

For staging purposes most experts now prefer the TNM system (Table 12.2) because it more accurately describes the extent of tumor involvement

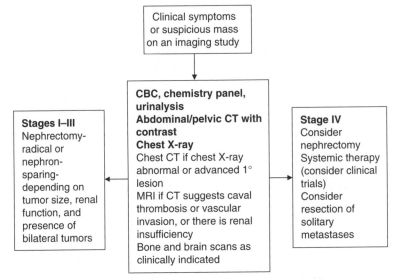

```
┌─────────────────────┐
│  Clinical symptoms  │
│  or suspicious mass │
│  on an imaging study│
└─────────────────────┘
           │
           ▼
```

CBC, chemistry panel, urinalysis
Abdominal/pelvic CT with contrast
Chest X-ray
Chest CT if chest X-ray abnormal or advanced 1° lesion
MRI if CT suggests caval thrombosis or vascular invasion, or there is renal insufficiency
Bone and brain scans as clinically indicated

Stages I–III
Nephrectomy- radical or nephron- sparing- depending on tumor size, renal function, and presence of bilateral tumors

Stage IV
Consider nephrectomy
Systemic therapy (consider clinical trials)
Consider resection of solitary metastases

Fig. 12.6 Suggested initial work-up. Courtesy of Dr. Arthur Patchefsky.

compared with the older Robson system (64). The TNM system emphasizes local and nodal spread and distant metastasis. The prognostic value of tumor extension into the renal vein or vena cava is still controversial; other adverse prognostic (e.g. biologic) factors that associate with vascular involvement may actually be of greater importance (65). The prognosis for patients with isolated

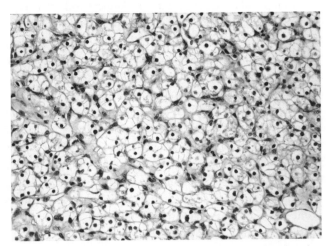

Fig. 12.7 Clear cell renal cancer. This photomicrograph shows the abundant clear cytoplasm typical of clear cell renal cancer. Courtesy of Dr. Arthur Patchefsky.

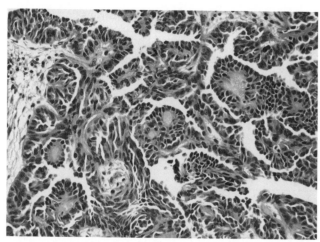

Fig. 12.8 Papillary renal cell cancer. This photomicrograph shows the typical cuboidal cells in papilla surrounding fibrovascular stalks. Courtesy of Dr. Arthur Patchefsky.

Table 12.2 TNM staging of renal cell carcinoma

Primary tumor (T)	
TX	Primary tumor cannot be assessed
T0	No evidence of primary tumor
T1	Tumor 7 cm or less in greatest dimension, limited to the kidney
T1a	Tumor 4 cm or less in greatest dimension, limited to the kidney
T1b	Tumor more than 4 cm but not more than 7 cm in greatest dimension, limited to the kidney
T2	Tumor more than 7 cm in greatest dimension, limited to the kidney
T3	Tumor extends into major veins or invades adrenal gland or perinephric tissues but not beyond Gerota's fascia
T3a	Tumor directly invades adrenal gland or perirenal and/or renal sinus fat but not beyond Gerota's fascia
T3b	Tumor grossly extends into the renal vein or its segmental (muscle containing) branches, or vena cava below diaphragm
T3c	Tumor grossly extends into vena cava above diaphragm or invades the wall of the vena cava
T4	Tumor invades beyond Gerota's fascia
Regional lymph nodes (N)	
NX	Regional lymph nodes cannot be assessed
N0	No regional lymph node metastases

Table 12.2 (*continued*) TNM staging of renal cell carcinoma

Regional lymph nodes (N)			
N1	Metastases in a single regional lymph node		
N2	Metastasis in more than one regional lymph node		

Distant metastasis (M)			
MX	Distant metastasis cannot be assessed		
M0	No distant metastasis		
M1	Distant metastasis		

Stage grouping			
Stage I	T1	N0	M0
Stage II	T2	N0	M0
Stage III	T1	N1	M0
	T2	N1	M0
	T3	N0	M0
	T3	N1	M0
	T3a	N0	M0
	T3a	N1	M0
	T3b	N0	M0
	T3b	N1	M0
	T3c	N0	M0
	T3c	N1	M0
Stage IV	T4	N0	M0
	T4	N1	M0
	Any T	N2	M0
	Any T	Any N	M1

Used with the permission of the American Joint Committee on Cancer (AJCC), Chicago, Illinois. The original source for this material is the *AJCC Cancer Staging Manual, Sixth Edition* (2002) published by Springer-Verlag New York, www.springer-ny.com.

renal vein extension, for example, is actually superior to that for patients with lymphatic metastasis.

Patient outcome correlates with stage. Increased use of medical imaging has resulted in significant stage migration with an increase in the number of earlier stage cases. Asymptomatic patients with incidentally discovered lower stage tumors have an improved outcome; five-year survival for patients with T1–T3 lesions without nodal involvement is 60–90% (62, 66–68). Nodal involvement (N1–N3) is an adverse finding with five-year survival around

15%. At the present time the disease is diagnosed with systemic metastases in up to a third of patients. All anatomic staging systems for kidney cancer suffer from the deficiency that a number of other variables have a critical impact on prognosis, including tumor grade and Eastern Cooperative Group Oncology (ECOG) performance status. In order to take these factors into account, alternative staging systems have been proposed (69), most notably the UISS/UCLA system (70). The latter system has undergone a prospective validation (71–72). What makes the UISS system particularly valuable is that it uses simple, readily available and inexpensive clinical data points and may be used to predict survival for all stage categories (local as well as metastatic disease). For non-metastatic patients, the key variables determining prognosis are Fuhrman's grade and ECOG performance status. For patients with metastatic disease, Fuhrman's grade, T stage (Table 12.1), number of symptoms, and nodal involvement are independent predictors for survival (70). Other prognostic factors include time from diagnosis to metastasis, location and number of metastatic sites, weight loss, whether the patient has had a nephrectomy, elevated LDH (>1.5-fold normal), and serum Ca^{++} >10 mg/dl (73). For reasons that remain unclear, patients requiring dialysis for renal cancer often have a poor outcome, inferior to that of patients with diabetes (74).

Surgical treatment

Radical nephrectomy has been the traditional surgical approach for the past half-century. The term radical nephrectomy generally implies perifascial resection of the kidney, peri-renal fat, regional lymph nodes, and ipsilateral adrenal gland and includes early ligation of the renal artery and excision of Gerota's fascia and its contents. Adrenalectomy is not mandatory if the adrenal gland is uninvolved radiographically (lower pole lesions) or at the time of surgery, as the adrenal has a separate blood supply from the kidney. Participation of a vascular surgery team is usually indicated if there is vena cava invasion on the pre-operative scan. The role and value of regional lymph node dissection in patients without enlarged nodes is a subject of continuing controversy.

Improvements in surgical management along with downward stage migration due to improved radiological imaging have created an expanding role for nephron-sparing surgery in the management of renal cancer. The small, incidentally detected tumor is particularly suited for nephron-sparing surgery. Indications for nephron-sparing surgery include: small tumors (less than 4.0 cm), bilateral tumors, solitary kidney (75), poorly functioning contralateral kidney, contralateral kidney threatened by present or future medical disease (diabetes, hypertension, and vascular disease), as well as a familial cancer syndrome predisposing to the eventual development of bilateral tumors (76). A functioning remnant kidney of at least 25% of the original kidney mass (i.e. half of a remaining single kidney) is needed to avoid dialysis and patients with a remnant kidney are at greater risk of proteinuria, glomerulopathy, and progressive renal failure (77). Three-dimensional spiral CT can be helpful in planning a partial nephrectomy and allowing conservation of the maximal amount of normal renal tissue while optimizing the chances to achieve negative surgical tumor margins (78).

Peri-operative morbidity for tumors that are 4.0 cm or less is similar to that for radical nephrectomy (79–81). Experts have speculated that future benefits may exist if one performs partial nephrectomies for small, localized renal cancers detected incidentally, because these cancers are usually discovered in a population that can anticipate prolonged survival and the eventual development of diseases such as diabetes mellitus, atherosclerosis, and intrinsic renal disease. This theory is supported by retrospective data indicating that partial nephrectomy protects patients against subsequent development of chronic kidney disease as compared with radical nephrectomy (82). Radical nephrectomy and nephron-sparing surgery do appear to be equally effective and potentially curative therapy for patients with single, small (less than 4 cm), localized renal cancers (80–81, 83). A large international prospective study comparing nephron-sparing surgery to radical nephrectomy is ongoing and survival data are eagerly anticipated. However, in advance of these data, the current trend is moving towards nephron-sparing surgery for appropriate renal masses (84–85).

The principal disadvantage of nephron-sparing surgery is a real increased risk of local recurrence, most likely due to unrecognized multi-focal cancer. The overall local recurrence rate after partial nephrectomy ranges from 0 to 12%, depending on patient selection factors, and is higher in patients with larger tumors (84). Local recurrence is a particular problem when contemplating nephron-sparing surgery for patients with VHL syndrome who have the highest incidence of post-operative tumor recurrence (up to 50%). However, given the fact that most of these patients will ultimately develop multiple tumors in both kidneys, nephron-sparing surgical treatment of these tumors, repeated as necessary, may allow patients to defer dialysis. Regardless of treatment, patients with VHL syndrome require very close follow-up; most will develop recurrent renal cancer (83).

More recent surgical innovations include cryosurgery and radiofrequency ablation (RFA) of small peripheral renal cell cancers; the latter has been shown to be feasible and safe (86). Laparoscopic nephrectomy is also promising for T1 and T2 lesions (87). A very important change in surgical practice resulted from the publication of two landmark randomized phase III trials conducted in the USA (Southwest Oncology Group, SWOG) and Europe (EORTC) that indicated a survival benefit for nephrectomy before interferon-α therapy for patients presenting with incurable, metastatic disease. Thus, nephrectomy followed by interferon-α therapy results in better survival among patients with metastatic renal cell cancer than does interferon-α therapy alone. Improvement in survival was greatest for patients with good performance status and lung metastases. Why nephrectomy before systemic immune therapy might promote improved survival is unknown (88–89). The precise role of cytoreductive nephrectomy is currently being re-evaluated in the current era of targeted therapy. Clinical trials both in Europe and the United States are under way. Until these results are known, however, the standard of care remains cytoreductive nephrectomy for most patients.

After nephrectomy for localized renal cell cancer, 20–30% of patients will relapse (90), most in the lung (50–60%). Median time to relapse is one to two years and most relapses (>85%) occur within three years. African American men are at higher risk of relapse than whites in the first five years (21). Experts recommend that patients with stage I or II disease (Table 12.1) be followed every six months for two years and annually thereafter for five years. At each visit, they should undergo a history and physical examination, chest X-ray, and serum chemistry evaluation. Abdominal CT scanning should be dictated by clinical symptoms. Patients with stage III disease are at a higher risk of relapse and should be seen more frequently (every four months for two years, every six months for three years, and then annually). Up to 50% of patients with stage III disease will relapse after surgery. Current follow-up guidelines are based on the concept that the risk of a second primary cancer is highest in the first five years after diagnosis (76). It turns out, however, that the relative risk of metachronous renal cell cancer after initial diagnosis is stable at long-term follow-up (i.e. the elevated risk never goes away). These findings imply that imaging of the contralateral kidney should not cease at 5-10 years but should continue for life. Follow-up recommendations also differ for patients who have had nephron-sparing surgery because their risk of a local recurrence is higher. The consensus is that patients with T1 disease do not require intensive radiographic surveillance. On the other hand, patients with T3 disease are at higher risk of recurrence and may benefit from CT surveillance. These are common-sense rather than evidence-based recommendations, however.

Medical treatment of advanced disease

Prior to 2005, the only approved treatment for renal cell carcinoma was the cytokine interleukin-2. Interferon-α was widely used off-label in the USA based on European data indicating a modest survival advantage (91–92).

Over the past decade, research into the biologic mechanisms of renal cell carcinoma has resulted in the development of an arsenal of new 'targeted agents' that disrupt key pathways in carcinogenesis. These agents have made their way through clinical trials and have yielded significant improvements in clinical benefit and overall survival in patients with advanced renal cell carcinoma. Despite these important advances curative systemic treatment remains largely elusive for most patients with advanced disease.

Although immunotherapy has largely fallen by the wayside in the treatment of renal cell carcinoma, it remains useful for a small subset of patients. The US Food and Drug Administration approved recombinant interleukin-2 (IL-2) for the treatment of metastatic renal cancer based upon the results of a multi-center series of 255 patients treated with high dose IL-2 alone (106). Toxicities of this treatment are considerable and include hypotension, cardiac arrhythmias, capillary leak syndrome, severe pruritus, renal impairment, and decreased blood counts. Complete responses occur in 7% of patients, and occur mainly in patients with lung or lymph nodes as the only sites of metastases. Another 15% of patients had partial responses. A long-term survival update showed a median survival of 16 months and a median duration of response of 54 months (range 3 to 107+). The most important finding of this and other studies of high dose IL-2 in advanced renal cell carcinoma is that complete responses, while occurring in a minority of patients, are highly durable with very few late relapses (93–95). Therefore, high dose interleukin-2 is still considered the only potentially curative systemic treatment for advanced renal cell carcinoma and for this reason, despite its marked toxicity, it is still indicated for a highly selected subset of healthy and motivated patients. Given the toxicity profile, high dose IL-2 is administered in an inpatient setting with intensive care unit monitoring and trained nursing and support staff. This treatment is offered only at a select number of specialized centers where trained physicians and appropriate support services are available.

Vascular endothelial growth factor (VEGF) pathway targeted agents

Agents targeting the VEGF pathway have recently become the mainstay of treatment for incurable clear cell renal cell carcinoma. There are several agents in this class, all with overlapping mechanisms of action, most of which have been evaluated in a randomized fashion with interferon alpha serving as the control arm. The majority of patients on these studies, including those on the control arms, received more than one targeted therapy over the course of their disease; therefore accurate assessment of effects on overall survival is hampered by significant cross-over effects. Overall, this class of agents has doubled the median survival of patients with incurable renal cell carcinoma from approximately one year to over two years.

Bevacizumab, a humanized monoclonal antibody to vascular endothelial growth factor (VEGF-A), was the first targeted therapy to show efficacy in the treatment of advanced renal cell carcinoma although it was not the first anti-angiogenic agent to receive regulatory approval for this disease. In a small phase 2 trial, bevacizumab showed an improvement in disease control compared to placebo in patients who had progressed after previous therapy with interleukin-2 (or had contraindications to standard interleukin-2 therapy). Patients receiving bevacizumab had a median time to progression of 4.8 months compared to 2.5 months in the placebo group (96). The majority of patients responding to bevacizumab had stabilization of their disease, with only 10% of patients achieving an objective response by RECIST (Response Evaluation Criteria in Solid Tumors) (97). In July 2009 the United States Food and Drug Administration (US FDA) approved bevacizumab for the treatment of kidney cancer when given in combination with interferon. The recommendation for the combination in the labeling reflects the way the agent was studied in two large randomized registration trials, one in the United States and the other in Europe. Both studies compared bevacizumab plus interferon to interferon alone in previously untreated patients. In these studies, the median progression free survival with bevacizumab plus interferon was approximately nine months with an overall response rate of about 30% compared with five months and 14%, respectively, for patients receiving interferon (98–99). The most common moderate to severe side effects were hypertension and proteinuria (known side effects of bevacizumab) and anorexia and fatigue (known side effects of interferon). The contribution of interferon to the response rate and survival outcomes is unclear because prospective data comparing the combination of bevacizumab and interferon to bevacizumab alone are lacking. Given that bevacizumab is the more active of the two agents based on single agent data, in addition to the unpleasant side effects with interferon, most patients in the USA in practice will likely receive bevacizumab as a single agent rather than in combination with interferon.

Sorafenib, a multi-targeted tyrosine kinase inhibitor targeting a spectrum of receptors including vascular endothelial growth factor receptor (VEGF-R2), platelet derived growth factor receptor (PDGFR), and RAF kinase was the first molecularly targeted agent to receive US FDA approval (2005) for the treatment of renal cell carcinoma. Approval was based on the results of a randomized phase III trial. This large multi-center study compared sorafenib to placebo in patients with clear cell carcinoma previously treated with cytokines (100).

A total of 903 patients were enrolled. Median progression-free survival was 5.5 months in the sorafenib group and 2.8 months in the placebo group. The overall objective response rate of ~10% was similar to that seen with single agent bevacizumab. The most common side effects from sorafenib were diarrhea, rash, fatigue, and skin reactions (hand-foot syndrome).

Sunitinib, another multi-targeted tyrosine kinase inhibitor, was approved by the US FDA one month after sorafenib. Sunitinib inhibits VEGF-R2 and PDGFR among other targets. The drug first showed promise in phase II studies in RCC and was ultimately assessed in a randomized phase III study comparing sunitinib to interferon alpha in previously untreated patients with metastatic clear cell renal carcinoma. Median progression-free survival was significantly longer in patients receiving sunitinib (11 months) compared to interferon alpha (5 months). The overall response rate was 31% in patients receiving sunitinib (101). Important side effects of sunitinib included diarrhea, vomiting, hypertension, and hand–foot syndrome. Subsequently, the results of an expanded access study were reported. These results describe the efficacy of sunitinib in a less homogeneous patient population. In this study, the overall response rate was 17% with a clinical benefit rate of 76%. Patients with poor prognostic features such as brain metastases and decreased functional status also showed benefit from sunitinib. Based on these results, especially the higher objective response rate, sunitinib is currently the standard of care for the initial treatment of patients with advanced clear cell renal cell carcinoma.

Pazopanib, the latest of the multi-functional tyrosine kinase inhibitors to enter the market, was approved in October 2009 based on data from a large randomized trial of pazopanib versus placebo conducted primarily in Eastern Europe showing a response rate of 30% and a median progression free survival of 9.2 months, compared with 3% and 4.2 months respectively for interferon (102). The mechanism of action is similar to the other tyrosine kinase inhibitors. The hypothesis that the toxicity profile of pazopanib may be superior to sunitinib is being tested in a large phase III trial of pazopanib versus sunitinib in the first-line setting.

Axitinib is yet another VEGF-targeted tyrosine kinase inhibitor currently in late phase studies seeking FDA approval. Evidence of axitinib's efficacy in clear cell renal cell carcinoma is impressive compared to similar agents, but these results come from two small non-randomized studies. The first study investigating axitinib in this disease was a phase II study in cytokine-refractory patients. Of 52 patients treated, 44% had an objective response by RECIST, and 4% had a complete response, yielding an overall response rate of 48%, the best noted to date in advanced renal cell carcinoma (103). Furthermore, this small but real percentage of complete responses has not been seen with the other VEGF-targeted agents. Evaluation of axitinib in the second-line setting also shows impressive efficacy, with a 23% response rate in patients previously treated with sorafenib or sorafenib and sunitinib (104). Axitinib is currently being evaluated for FDA approval in a phase III randomized study comparing axitinib with sorafenib in the second-line setting.

In general, the toxicity profiles of the multi-targeted tyrosine kinase inhibitors are similar. Common side effects include hypertension, stomatitis, taste changes, fatigue, diarrhea, cytopenias, desquamation and tenderness of the skin of the hands and feet (hand–foot syndrome), delayed wound healing, and hypothyroidism (98, 102–103, 105). Bevacizumab is noted for prominent vascular-associated side effects such as poor wound healing, hypertension, proteinuria, and hemorrhage, but typically does not cause the off-target toxicities noted with the tyrosine kinase inhibitors. These toxicities are discussed in detail in Chapter 6, on biologic therapies for cancer. If side effects are severe, treatment is typically withheld until symptoms improve, and patients may be restarted at a lower dose or on an alternate schedule. For sunitinib, for example, side effects can often be mitigated by altering the schedule to two weeks on, one week off, instead of the conventional four weeks on, two weeks off schedule. Treatment with these agents has also been associated with an increased risk of cardiac events. In a recent observational study of patients with RCC treated with sunitinib or sorafenib with careful cardiac monitoring, approximately 10% had a serious cardiac event such as myocardial damage or arrhythmia (115). If properly recognized and managed, however, permanent cardiac sequelae are infrequent.

mTor Inhibitors

The mTOR inhibitors temsirolimus and everolimus represent another class of agent used for the treatment of metastatic renal cell carcinoma. Temsirolimus (CCI-779), the first mTOR inhibitor to be evaluated for the treatment of cancer, was FDA approved in 2007 for patients with advanced or metastatic RCC. Everolimus (RAD001) has been evaluated in patients with metastatic RCC whose disease has progressed after treatment with sunitinib or sorafenib, and was approved by the FDA for this indication in March of 2009. Ridaforolimus (formerly deforolimus) is currently in clinical trials for cancer but has yet to be evaluated in RCC.

Temsirolimus is an intravenously administered mTOR inhibitor. Early on in the clinical development of temsirolimus, anti-tumor efficacy was seen in patients with RCC (116–117). During these early dose-finding studies, a formal maximum tolerated dose was never reached. Ultimately, a lower dose of temsirolimus (25 mg) seemed to be as effective as the higher doses and was better tolerated over multiple cycles, and therefore selected for subsequent studies (106). In phase II studies of temsirolimus, patients with three or more predictors of poor prognosis according to the Memorial Sloan-Kettering Cancer Center (MSKCC) risk model had a median overall survival (OS) of 8.2 months. This survival is significantly shorter than the median OS of patients with fewer risk factors (approximately 23 months), but longer than would be expected for patients with multiple adverse prognostic factors treated with interferon in the first-line setting (95, 119). Based on these results, the Global Advanced Renal Cell Carcinoma (Global ARCC) Trial was designed to deter-mine whether temsirolimus as a single agent or in combination with interferon alpha would improve the OS of patients with advanced, poor prognosis RCC (107). Study enrollment was limited to a poor prognosis population, defined using criteria based on the MSKCC risk model. In this study, 626 patients were randomized to one of three treatment groups: temsirolimus, 25 mg intrave-nously (IV) each week; interferon alpha, three million units (MU) subcutane-ously (SC) 3 times weekly (escalating to 18 MU SC three times weekly or maximum tolerated dose), or a combination of temsirolimus, 15 mg IV weekly, and interferon alpha, 6 MU SC 3 times weekly (121). Median overall survival for the groups receiving temsirolimus, interferon, and the combination groups was 10.9, 7.3, and 8.4 months, respectively. Overall survival was greater for patients who received single-agent temsirolimus compared with those receiv-ing interferon alone (hazard ratio for death, 0.73; 95% confidence interval, 0.58–0.92; P = .008).

Everolimus is an orally bioavailable mTOR inhibitor. Similar to the early temsirolimus dose-finding studies, no maximum tolerated dose was reached, and clinical benefit was found at all dose levels studied (108). The phase III trial establishing the utility of everolimus in renal cell carcinoma was an interna-tional, multi-center study that compared everolimus to placebo in the second-line setting after disease progression on sunitinib, sorafenib, or both (123) Four hundred and ten (410) patients were randomized in a 2:1 ratio to receive either everolimus at 10 mg/day or placebo in a double blind fashion. Unblinding was permitted at time of progression, and crossover to everolimus was offered to patients who had received placebo. Progression free survival was the pri-mary endpoint. The median progression free survival was 4.0 months for the everolimus group and 1.9 months for the placebo group (p<0.001). Only three patients (1%) had an objective response to everolimus by RECIST. Overall survival was not significantly different between the two groups, a finding that is likely confounded by the fact that most patients (79%) in the placebo group crossed over to receive everolimus at progression. Predefined subgroups included stratification by MSKCC risk criteria (73), prior treatment, age, gender, and geographic region. All subgroups derived a progression-free survival benefit from everolimus as compared with placebo. These results indicate that everolimus provides a modest benefit with respect to progression free survival for patients previously treated with VEGF-targeted therapies.

Hyperglycemia and hyperlipidemia are commonly observed side effects of treatment with mTOR inhibitors, reflecting blockade of the main signaling conduits for insulin and insulin-like growth factor. Other common toxicities for the class include fatigue, stomatitis, diarrhea, anemia, thrombocytopenia, rash, and peripheral edema. Less common effects include renal insufficiency, interstitial pneumonitis, and neutropenia (73, 106, 108–111).

Special situations

Treatment of patients with renal insufficiency

Renal insufficiency is relatively common in patients with renal cell carcinoma, as many of them are older and most have had one kidney resected. The excretion of the newer targeted therapy agents (multi-targeted TKIs and the rapamycin analogs) is mostly in feces with only a small percentage of drug cleared in the urine. Currently available data based on small-case series indicates that sunitinib, sorafenib, and temsirolimus will reach therapeutic levels and are safe at full doses in patients with renal insufficiency including patients on hemodialysis (112–113). Further studies will help better define the use of these agents in patients with renal failure.

Treatment of patients with advanced non-clear cell renal cell carcinoma

Clear cell RCC accounts for approximately 80% of all kidney cancer diagnoses. Other histologies comprising the remaining 20% of diagnoses include papillary, chromophobe, sarcomatoid, collecting duct and medullary (see Table 12.1). Each of these has a different biological behavior and treatment recommendations vary for each. Sarcomatoid, medullary, and collecting duct renal cell carcinomas are usually treated with chemotherapy. Medullary and collecting duct tumors respond to typical bladder cancer regimens (114–115). Sarcomatoid renal cell carcinoma is usually treated with doxorubicin and gemcitabine, agents active in sarcoma and urothelial carcinomas respectively (116). Chromophobe renal cell carcinoma has an indolent biology and can often be observed, though responses have been seen with sunitinib and sorafenib (117). Papillary renal cell carcinoma has historically been difficult to treat, as it is refractory to cytokine therapies.

Unfortunately, non-clear cell renal cell carcinomas have been largely excluded from clinical trials investigating the new targeted therapies. A notable exception to this is the phase III study of temsirolimus, which included patients with non-clear cell histologies. Efficacy in the non-clear cell group as a whole was assessed in a planned subgroup analysis revealing that the overall survival advantage for temsirolimus was similar to that seen in patients with clear cell renal cell carcinoma (107). As a result, current guidelines recommend temsirolimus as first-line treatment for non-clear cell renal cell carcinoma regardless of MSKCC risk category. The expanded access study of sunitinib included non-clear cell patients as well, with a reported response rate of 11% (105). In both these studies, however, the different non-clear cell histologies were not evaluated separately. Given the biologic diversity within this category, it is difficult to draw any firm conclusions for a given patient with a distinct non-clear cell histology. Further complicating the issue is that both papillary and sarcomatoid renal cell carcinomas frequently have a clear cell component. Depending on the histology of the metastases—and biopsy is not always performed to establish this—they may behave more like clear cell than non-clear cell depending on which component has metastasized or predominates.

Data are beginning to emerge from a few studies investigating molecularly targeted therapies in specific histologies. In papillary renal cell carcinoma, for example, two small prospective studies show no responses to sunitinib (118–119).

Table 12.3 Randomized Phase III Trials of Targeted Agents in Patients with Metastatic Renal Cell Carcinoma

Trial	Setting	No. of Patients	Endpoint	Benefit in Targeted Therapy
Sorafenib vs. Placebo[5]	Second-line after cytokines, MSKCC poor/intermediate-risk groups	903	PFS	Yes
Sunitinib vs. Interferon[6]	First-line, all MSKCC risk groups	750	PFS	Yes
Temsirolimus vs. Interferon[7]	First-line, modified MSKCC poor-risk group only	626	Survival	Yes
Bevacizumab + Interferon vs. Interferon[8]	First-line, all MSKCC risk groups	649	PFS	Yes
Everolimus vs. Placebo[9]	Second-line after VEGF-targeted therapy, all MSKCC risk groups	410	PFS	Yes

Abbreviations: MSKCC = Memorial Sloan-Kettering Cancer Center; PFS = progression-free survival; VEGF = vascular endothelial growth factor.
Reproduced with permission from Molina AM, Motzer RJ. Current algorithms and prognostic factors in the treatment of metastatic carcinoma. *Clin Genitourin Cancer*. 2008 Dec; **6**(3): s7–s13.

Future studies will investigate various c-met targeted agents currently in development as treatment for papillary renal cell carcinoma, given the known activation of c-Met in this disease. A study combining gemcitabine chemotherapy with sunitinib is being developed to treat patients with sarcomatoid or mixed clear cell and sarcomatoid renal cell carcinoma.

Ongoing areas of investigation

Given the relatively recent approvals of multiple new agents for renal cell carcinoma, many questions remain as to how to best use these agents. Multiple small studies have investigated the obvious question of using these agents in combination. A four-arm randomized study of all three possible combinations of bevacizumab, temsirolimus, and sorafenib vs. a fourth arm of bevacizumab alone in the first-line setting is ongoing. Another question is the issue of sequence of the available agents, i.e. which agents should be used in the first-line setting and which are active in the second-line setting. Currently these drugs are used in the setting in which they were studied and for which they are approved (see Table 12.3 (120)). Ongoing trials are looking at whether the sequence of administration influences overall survival. A third question of ongoing interest is whether these drugs are useful in the adjuvant setting. Several large studies in the United States and Europe are addressing the efficacy of sorafenib and sunitinib in this setting, though it will likely be years before results of these are available. Currently, combination therapy and adjuvant therapy are not recommended outside of a clinical trial. Central to all of these questions is the issue of cost. All targeted therapies for renal cell carcinoma are expensive, and the cost per quality-adjusted life year (QALY) is prohibitive in some health care systems (121). As a result, access to these treatments is not universal. Expanding use into the adjuvant setting and combining agents will likely require that significant incremental benefit be shown in order to justify the cost of treatment.

References

1 Parkin DM, Bray F, Ferlay J, Pisani P (2005). Global cancer statistics, 2002. *CA Cancer J Clin* **55**: 74–108.

2 Horner MJ RL, Krapcho M, Neyman N, Aminou R, Howlader N, et al. (2009). SEER Cancer Statistics Review, 1975–2006. Bethesda, http://seer.cancer.gov/csr/1975_2006/.

3 Motzer RJ, Bander NH, Nanus DM (1996). Renal-cell carcinoma. *N Engl J Med* **335**: 865–75.

4 Jemal A, Siegel R, Ward E, Hao Y, Xu J, Thun MJ (2009). Cancer statistics, 2009. *CA Cancer J Clin* **59**(4): 225–49.

5 Jayson M, Sanders H (1998). Increased incidence of serendipitously discovered renal cell carcinoma. *Urology* **51**: 203–5.

6 Gold PJ, Fefer A, Thompson JA (1996). Paraneoplastic manifestations of renal cell carcinoma. *Semin Urol Oncol* **14**: 216–22.

7 Grimaldi G, Reuter V, Russo P (1998). Bilateral non-familial renal cell carcinoma. *Ann Surg Oncol* **5**: 548–52.

8 Wunderlich H, Schlichter A, Zermann D, Reichelt O, Kosmehl H, Schubert J (1999). Multifocality in renal cell carcinoma: A bilateral event? *Urol Int* **63**: 160–3.

9 Henriksson C, Geterud K, Aldenborg F, Zachrisson BF, Pettersson S (1992). Bilateral asynchronous renal cell carcinoma. Computed tomography of the contralateral kidney 10–43 years after nephrectomy. *Eur Urol* **22**: 209–12.

10 McLaughlin JK, Lindblad P, Mellemgaard A, McCredie M, Mandel JS, Schlehofer B, et al. (1995). International renal-cell cancer study. I. Tobacco use. *Int J Cancer* **60**: 194–8.

11 Bergstrom A, Hsieh CC, Lindblad P, Lu CM, Cook NR, Wolk A (2001). Obesity and renal cell cancer—a quantitative review. *Br J Cancer* **85**: 984–90.

12 Lindblad P, Mellemgaard A, Schlehofer B, Adami HO, McCredie M, McLaughlin JK, et al. (1995). International renal-cell cancer study. V. Reproductive factors, gynecologic operations and exogenous hormones. *Int J Cancer* **61**: 192–8.

13 McLaughlin JK, Gao YT, Gao RN, Zheng W, Ji BT, Blot WJ, et al. (1992). Risk factors for renal-cell cancer in Shanghai, China. *Int J Cancer* **52**: 562–5.

14 Hiatt RA, Tolan K, Quesenberry Jr CP (1994). Renal cell carcinoma and thiazide use: a historical, case-control study (California, USA). *Cancer Causes Control* **5**: 319–25.

15 Hole DJ, Hawthorne VM, Isles CG, McGhee SM, Robertson JW, Gillis CR, et al. (1993). Incidence of and mortality from cancer in hypertensive patients. *BMJ* **306**: 609–11.

16 Yu MC, Mack TM, Hanisch R, Cicioni C, Henderson BE (1986). Cigarette smoking, obesity, diuretic use, and coffee consumption as risk factors for renal cell carcinoma. *J Natl Cancer Inst* **77**: 351–6.

17 Yuan JM, Castelao JE, Gago-Dominguez M, Ross RK, Yu MC (1998). Hypertension, obesity and their medications in relation to renal cell carcinoma. *Br J Cancer* **77**: 1508–13.

18 Benichou J, Chow WH, McLaughlin JK, Mandel JS, Fraumeni Jr JF (1998). Population attributable risk of renal cell cancer in Minnesota. *Am J Epidemiol* **148**: 424–30.

19 Armstrong B, Doll R (1975). Environmental factors and cancer incidence and mortality in different countries, with special reference to dietary practices. *Int J Cancer* **15**: 617–31.

20 Moyad MA (2001). Review of potential risk factors for kidney (renal cell) cancer. *Semin Urol Oncol* **19**: 280–93.

21 Rabbani F, Herr HW, Almahmeed T, Russo P (2002). Temporal change in risk of metachronous contralateral renal cell carcinoma: influence of tumor characteristics and demographic factors. *J Clin Oncol* **20**: 2370–5.

22 Chow WH, Devesa SS, Warren JL, Fraumeni Jr JF (1999). Rising incidence of renal cell cancer in the United States. *JAMA* **281**: 1628–31.

23 Hii SI, Nicol DL, Gotley DC, Thompson LC, Green MK, Jonsson JR (1998). Captopril inhibits tumour growth in a xenograft model of human renal cell carcinoma. *Br J Cancer* **77**: 880–3.

24 Chow WH, Gridley G, Fraumeni Jr JF, Jarvholm B (2000). Obesity, hypertension, and the risk of kidney cancer in men. *N Engl J Med* **343**: 1305–11.

25 Gago-Dominguez M, Yuan JM, Castelao JE, Ross RK, Yu MC (2001). Family history and risk of renal cell carcinoma. *Cancer Epidemiol Biomarkers Prev* **10**: 1001–4.

26 Schlehofer B, Pommer W, Mellemgaard A, Stewart JH, McCredie M, Niwa S, et al. (1996). International renal-cell-cancer study. VI. the role of medical and family history. *Int J Cancer* **66**: 723–6.

27 Conaway RC, Conaway JW (2002). The von Hippel–Lindau tumor suppressor complex and regulation of hypoxia-inducible transcription. *Adv Cancer Res* **85**: 1–12.

28 Bretan Jr PN, Busch MP, Hricak H, Williams RD (1986). Chronic renal failure: a significant risk factor in the development of acquired renal cysts and renal cell carcinoma. Case reports and review of the literature. *Cancer* **57**: 1871–9.

29 MacDougall ML, Welling LW, Wiegmann TB (1987). Renal adenocarcinoma and acquired cystic disease in chronic hemodialysis patients. *Am J Kidney Dis* **9**: 166–71.

30 Ikeda R, Tanaka T, Moriyama MT, Kawamura K, Miyazawa K, Suzuki K (2002). Proliferative activity of renal cell carcinoma associated with acquired cystic disease of the kidney: comparison with typical renal cell carcinoma. *Hum Pathol* **33**: 230–5.

31 Rubio Briones J, Regalado Pareja R, Sanchez Martin F, Chechile Toniolo G, Huguet Perez J, Villavicencio Mavrich H (1998). Incidence of tumoural pathology in horseshoe kidneys. *Eur Urol* **33**: 175–9.

32 McLaughlin JK, Lipworth L (2000). Epidemiologic aspects of renal cell cancer. *Semin Oncol* **27**: 115–23.

33 Anttila A, Pukkala E, Sallmen M, Hernberg S, Hemminki K (1995). Cancer incidence among Finnish workers exposed to halogenated hydrocarbons. *J Occup Environ Med* **37**: 797–806.

34 Lynge E, Anttila A, Hemminki K (1997). Organic solvents and cancer. *Cancer Causes Control* **8**: 406–19.

35 Mandel JS, McLaughlin JK, Schlehofer B, Mellemgaard A, Helmert U, Lindblad P, et al. (1995). International renal-cell cancer study. IV. Occupation. *Int J Cancer* **61**: 601–5.

36 Cooper PH, Waisman J (1973). Tubular differentiation and basement-membrane production in a renal adenoma: ultrastructural features. *J Pathol* **109**: 113–21.

37 Schraml P, Struckmann K, Hatz F, Sonnet S, Kully C, Gasser T, et al. (2002). VHL mutations and their correlation with tumour cell proliferation, microvessel density, and patient prognosis in clear cell renal cell carcinoma. *J Pathol* **196**: 186–93.

38 Kovacs G, Akhtar M, Beckwith BJ, Bugert P, Cooper CS, Delahunt B, et al. (1997). The Heidelberg classification of renal cell tumours. *J Pathol* **183**: 131–3.

39 Storkel S, Eble JN, Adlakha K, Amin M, Blute ML, Bostwick DG, et al. (1997). Classification of renal cell carcinoma: Workgroup No. 1. Union Internationale Contre le Cancer (UICC) and the American Joint Committee on Cancer (AJCC). *Cancer* **80**: 987–9.

40 Van Poppel H, Nilsson S, Algaba F, Bergerheim U, Dal Cin P, Fleming S, et al. (2000). Precancerous lesions in the kidney. *Scand J Urol Nephrol Suppl* **205**: 136–65.

41 Reuter VE, Presti Jr JC (2000). Contemporary approach to the classification of renal epithelial tumors. *Semin Oncol* **27**: 124–37.

42 Davis Jr CJ, Mostofi FK, Sesterhenn IA (1995). Renal medullary carcinoma. The seventh sickle cell nephropathy. *Am J Surg Pathol* **19**: 1–11.

43 Motzer RJ, Bacik J, Mariani T, Russo P, Mazumdar M, Reuter V (2002). Treatment outcome and survival associated with metastatic renal cell carcinoma of non-clear-cell histology. *J Clin Oncol* **20**: 2376–81.

44 Bodmer D, Van Den Hurk W, Van Groningen JJ, Eleveld MJ, Martens GJ, Weterman MA, et al. (2002). Understanding familial and non-familial renal cell cancer. *Hum Mol Genet* **11**: 2489–98.

45 Latif F, Tory K, Gnarra J, Yao M, Duh FM, Orcutt ML, et al. (1993). Identification of the von Hippel–Lindau disease tumor suppressor gene. *Science* **260**: 1317–20.

46 Gorospe M, Egan JM, Zbar B, Lerman M, Geil L, Kuzmin I, et al. (1999). Protective function of von Hippel-Lindau protein against impaired protein processing in renal carcinoma cells. *Mol Cell Biol* **19**: 1289–300.

47 Horton WA, Wong V, Eldridge R (1976). Von Hippel–Lindau disease: clinical and pathological manifestations in nine families with 50 affected members. *Arch Intern Med* **136**: 769–77.

48 Nelson JB, Oyasu R, Dalton DP (1994). The clinical and pathological manifestations of renal tumors in von Hippel–Lindau disease. *J Urol* **152**: 2221–6.

49 Linehan WM, Lerman MI, Zbar B (1995). Identification of the von Hippel–Lindau (VHL) gene. Its role in renal cancer. *JAMA* **273**: 564–70.

50 Cohen AJ, Li FP, Berg S, Marchetto DJ, Tsai S, Jacobs SC, et al. (1979). Hereditary renal-cell carcinoma associated with a chromosomal translocation. *N Engl J Med* **301**: 592–5.

51 Zbar B, Lerman M (1998). Inherited carcinomas of the kidney. *Adv Cancer Res* **75**: 163–201.

52 Duffy K, Al-Saleem T, Karbowniczek M, Ewalt D, Prowse AH, Henske EP (2002). Mutational analysis of the von hippel lindau gene in clear cell renal carcinomas from tuberous sclerosis complex patients. *Mod Pathol* **15**: 205–10.

53 Brauch H, Weirich G, Brieger J, Glavac D, Rodl H, Eichinger M, et al. (2000). VHL alterations in human clear cell renal cell carcinoma: association with advanced tumor stage and a novel hot spot mutation. *Cancer Res* **60**: 1942–8.

54 Kondo K, Yao M, Yoshida M, Kishida T, Shuin T, Miura T, et al. (2002). Comprehensive mutational analysis of the VHL gene in sporadic renal cell carcinoma: relationship to clinicopathological parameters. *Genes Chromosomes Cancer* **34**: 58–68.

55 Gallou C, Joly D, Mejean A, Staroz F, Martin N, Tarlet G, et al. (1999). Mutations of the VHL gene in sporadic renal cell carcinoma: definition of a risk factor for VHL patients to develop an RCC. *Hum Mutat* **13**: 464–75.

56 de Paulsen N, Brychzy A, Fournier MC, Klausner RD, Gnarra JR, Pause A, et al. (2001). Role of transforming growth factor-alpha in von Hippel–Lindau (VHL)(-/-) clear cell renal carcinoma cell proliferation: a possible mechanism coupling VHL tumor suppressor inactivation and tumorigenesis. *Proc Natl Acad Sci USA* **98**: 1387–92.

57 Majhail NS, Urbain JL, Albani JM, Kanvinde MH, Rice TW, Novick AC, et al. (2003). F–18 fluorodeoxyglucose positron emission tomography in the evaluation of distant metastases from renal cell carcinoma. *J Clin Oncol* **21**: 3995–4000.

58 Bretheau D, Lechevallier E, de Fromont M, Sault MC, Rampal M, Coulange C (1995). Prognostic value of nuclear grade of renal cell carcinoma. *Cancer* **76**: 2543–9.

59 Fuhrman SA, Lasky LC, Limas C (1982). Prognostic significance of morphologic parameters in renal cell carcinoma. *Am J Surg Pathol* **6**: 655–63.

60 Thrasher JB, Paulson DF (1993). Prognostic factors in renal cancer. *Urol Clin North Am* **20**: 247–62.

61 Elson PJ, Witte RS, Trump DL (1988). Prognostic factors for survival in patients with recurrent or metastatic renal cell carcinoma. *Cancer Res* **48**: 7310–3.

62 Tsui KH, Shvarts O, Smith RB, Figlin R, de Kernion JB, Belldegrun A (2000). Renal cell carcinoma: prognostic significance of incidentally detected tumors. *J Urol* **163**(2): 426–30.

63 Medeiros LJ, Gelb AB, Weiss LM (1988). Renal cell carcinoma. Prognostic significance of morphologic parameters in 121 cases. *Cancer* **61**: 1639–51.

64 Gettman MT, Blute ML, Spotts B, Bryant SC, Zincke H (2001). Pathologic staging of renal cell carcinoma: significance of tumor classification with the 1997 TNM staging system. *Cancer* **91**: 354–61.

65 Ficarra V, Righetti R, D'Amico A, Rubilotta E, Novella G, Malossini G, et al. (2001). Renal vein and vena cava involvement does not affect prognosis in patients with renal cell carcinoma. *Oncology* **61**: 10–5.

66 Bos SD, Mellema CT, Mensink HJ (2000). Increase in incidental renal cell carcinoma in the northern part of the Netherlands. *Eur Urol* **37**: 267–70.

67 Katusin D, Uzarevic B, Petrovecki M, Mlinac-Lucijanic M, Marusic M, Marekovic Z (2000). Clinical, histopathological and flow-cytometric properties of incidental renal cell carcinomas. *Urol Res* **28**: 52–6.

68 Patard JJ, Rodriguez A, Rioux-Leclercq N, Guille F, Lobel B (2002). Prognostic significance of the mode of detection in renal tumours. *BJU Int* **90**: 358–63.

69 Frank I, Blute ML, Cheville JC, Lohse CM, Weaver AL, Zincke H (2002). An outcome prediction model for patients with clear cell renal cell carcinoma treated with radical nephrectomy based on tumor stage, size, grade and necrosis: the SSIGN score. *J Urol* **168**: 2395–400.

70 Zisman A, Pantuck AJ, Dorey F, Chao DH, Gitlitz BJ, Moldawer N, et al. (2002). Mathematical model to predict individual survival for patients with renal cell carcinoma. *J Clin Oncol* **20**: 1368–74.

71 Zisman A, Pantuck AJ, Figlin RA, Belldegrun AS (2001). Validation of the UCLA integrated staging system for patients with renal cell carcinoma. *J Clin Oncol* **19**: 3792–3.

72 Zisman A, Pantuck AJ, Dorey F, Said JW, Shvarts O, Quintana D, et al. (2001). Improved prognostication of renal cell carcinoma using an integrated staging system. *J Clin Oncol* **19**: 1649–57.

73 Motzer RJ, Mazumdar M, Bacik J, Berg W, Amsterdam A, Ferrara J (1999). Survival and prognostic stratification of 670 patients with advanced renal cell carcinoma. *J Clin Oncol* **17**: 2530–40.

74 Stiles KP, Moffatt MJ, Agodoa LY, Swanson SJ, Abbott KC (2003). Renal cell carcinoma as a cause of end-stage renal disease in the United States: patient characteristics and survival. *Kidney Intl* **64**: 247–53.

75 Ghavamian R, Cheville JC, Lohse CM, Weaver AL, Zincke H, Blute ML (2002). Renal cell carcinoma in the solitary kidney: an analysis of complications and outcome after nephron sparing surgery. *J Urol* **168**: 454–9.

76 Motzer RJ, Agarwal N, Beard C, Bolger GB, Boston B, Carducci MA, et al. (2009). NCCN clinical practice guidelines in oncology: kidney cancer. *J Natl Compr Canc Netw* **7**: 618–30.

77 Novick AC, Gephardt G, Guz B, Steinmuller D, Tubbs RR (1991). Long-term follow-up after partial removal of a solitary kidney. *N Engl J Med* **325**: 1058–62.

78 Leder RA, Nelson RC (2001). Three-dimensional CT of the genitourinary tract. *J Endourol* **15**: 37–46.

79 Lee CT, Katz J, Shi W, Thaler HT, Reuter VE, Russo P (2000). Surgical management of renal tumors 4 cm. or less in a contemporary cohort. *J Urol* **163**: 730–6.

80 Patard JJ, Pantuck AJ, Crepel M, Lam JS, Bellec L, Albouy B, et al. (2007). Morbidity and clinical outcome of nephron-sparing surgery in relation to tumour size and indication. *Eur Urol* **52**: 148–54.

81 Van Poppel H, Da Pozzo L, Albrecht W, Matveev V, Bono A, Borkowski A, et al. (2007). A prospective randomized EORTC intergroup phase 3 study comparing the complications of elective nephron-sparing surgery and radical nephrectomy for low-stage renal cell carcinoma. *Eur Urol* **51**: 1606–15.

82 Huang WC, Levey AS, Serio AM, Snyder M, Vickers AJ, Raj GV, et al. (2006). Chronic kidney disease after nephrectomy in patients with renal cortical tumours: a retrospective cohort study. *Lancet Oncol* **7**: 735–40.

83 Novick AC (1998). Nephron-sparing surgery for renal cell carcinoma. *Br J Urol* **82**: 321–4.

84 Touijer K, Jacqmin D, Kavoussi LR, Montorsi F, Patard JJ, Rogers CG, et al. (2010). The expanding role of partial nephrectomy: a critical analysis of indications, results, and complications. *Eur Urol* **57**: 214–20 (epub. 20 Oct 2009).

85 Miller DC, Hollingsworth JM, Hafez KS, Daignault S, Hollenbeck BK (2006). Partial nephrectomy for small renal masses: an emerging quality of care concern? *J Urol* **175**: 853–7, discussion 8.

86 de Baere T, Kuoch V, Smayra T, Dromain C, Cabrera T, Court B, et al. (2002). Radio frequency ablation of renal cell carcinoma: preliminary clinical experience. *J Urol* **167**: 1961–4.

87 Matin SF, Gill IS, Worley S, Novick AC (2002). Outcome of laparoscopic radical and open partial nephrectomy for the sporadic 4 cm. or less renal tumor with a normal contralateral kidney. *J Urol* **168**: 1356–9, discussion 9–60.

88 Flanigan RC, Salmon SE, Blumenstein BA, Bearman SI, Roy V, McGrath PC, et al. (2001). Nephrectomy followed by interferon alfa–2b compared with interferon alfa–2b alone for metastatic renal-cell cancer. *N Engl J Med* **345**: 1655–9.

89 Mickisch GH, Garin A, van Poppel H, de Prijck L, Sylvester R (2001). Radical nephrectomy plus interferon-alfa-based immunotherapy compared with interferon alfa alone in metastatic renal-cell carcinoma: a randomised trial. *Lancet* **358**: 966–70.

90 Sandock DS, Seftel AD, Resnick MI (1995). A new protocol for the followup of renal cell carcinoma based on pathological stage. *J Urol* **154**: 28–31.

91 Medical Research Council Renal Cancer Collaborators (1999). Interferon-alpha and survival in metastatic renal carcinoma: early results of a randomised controlled trial. *Lancet* **353**: 14–17.

92 Pyrhonen S, Salminen E, Ruutu M, Lehtonen T, Nurmi M, Tammela T, et al. (1999). Prospective randomized trial of interferon alfa-2a plus vinblastine versus vinblastine alone in patients with advanced renal cell cancer. *J Clin Oncol* **17**: 2859–67.

93 Belldegrun AS, Klatte T, Shuch B, LaRochelle JC, Miller DC, Said JW, et al. (2008). Cancer-specific survival outcomes among patients treated during the cytokine era of kidney cancer (1989–2005): a benchmark for emerging targeted cancer therapies. *Cancer* **113**: 2457–63.

94 Klapper JA, Downey SG, Smith FO, Yang JC, Hughes MS, Kammula US, et al. (2008). High-dose interleukin-2 for the treatment of metastatic renal cell carcinoma : a retrospective analysis of response and survival in patients treated in the surgery branch at the National Cancer Institute between 1986 and 2006. *Cancer* **113**: 293–301.

95 Fyfe G, Fisher RI, Rosenberg SA, Sznol M, Parkinson DR, Louie AC (1995). Results of treatment of 255 patients with metastatic renal cell carcinoma who received high-dose recombinant interleukin-2 therapy. *J Clin Oncol* **13**: 688–96.

96 Yang JC, Haworth L, Sherry RM, Hwu P, Schwartzentruber DJ, Topalian SL, et al. (2003). A randomized trial of bevacizumab, an anti-vascular endothelial growth factor antibody, for metastatic renal cancer. *N Engl J Med* **349**: 427–34.

97 Eisenhauer EA, Therasse P, Bogaerts J, Schwartz LH, Sargent D, Ford R, et al. (2009). New response evaluation criteria in solid tumours: revised RECIST guideline (version 1.1). *Eur J Cancer* **45**: 228–47.

98 Escudier B, Pluzanska A, Koralewski P, Ravaud A, Bracarda S, Szczylik C, et al. (2007). Bevacizumab plus interferon alfa-2a for treatment of metastatic renal cell carcinoma: a randomised, double-blind phase III trial. *Lancet* **370**: 2103–11.

99 Rini BI, Halabi S, Rosenberg JE, Stadler WM, Vaena DA, Ou SS, et al. (2008). Bevacizumab plus interferon alfa compared with interferon alfa monotherapy in patients with metastatic renal cell carcinoma: CALGB 90206. *J Clin Oncol* **26**: 5422–8.

100 Escudier B, Eisen T, Stadler WM, Szczylik C, Oudard S, Staehler M, et al. (2009). Sorafenib for treatment of renal cell carcinoma: Final efficacy and safety results of the phase III treatment approaches in renal cancer global evaluation trial. *J Clin Oncol* **27**: 3312–8.

101 Motzer RJ, Hutson TE, Tomczak P, Michaelson MD, Bukowski RM, Oudard S, et al. (2009). Overall survival and updated results for sunitinib compared with interferon alfa in patients with metastatic renal cell carcinoma. *J Clin Oncol* **27**: 3584–90.

102 Sternberg CN, Szczylik C, Lee E, Salman PV, Mardiak J, Davis ID, et al. (2009). A randomized, double-blind phase III study of pazopanib in treatment-naive and cytokine-pretreated patients with advanced renal cell carcinoma (RCC). *J Clin Oncol* (meeting abstracts) **27**: 5021ff.

103 Rixe O, Bukowski RM, Michaelson MD, Wilding G, Hudes GR, Bolte O, et al. (2007). Axitinib treatment in patients with cytokine-refractory metastatic renal-cell cancer: a phase II study. *Lancet Oncol* **8**: 975–84.

104 Rini BI, Wilding G, Hudes G, Stadler WM, Kim S, Tarazi J, et al. (2009). Phase II study of axitinib in sorafenib-refractory metastatic renal cell carcinoma. *J Clin Oncol* **27**: 4462–8.

105 Gore ME, Szczylik C, Porta C, Bracarda S, Bjarnason GA, Oudard S, et al. (2009). Safety and efficacy of sunitinib for metastatic renal-cell carcinoma: an expanded-access trial. *Lancet Oncol* **10**: 757–63.

106 Atkins MB, Hidalgo M, Stadler WM, Logan TF, Dutcher JP, Hudes GR, et al. (2004). Randomized phase II study of multiple dose levels of CCI-779, a novel mammalian target of rapamycin kinase inhibitor, in patients with advanced refractory renal cell carcinoma. *J Clin Oncol* **22**: 909–18.

107 Hudes G, Carducci M, Tomczak P, Dutcher J, Figlin R, Kapoor A, et al. (2007). Temsirolimus, interferon alfa, or both for advanced renal-cell carcinoma. *N Engl J Med* **356**: 2271–81.

108 O"Donnell A, Faivre S, Burris 3rd HA, Rea D, Papadimitrakopoulou V, Shand N, et al. (2008). Phase I pharmacokinetic and pharmacodynamic study of the oral mammalian target of rapamycin inhibitor everolimus in patients with advanced solid tumors. *J Clin Oncol* **26**: 1588–95.

109 Hidalgo M, Buckner JC, Erlichman C, Pollack MS, Boni JP, Dukart G, et al. (2006). A phase I and pharmacokinetic study of temsirolimus (CCI–779) administered intravenously daily for 5 days every 2 weeks to patients with advanced cancer. *Clin Cancer Res* **12**: 5755–63.

110 Mita MM, Mita AC, Chu QS, Rowinsky EK, Fetterly GJ, Goldston M, et al.(2008). Phase I trial of the novel mammalian target of rapamycin inhibitor deforolimus (AP23573; MK-8669) administered intravenously daily for 5 days every 2 weeks to patients with advanced malignancies. *J Clin Oncol* **26**: 361–7.

111 Raymond E, Alexandre J, Faivre S, Vera K, Materman E, Boni J, et al. (2004). Safety and pharmacokinetics of escalated doses of weekly intravenous infusion of CCI-779, a novel mTOR inhibitor, in patients with cancer. *J Clin Oncol* **22**: 2336–47.

112 Lunardi G, Armirotti A, Nicodemo M, Cavallini L, Damonte G, Vannozzi MO, et al. (2009). Comparison of temsirolimus pharmacokinetics in patients with renal cell carcinoma not receiving dialysis and those receiving hemodialysis: a case series. *Clin Ther* **31**: 1812–9.

113 Khan G, Golshayan A, Elson P, Wood L, Garcia J, Bukowski R, et al. (2010). Sunitinib and sorafenib in metastatic renal cell carcinoma patients with renal insufficiency. *Ann Oncol* **21**: 1618–22.

114 Rathmell WK, Monk JP (2008). High-dose-intensity MVAC for advanced renal medullary carcinoma: report of three cases and literature review. *Urology* **72**: 659–63.

115 Oudard S, Banu E, Vieillefond A, Fournier L, Priou F, Medioni J, et al. (2007). Prospective multicenter phase II study of gemcitabine plus platinum salt for metastatic collecting duct carcinoma: results of a GETUG (Groupe d'Etudes des Tumeurs Uro-Genitales) study. *J Urol* **177**: 1698–702.

116 Nanus DM, Garino A, Milowsky MI, Larkin M, Dutcher JP (2004). Active chemotherapy for sarcomatoid and rapidly progressing renal cell carcinoma. *Cancer* **101**: 1545–51.

117 Choueiri TK, Plantade A, Elson P, Negrier S, Ravaud A, Oudard S, et al. (2008). Efficacy of sunitinib and sorafenib in metastatic papillary and chromophobe renal cell carcinoma. *J Clin Oncol* **26**: 127–31.

118 Plimack ER, Jonasch E, Bekele BN, Smith LA, Araujo JC, Tannir NM (2008). Sunitinib in non-clear cell renal cell carcinoma (ncc-RCC): A phase II study. *J Clin Oncol* (meeting abstracts) **26**: 5112ff.

119 Ravaud A, Oudard S, Gravis-Mescam G, Sevin E, Zanetta S, Theodore C, et al. (2009). First-line sunitinib in type I and II papillary renal cell carcinoma (PRCC): SUPAP, a phase II study of the French Genito-Urinary Group (GETUG) and the Group of Early Phase trials (GEP). *J Clin Oncol* (meeting abstracts) **27**: 5146ff.

120 Molina AM, Motzer RJ (2008). Current algorithms and prognostic factors in the treatment of metastatic renal cell carcinoma. *Clin Genitourin Cancer* **6**: s7–s13.

121 Thompson Coon J, Hoyle M, Green C, Liu Z, Welch K, Moxham T, et al. (2010). Bevacizumab, sorafenib tosylate, sunitinib and temsirolimus for renal cell carcinoma: a systematic review and economic evaluation. *Health Technol Assess* **14**: 1–184, iii–iv.

Chapter 13

Cancer after renal transplantation

Kadiyala V. Ravindra, Michael Marvin, and
Joseph F. Buell

Case report

A 35-year-old man presented with von Hippel–Lindau disease and hematuria. A computed
tomography (CT) scan identified two large central tumors in his kidneys. Following bilateral laparoscopic nephrectomy, the tumors were identified to be 3 and 5 cm Fuhrman grade
2 renal cell carcinomas. He was started on hemodialysis and evaluated by the local transplant
center, where a five-year interval from operation to transplantation was recommended. Five
years later, he received a deceased donor renal transplant from an Epstein–Barr virus (EBV)
positive organ donor. He was maintained on tacrolimus, mycophenolate mofetil, and prednisone. After 12 months of receiving his transplant, he noticed a large mass in his neck,
which was shown to be a monomorphic EBV+, CD20+, B-cell lymphoma. A CT scan of the
chest, abdomen, and the pelvis identified nodal disease in the iliac fossa and para-aortic
regions. A renal allograft biopsy demonstrated the presence of post-transplant proliferative
disease (PTLD). Mycophenolate mofetil was discontinued and his tacrolimus decreased by
50% percent. A repeat CT scan at six weeks revealed the nodal disease regressed, and at ten
weeks showed complete resolution. A repeat biopsy of the allograft showed no PTLD; however, a Banff grade I rejection was present, which was treated with local allograft irradiation.
At one-year post-PTLD the patient had a normal serum creatinine and CT scans. This case
illustrates the oncogenic potential of immunosuppression associated with transplantation.

Introduction

Most conditions associated with a state of profound immune suppression are
associated with an increased risk of malignancy. Individuals with known congenital defects of antibody production or immune response mechanisms have
higher incidences of non Hodgkin's lymphoma, leukemias, and other malignancies. In states of acquired immunodeficiencies, such as the acquired immunodeficiency syndrome (AIDS), higher incidences of skin and lymphoid
malignancies (such as Kaposi's sarcoma and non Hodgkin's lymphoma) exist.
Immunosuppressed transplant recipients have a three- to fourfold overall
increased risk of cancer, with some individual cancers having risk increases a
hundredfold or greater over the general population (1–2).

The improved survival with solid organ transplantation has brought focus on the long term adverse sequelae of immunosuppression—the most serious being post-transplant neoplasia. Malignancy after transplantation is now the third leading cause of mortality in kidney transplant recipients (3). Malignancy is projected to surpass cardiovascular disease as the leading cause of death in these patients in the next two decades (4). The effect of immunosuppression has been thought to be cumulative, with the occurrence of the malignancy reaching 20% in all solid organ recipients by 20 years post-transplantation. In 2004, malignancy was the cause of mortality in 7% of kidney transplant recipients in the US (US Renal Data System (USRDS) 2006 annual data report). Post-transplant mortality associated with de novo cancers is high—ten-year survival in patients with malignancy being 57% compared with 93% in those without cancer (5).

A large cohort study from Australia and New Zealand demonstrated the site-specific cancer risk for kidney transplant recipients (Table 13.1 and Fig. 13.1) (6). Cancer rates amongst kidney recipients are similar to those of non-transplanted people 20 to 30 years older (6).

Malignancies that are more commonly seen in the general population, such as lung, colon, and breast cancer, do not appear with a greatly increased frequency in the transplant population. In contrast, malignancies that are virally driven have the highest increased incidence. These include post-transplant lymphoproliferative disease (PTLD, Epstein–Barr virus), Kaposi's sarcoma (human herpesvirus-8), and cervical and vulvar cancers (human papillomavirus).

The most common malignancies encountered in the post-transplant setting are non-melanoma skin cancers (NMSCs—up to 80%), PTLD (5–10%), and Kaposi's sarcoma (<5%). Among the skin cancers, squamous cell cancer (SCC) is the commonest subtype with an incidence 65–250 times higher than in the general population (7). Several differences have been noted between the skin malignancies appearing in immunosuppressed patients and those found in the general population. Skin malignancies in kidney transplant recipients tend to occur at earlier ages, occur in multiple sites, and often have multiple recurrences (8–9). The transplant patients also demonstrate a higher incidence of squamous cell cancers compared to basal cell cancers (10). Even in non-skin cancers a higher incidence of malignancy has been observed. In a recent single-center study of almost 2000 kidney transplant recipients, a calculated relative risk of 1.4 was observed when compared to the general population (11).

The Israel Penn International Transplant Tumor Registry (IPITTR) has accrued data on transplant-related malignancies for over 30 years (Fig. 13.2). Following Dr. Penn's death in 1999, the Registry was renamed in his honor, and the data was computerized, thereby preserving his vision. The IPITTR

Table 13.1 Site-specific cancer risk for kidney transplant recipients, by age and sex

Age at cancer diagnosis	<35 years			35–44 years			45–54 years			≥55 years		
	O*	E*	SRR (95% CI)	O*	E*	SRR (95% CI)	O*	E*	SRR (95% CI)	O*	E*	SRR (95% CI)
Female												
Breast	4	1.28	3.12 (1.17, 8.31)	11	7.80	1.41 (0.78, 2.51)	30	19.23	1.56 (1.08, 2.21)	34	37.31	0.91 (0.65, 1.27)
olorectal	3	0.22	13.51 (4.34, 41.61)	8	1.16	6.88 (3.44, 13.75)	18	4.91	3.66 (2.31, 5.82)	45	19.88	2.26 (1.69, 3.03)
Melanoma	6	1.90	3.17 (1.42, 7.04)	7	3.25	2.46 (1.23, 4.93)	18	4.90	3.88 (2.47, 6.08)	33	8.93	3.70 (2.63, 5.20)
Lung	0	0.04	.	0	0.38	.	8	1.97	4.06 (2.03, 8.11)	30	10.08	2.98 (2.08, 4.26)
Lymphoma†	19	0.51	37.30 (23.79, 58.48)	11	0.75	14.67 (8.13, 26.50)	16	1.61	9.95 (6.09, 16.24)	33	5.23	6.30 (4.48, 8.87)
Male												
Prostate	0	0.00	.	0	0.13	.	2	4.02	0.50 (0.12, 1.98)	43	47.87	0.90 (0.64, 1.20)
Colorectal	0	0.33	.	13	1.93	6.73 (3.91, 11.60)	11	8.67	1.27 (0.70, 2.29)	37	33.14	1.12 (0.81, 1.54)
Lung	1	0.08	11.81 (1.66, 83.83)	4	0.80	5.03 (1.89, 13.39)	13	5.45	2.39 (1.39, 4.11)	48	27.85	1.72 (1.30, 2.29)
Melanoma	10	2.13	4.69 (2.53, 8.72)	20	4.57	4.38 (2.82, 6.79)	23	8.34	2.74 (1.82, 4.12)	46	15.54	3.15 (2.38, 4.17)
Lymphoma†	25	1.09	23.03 (15.56, 34.09)	23	1.85	12.43 (8.26, 18.71)	31	3.42	9.06 (6.37, 12.88)	50	7.57	6.61 (5.01, 8.72)

*O = observed incident cancers, in ANZDATA cohort, between 1980 and 2002

E = expected number of incident cancers in Australian and New Zealand general population of the same age and sex distribution, occurring over the same calendar years

†Lymphoma classified in the general and transplanted populations to include Hodgkin's and non Hodgkin's lymphoma. Comparison is made only with incidence in the Australian general population, as comparable lymphoma data was not available for New Zealand.

From Webster et al. (6)

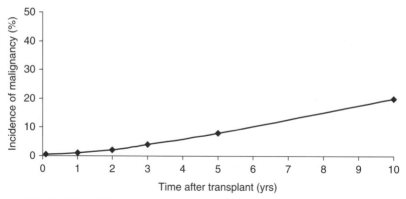

Fig. 13.1 Fig 13.1a: Site-specific cancer risk for kidney transplant recipients, by age and sex.

now provides over 300 consult services per year to transplant centers and oncologists worldwide.

Mechanisms of cancer development

The different mechanisms thought to play a crucial role in the development of neoplasia after transplantation include (12):

1 Impaired immune surveillance and antiviral activity due to the immuno-suppressive agents;

2 Chronic antigen stimulation of the graft;

3 Reactivation of latent oncogenic viruses; and

4 Oncogenicity directly related to the immunosuppressive drugs.

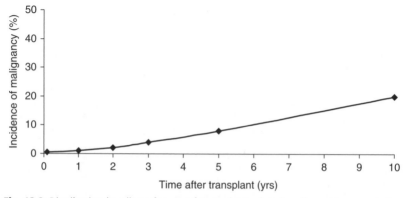

Fig. 13.2 Distribution by allograft type of transplant-related malignancies reported to the Israel Penn International Transplant Tumor Registry (IPITTR).

Immunosuppression and carcinogenesis

Long-term graft survival following solid organ transplantation requires continuous immunosuppressive therapy. The first immunosuppressive regimen in transplantation consisted of azathioprine and corticosteroids (2) with polyclonal anti-lymphocyte antibody therapy being introduced in the 1960s. Cyclosporine and the murine monoclonal antibody OKT3, which were introduced in the early 1980s, greatly enhanced organ transplant survival. The United States Food and Drug Administration (FDA) has subsequently approved the use of a number of immunosuppressive agents, including tacrolimus, mycophenolate mofetil, humanized IL-2 antibodies (basiliximab and daclizumab), thymoglobulin, and rapamycin.

Impaired immune surveillance

The immune system is thought to be essential in the surveillance and elimination of malignant cells. Impairment or loss of immuno-surveillance is thought to be a proximate cause of cancer in immunodeficient patients. Immunologists have demonstrated the importance of the immune response in reducing malignancy incidence and/or its progression (1, 13). Treatment of metastatic melanoma and/or renal cell cancer with systemic interleukin-2 (IL-2) has resulted in complete remission for a significant proportion of patients (13). Syndromes associated with immune-related malignancies include congenital immune deficiencies, such as combined immunodeficiency, or acquired immune deficiencies, such as AIDS. Patients afflicted with these syndromes are at risk of developing skin cancers, lymphomas, Kaposi's sarcoma, or Merkel cell cancer.

Oncogenic viruses

A number of viruses with oncogenic potential have been described, a few of which assume clinical importance in immunosuppressed patients. The association between Epstein–Barr virus and Burkitt's lymphoma has long been established (4). Early in the cyclosporine era, the association of EBV with post-transplant lymphoproliferative disorder was identified (14). This work also established the association of calcineurin inhibitors and the anti-lymphocyte agents with inhibition of certain T-cell functions, enabling either unrestricted B-cell proliferation in response to a primary viral infection or the reactivation of a latent virus (14–15). With the majority of adult and pediatric PTLD cases being EBV+, immunosuppression reduction in early cases of PTLD has proven successful.

A similar association between human papillomavirus and cervical cancer has been established in the general population (16). Recent work has demonstrated the efficacy of the HPV vaccination for the prevention of cervical cancer (17). Work from the IPITTR associated serotype positivity, specifically serotype 18 of the HPV, with the development of vulvar carcinoma in solid organ transplant recipients (18).

Human herpesvirus, particularly HHV-8, has long been associated with the development of Kaposi's sarcoma (19–20). Kaposi's sarcoma, which occurs in both endemic and non-endemic forms, has proven responsive to immunomodulation.

Neoplastic effects of immunosuppressive drugs

1 Calcineurin inhibitors (CNIs): Cyclosporine was assumed to cause cancer by inhibiting T-lymphocyte-mediated immune surveillance. It has now been shown to increase TGF-β levels which has a direct neoplastic effect (15). Other mechanisms include enhanced expression of vascular endothelial growth factor (VEGF) (21) and up-regulation of IL-6 which increases growth of EBV transformed B cells (22). Tacrolimus enhances cancer by similar mechanisms.

2 Corticosteroids: These agents are widely used in most immunosuppression protocols. The enhanced risk of skin cancers with long-term steroid use even in the non-transplant setting has been established (23). These agents thus play a role in the transplant population.

3 Antimetabolites: Azathioprine, a purine analog, has been demonstrated to produce chromosomal injury in animal models (2). In a human trial examining peripheral blood smears from patients treated with cyclosporine or azathioprine for more than one year, 31 of 50 subjects receiving azathioprine displayed chromosome aberrations, compared to 17 of 25 subjects that received cyclosporine. This chromosomal damage has been thought to result in sporadic malignancies in high-turnover tissue, such as skin and lymphoid cells.

4 Mycophenolate mofetil (MMF) has largely replaced azathioprine as an adjunct agent in most immunosuppression regimes (24). Several phase III randomized double-blind trials have established equivalence in the incidence of post-transplant malignancy with the use of cyclosporine, tacrolimus, and MMF (24–27). Some data suggest that MMF may increase tumor invasiveness (28) while other data contradict this (29).

5 mTOR inhibitors: Sirolimus (Rapamycin), another immunosuppressive agent recently approved by the FDA, was initially investigated for its anti-neoplastic activity. Rapamycin has demonstrated in vitro and in vivo activity against multiple types of solid organ malignancies (30). The mechanisms thus far shown might involve a reduction in TGF-β and VEGF levels. Everolimus has demonstrated an anti-proliferative effect on EBV-transformed B cells by a reduction in IL-10 levels. Replacement of calcineurin inhibitors (CNIs) with sirolimus in renal transplant recipients with malignancy has been reported to result in complete regression of Kaposi's sarcoma and PTLD (31). A recent five-year randomized controlled trial has shown that sirolimus (as compared with cyclosporine) resulted in a lower relative risk of developing skin cancer with a delayed median time to first skin cancer and a reduced incidence of non-skin cancers (32). The overall incidence of cancer in transplant patients maintained on rapamycin does appear lower than that for patients maintained on a calcineurin inhibitors, antimetabolites, and prednisone.

Classification and distribution of transplant-related malignancies

Transplant-related malignancies can be classified into three broad categories (Table 13.2).

1 Donor-transmitted malignancy: a malignancy transferred to an organ recipient through the donor allograft. The donor source may be confirmed through a genetic analysis or (by) other means.

2 Recurrence of the pre-existing recipient malignancy: Immunosuppression in patients that were treated earlier for malignancy may increase the incidence of recurrence or diminish the interval to the tumor recurrence.

3 De novo malignancy: Tumors that occur after transplantation in patients without pre-existing histories of the specific malignancy.

Donor-transmitted malignancy

Early experiences in transplantation, prior to the brain death laws, were associated with relatively frequent use of organs from donors with active malignancies (33). Recognition of the potential for malignancy transmission by organ transplantation decreased the use of donors with malignancy histories. As a result, donor-transmitted malignancies today are infrequently encountered.

The most commonly encountered tumors in eligible donors are those of the central nervous system (CNS) (34–36). The CNS tumors in donors continue

Table 13.2 Author's treatment recommendations

Diesease	Treatment recommendations[a]
Non-melanoma skin cancers	Immunosuppression reduction Surgical excision (depending on site and extent of tumor
PTLD	
Early lesions	Monitor after immunosuppression reduction;if no response (or progression) after 3 months,treat with rituximab,375 mg/m^2 weekly for four treatments
Monomorphic B-cell, EBV present	Rituximab,375 mg/m^2 weekly for four treatment R-CHOP or R-ESHAP if no on disease progression
Monomorphic B-cell, no EBV present	R-CHOP or R-ESHAP
Monomorphic T-cell	CHOP or R-ESHAP
Hodgkin's lymphoma-like	R-CHOP or R-ESHAP
Kaposi's sarcoma	Immunosuppression reduction Switch to sirolimus
Single lesion	Surgical resection
Multiple lesions	Monitor, as these treatment provide limited response of short duration
Metastatic to organs	Poor response with standard therapy Clinical trial is the most reasonable option

[a]Treatment for allthese tumors should begin with modulation of the immunosuppressive. Close monitoring is necessary to prevent loss of graft while attempting to affectthe malignancy.

Abbreviations: CHOP, cyclophosphamide, doxorubicin, vincristine, and prednisone; EBV, Epstein-Barr virus; ESHAP, etoposide, methylprednisolone, cytarabine, and cisplatin; PTLD, post-transplant lymphoproliferative disorder; R-CHOP, rituximab plus CHOP; R-Eshap, rituximab plus ESHAP.

to present challenges that reduce the use of their organs. A recent study from the IPITTR evaluated risk factors involved in donor transmission. In their series, an overall CNS tumor transmission rate of 23% was observed, and several risk factors for tumor transmission were identified: high-grade tumors, ventriculoperitoneal and ventriculoatrial shunts, craniotomy, and external radiation (37). When no identifiable risk factor was found, the incidence of donor transmission was only 7%. In the presence of one or more risk factors, the incidence of tumor transmission increased to 53% (37) (Fig. 13.3).

IPITTR experience with transmission of non-CNS donor tumors

Malignant melanoma and choriocarcinoma are among the non-CNS tumors with the highest overall rates of donor transmission and transmission to metastatic sites (35, 38) (Fig. 13.4). Choriocarcinoma, a gynecologic

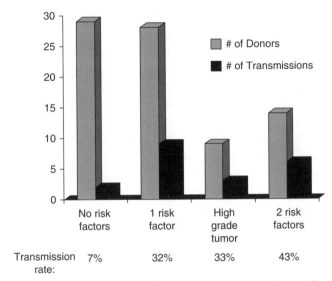

Fig. 13.3 Impact of donor risk factors (high-grade tumor, extensive crainiotomy, and peritoneal shunt) on transmission rates of CNS malignancy to solid organ recipients.

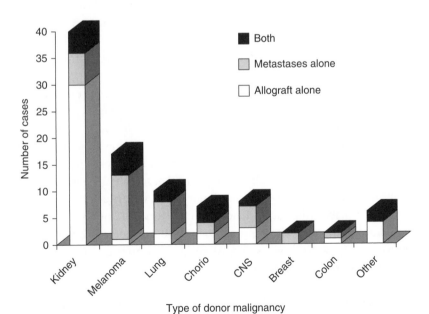

Fig. 13.4 Distribution of sites of donor tumor transmission segregated by individual donor tumor histology.

malignancy, has a transmission rate of 93%, with a 64% mortality rate. In non-immunosuppressed patients, malignant melanoma has been seen to recur up to 15 years after spontaneous resolution or surgical excision of superficial lesions. Melanoma recurrence has also been observed, when organs from the donors with a distant history of melanoma were used. Similar to choriocarcinoma, the malignant melanoma demonstrates a 74% tumor transmission rate with a resulting 58% mortality (38).

The IPITTR has reported on the utilization of 14 donor organs whose renal cell carcinomas (RCC) were excised at the time of harvesting immediately prior to implantation (38–40).The mean size of the excised RCC was 2.1 cm (range 0.5–4.1 cm). All lesions were graded as Fuhrman 1/4 or 2/4. There was no tumor transmission identified in any of these patients. In a later IPITTR study examining 70 donors with RCC, 43 (61%) of the donor organs resulted in malignancy transmission to the recipient (41). The majority of these RCC transmissions, which were confined to the allograft, were discovered between three months and three years after the transplantation. The resulting patient mortality (15%) was indicative of the less aggressive biologic activity of RCC, compared to melanoma or choriocarcinoma (Fig. 13.5). The study suggested that the organs from donors with low-grade RCC without extra capsular or vascular invasion could be utilized with a low risk of transmission.

Lung cancer remains one of the most common causes of cancer-related mortality in the United States. Utilization of organs from donors with a historic or active lung malignancy resulted in a 43% tumor transmission rate, with a corresponding 32% mortality rate (42). The use of organs from donors with a history of lung cancer should be avoided.

An overall transmission rate of 19% was experienced with the use of organs from donors with a history of colon cancer. Data presented at a consensus conference of the American Society of Transplant Surgeons cited the incidence of nodal or metastatic disease in kidney recipients from donors with T1 colon cancer to be less than 1%. In T2 and T3 lesions, the incidence was found to increase, with survival decreasing until a period of seven years post resection. It was concluded that the risk of using donors with a history of T1 colon cancer appears acceptable, while using donors with a history of T2 or T3 colon cancer should be approached with caution, but only after completing a minimum seven-year disease-free wait period. All recipients who had tumor transmission were treated with the standard therapy, and remained alive in remission at the last follow-up.

Little data exists on the use of organs from donors with a historic or active breast malignancy (42). A recent IPITTR review, which looked at seven donors with breast cancer, identified a tumor transmission rate of 29%. Tumor transmission

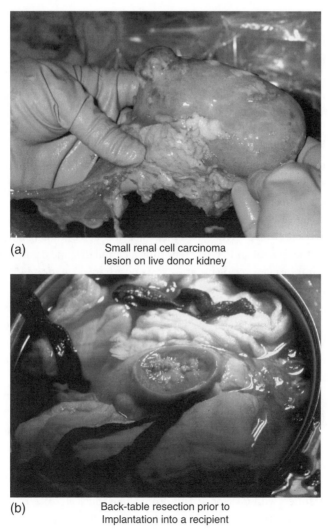

(a)   Small renal cell carcinoma
               lesion on live donor kidney

(b)   Back-table resection prior to
               Implantation into a recipient

Fig. 13.5 Utilization of a donor organ after local excision of a low Fuhrman-grade renal cell carcinoma by back-table resection (a) Small renal cell carcinoma lesion on live donor kidney. (b) Back-table resection prior to Implantation into a recipient.

was found in cases involving invasive breast cancer, but not with cases of in situ disease, such as ductal carcinoma in situ (DCIS), and lobular carcinoma in situ (LCIS). As with melanoma, breast cancer has a notorious reputation for late and aggressive recurrences. Consequently, the use of donors with a history of breast cancer should be limited to those with the non-invasive forms, such as DCIS or LCIS, and with low-stage invasive lesions with an extended disease-free interval.

Recipient de novo malignancies

While malignancies of the lung, colon, prostate, and breast occur in the transplant population with a frequency similar to that seen in the general population, virally driven malignancies (PTLD, Kaposi's sarcoma, cervical, and vaginal cancer) occur in solid organ transplant recipients with a substantially greater frequency.

Skin cancers

Skin cancers are the most common de novo malignancy among immunosuppressed transplant recipients, accounting for nearly 40% of all the malignancies (1, 43). In the transplant population, the development of skin malignancies appears to correlate with the duration of immunosuppression (9, 44). Several studies have confirmed an increased incidence of cutaneous malignancies over time, with the Australian Registry reporting a cumulative incidence of 66% in solid organ transplant recipients at 24 years post transplantation (45). A similar report from the Netherlands also noted a linear increase in the incidence of skin malignancies, with an incidence of 40% at 20 years (43). The difference in the magnitude of risk in these two populations may be due to the differences in the exposure to sun between the two countries.

The type and biologic activity of skin cancers in the transplant population differ from those in the general population. Basal cell cancers are the most common skin cancers in the general population, outnumbering squamous cell cancers five to one. In the general population, skin cancers account for only 1–2% of all cancer-related deaths, with the majority of them occurring from melanoma. In the transplant population, squamous cell carcinoma is the most commonly encountered skin cancer, occurring at a ratio to basal cell carcinoma of 2 to 110. Skin cancer accounts for almost 5% of the transplant population mortalities, with 60% occurring from squamous cell cancer, 30% from malignant melanoma, 8% from Merkel cell, and 2% from basal cell cancer (10). The mean age of development of any skin cancer among the transplant recipients is 30 years, compared to 65 years in the general population. The skin cancers encountered in the transplant population are much more aggressive than those in the general population, and are frequently multi-centric in origin. Lymph node metastasis has been reported in approximately 6% of the transplant patients, with mortality resulting from the dissemination of skin cancer in approximately 5% of cases (11). Except for cases involving malignant melanoma, lymph node metastasis and death from skin cancers are rare in the general population. Thus, the frequency of squamous cell cancer in the transplant population is estimated to be between 40 and 250 times greater than that of the general population, with these cancers appearing more aggressive and presenting at an earlier age than in the general population (9, 11, 44). Similarly, malignant melanoma is encountered with a frequency five times that experienced in the general population (10). As with the general population, the rate of survival correlates directly with the Clark and Breslow levels (11).

Merkel cell cancer is a rare skin malignancy that acts much like an aggressive, high-grade sarcoma. With fewer than 2000 cases reported in the literature, a surprisingly high proportion (n = 40: 5%) has been identified in transplant recipients. Tumor recurrence is almost universal with Merkel cell cancer, and is associated with high mortality in transplant recipients (46).

The prevention of these cancers involves periodic full-skin examination by a physician. Studies have demonstrated a possible beneficial role for systemic retinoid chemoprophylaxis in transplant recipients. A review of nine studies reported fewer skin cancers in patients while on oral retinoids but a rebound effect of higher numbers of non-melanoma skin cancers and keratotic lesions upon cessation of therapy (47).

Post-transplant lymphoproliferative disorder

Post-transplant lymphoproliferative disorder (PTLD) is a lymphoid-derived malignancy unique to transplant recipients (1, 48). The term PTLD encompasses a wide spectrum, ranging from infectious mononucleosis to malignant lymphoma. Early experiences with PTLD noted an association between the Epstein–Barr virus and the development of PTLD (14). The incidence of PTLD varies with the organ: kidney–2.3%, liver—2.8%, heart–lung—5.8%, heart—6.3%,

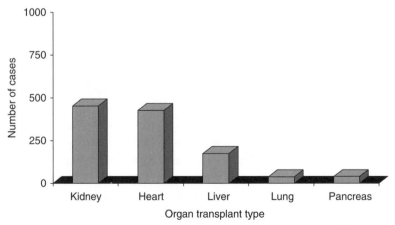

Fig. 13.6 Distribution of allograft types where posttransplant lymphoproliferative disorder (PTLD) cases were reported to the Israel Penn International Transplant Registry (IPITTR).

and small bowel—20%49. It is the most common malignancy in pediatric transplantation (50).

The IPITTR has provided analyses of the largest series of PTLD in kidney, pancreas, liver, and cardiac transplant recipients reported to date (51–52) (Fig. 13.6). A recent review from the IPITTR examined 402 cases of PTLD in renal transplant recipients (48).

The mean age of those who developed PTLD was 42 ± 16. Most tumors were B-cell predominant (86%), EBV + (81%), and monoclonal (64%). The PTLD presentation was variable, with an even distribution between a single-site and a multiple-site presentation. The majority of patients showed extra-allograft PTLD involvement, with 9% having allograft involvement and 13% having combined extra-renal and allograft involvement.

Sites of involvement include the lymph nodes, spleen, central nervous system, liver, lung, kidney, and the intestine. Overall five-year survival was 40%, with deaths resulting from progressive PTLD (58%), cardiac-related causes (16%), sepsis (14%), and other causes (16%). Patients with isolated allograft involvement did far better than those with the combined allograft and extra-renal involvement, having a five-year survival of 68%, compared to 36%; p <0.026. Extra-renal PTLD was associated with a lower five-year patient survival than PTLD of the allograft (68% vs. 34%; p <0.02). In a recent multivariate analysis of renal transplant PTLD patients, a survival advantage was observed for those with single-site versus multiple-site involvement of disease (47% vs. 27%; p <0.001) and for children (p <0.001)48. Survival was not influenced by gender, race, B-cell predominance, EBV positivity, antibody-based immunosuppression, calcineurin inhibitors, or azathioprine.

Early polymorphic lymphomas are generally EBV positive and respond to reduction of immunosuppression whereas late monomorphic lesions are EBV negative and have a worse prognosis. Periodic monitoring of EBV viral load has proved beneficial among pediatric liver transplant recipients in reducing the incidence from 16 to 2% (53). Antiviral therapy used for CMV prophylaxis (ganciclovir and anti-CMV globulin) has been shown to reduce the incidence of PTLD (54–55). Other studies have refuted this finding (56).

Treatment of PTLD may include, immunosuppression reduction (ISR), surgical excision, and/or administration of systemic chemotherapy, or biologic agents (51, 54). Case reports suggest that change of immunosuppression to sirolimus can induce complete remission of the disease (57). The presence of poor prognostic signs, including aggressive tumor histology, indicates the need for multi-agent systemic chemotherapy (51). When tumor fails to respond to reduction of immunosuppression alone chemotherapy is used. The most frequently used regimen is cyclophosphamide, doxorubicin, vincristine, and prednisone (CHOP). A recent study reported a 65% overall response rate with the regimen (58). Owing to the treatment-related morbidity of the above regimen, the use of less toxic agents such as rituximab (an anti-CD20 monoclonal antibody) has become more common. A phase II study reported a 64% response rate with the agent, similar to that of CHOP from previous studies but the agent was better tolerated (59). Other agents that have been used include interferon-α and interleukin-6. Adoptive T-cell immunotherapy using EBV-specific cytotoxic T-lymphocytes (CTLs) has been used successfully in EBV-positive PTLD (60). A recent review on malignancy after solid organ transplantation elegantly outlined the current management guidelines for the management of PTLD (Table 13.3) (61).

Kaposi's sarcoma

Kaposi's sarcoma (KS), a rare malignancy that has been linked to the human herpesvirus-8 (HHV-8), is more commonly seen among people of Arabic, African, Italian, Jewish or Greek ancestry (19, 62). The presentation of KS can be grouped into four categories: (1) endemic occurrence in the Mediterranean region of the world; (2) sporadic occurrence in the Western hemisphere; (3) occurrence within the AIDS population; and (4) occurrence within the transplant population. In the Western hemisphere, prior to the appearance of AIDS, KS was rarely seen. The pathogenesis of KS is related to human herpesvirus-8 infection.

Recent Organ Procurement and Transplantation Network (OPTN) data suggests an overall incidence of 8.8 cases of KS per 100,000 person-years in the

Table 13.3 Multivariate risk analysis of posttransplant lymphoproliferative disorder (PTLD) in kidney transplant recipients, with their representative odds ratios and survival rates

Variable	Survival	Odds ratio	p Value
Sites Single vs. Multiple	47% vs. 27%	2.62	0.0008
b-Cell (yes/no)	49% vs. 33%	1.9	not significant
ATG/ALG, OKT3	44% vs. 35%	1.5	not significant
EBV (yes/no)	54% vs. 50%	1.2	not significant
Gender Female vs. Male	45% vs. 42%	1.1	not significant
Race White vs. Black	45% vs. 45%	1.0	not significant
Age at Diagnosis	A one year increase in age increased odds of death by 1.02.	1.02	0.0004

transplant population (63). Most occurrences of KS found within the transplant population have cutaneous involvement (60%) (19, 52). The remaining cases have either isolated visceral involvement or a combined cutaneous and visceral involvement (40%). Cases involving KS with isolated cutaneous involvement generally have greater survival rate than cases with visceral involvement. Early aggressive therapeutic intervention, in the form of surgical resection, adjuvant chemotherapy, and ISR, is indicated in cases with visceral involvement (19, 54). When KS is suspected, a careful evaluation, including a visual inspection of the oral cavity and an endoscopic examination of the upper and lower GI tracts, should be conducted. Since KS may also present as a diffuse pulmonary infiltrate, a CT scan of the chest and abdomen is also necessary.Surgical resection of isolated lesions has been reported (64). Reduction of immunosuppression has improved outcomes only in those with isolated cutaneous disease. Recurrent disease requires treatment with chemotherapy including ABV (doxorubicin, bleomycin, and vincristine) or Paclitaxel (65–66).

Gynecologic cancer

The distribution of female malignancies in the transplant recipients is similar to that in the general population with a single exception: the incidence of ovarian cancer in the transplant population is less than that found in the general population. Ovarian cancer in the transplant population presents at an earlier age and is often detected at a later stage, compared to that identified in the general population.

Cervical and vulvar cancers, in contrast to ovarian cancer, are more frequently encountered in the transplant population than in the general population (1, 18, 67). Two separate epidemiological studies described a 14–16-fold increase in the incidence of in situ cervical carcinoma in kidney transplant patients compared to the general population (1, 18). An earlier report linked two HPV serotypes (16 and 18) to the development of cervical cancer in solid organ transplant recipients (18). Differences in the biologic activity of vulvar and cervical cancer in transplant recipients has been noted, with a higher incidence of multi-focal disease and tumor recurrence being observed among this population. This is similar to the experience with skin cancer in the solid organ transplant recipients (1, 44).

Renal cell cancer

Most native kidney renal cell carcinomas (RCC) in the renal transplant recipients are discovered incidentally, either during radiographic investigation or during a nephrectomy performed for unrelated pathology (38). In a recent review of 160 cases of de novo RCC, the mean age at diagnosis was 51 years, and the median time from transplant to malignancy diagnosis was 61 months (68). The majority of these tumors were native RCC, with only 11 (less than 10%) identified in the renal allograft. Eighty percent were unilateral lesions; 87% were successfully managed surgically. Thirty percent of the patients presented with advanced stage III or IV tumors, and 20% of the patients developed metastatic disease. Correspondingly, there was a 53% mortality rate, with a median survival of 4.7 months. Seven percent of the patients experienced a recurrence after a disease-free interval, with a resulting 64% mortality after a median survival time of 30 months.

Colon cancer

A recent analysis based on the surveillance, epidemiology, and end results (SEER) data demonstrated an increased incidence of colon cancer in the immunosuppressed population compared to the general population. In a separate analysis performed by the IPITTR, data from 150 transplant recipients with colorectal cancer (CRC) were compared with data from the National Cancer Institute (NCI) SEER database. The majority were renal transplant recipients (62%), followed by cardiac recipients (20%), and liver transplant recipients (18%). The median age at transplantation was 54 years, with a median age at diagnosis of CRC of 59 years, which was much younger than the median age of 72 years of age for the general population in the SEER database.

Transplant recipients who received azathioprine had shorter intervals from trans-plant to CRC diagnosis than those who did not receive azathioprine (34 vs. 63 months; p <0.04), however, no difference in survival was noted. A significant decrease in five-year survival among the kidney transplant recipients with stage I–III tumors was observed when compared to general population patients in the (NCI) SEER database. For lesions classified as the Duke's stage A or B, the survival was 74% versus 90%; for the Duke's stage C lesions, it was 20% versus 65%; and for the Duke's stage D, it was 0% versus 9% for the kidney transplant patients compared to the general population. The decreased time interval from transplant to presentation of CRC in the cadaveric kidney recipients receiving azathioprine suggests that the type of immunosuppression may affect the development of de novo CRC. Decreased five-year survival rates and a diagnosis of CRC at an early median age in transplant patients suggest that post-transplant colorectal screening programs are warranted.

Recurrence of pre-existing malignancyAs the number of older patients undergoing evaluation for transplantation increases, there will be an accompanying rise in the number of candidates who have either an active or a historic malignancy. Data concerning the risk of recurrence of pre-existing malignancies must be defined in order to recommend safe intervals between cancer therapy and transplantation.

Previous IPITTR recommendations were based on 1137 transplant recipients who had historic or active malignancies at the time of transplantation (41–2, 69). Two hundred and thirty-nine patients experienced recurrent disease (21%). The effect of interval waiting times was readily apparent, with 54% (128 cases) of tumor recurrences occurring in patients with less than a two-year interval from cancer treatment to transplantation. In those patients undergoing a two-to-five-year wait interval, the percentage decreased to 33% (80 cases). Beyond five years, the recurrence rate declined to 13%.

Tumors with low recurrence rates

Incidentally discovered RCC was found to have the lowest incidence (<7%) of tumor recurrence (69). An initial series of the RCC discovered incidentally at the time of bilateral nephrectomy demonstrated no recurrences. All of the lesions in the series were small asymptomatic tumors that were discovered during routine bilateral nephrectomy prior to transplantation. These findings lie in stark contrast to the almost 25% recurrence rate encountered with RCC that presented symptomatically or demonstrated evidence of extra capsular or neurovascular involvement.*

Patients with a history of either uterine or cervical cancer have low recurrence rates, and when transplanted after a two-to-five-year wait period did not experience any tumor recurrences. Several tumors were identified in individuals who underwent a five-to-ten-year wait. Most, if not all, of these reported recurrences might have, in fact, been ongoing primary lesions that occurred under the immunosuppression. In men, a few cases of recurrent testicular cancer were noted. This was especially true in cases of early-stage disease, where no recurrences were observed. The majority of these patients were transplanted prior to a five-year wait interval. Lastly, thyroid cancer also saw few tumor recurrences, with Hürthle cell and low-grade papillary carcinomas being among the varieties with the lowest incidence of recurrence.

Tumors with intermediate recurrence rates

Tumors having an intermediate (8–22%) incidence of recurrence included lymphoma, Wilms' tumor, prostate and colon cancers, and melanoma (69). The majority of patients with these cancers had undergone waiting times greater than five years. Colon and prostate cancer patients suffer tumor recurrence based on the stage of the tumor.

Tumors with high recurrence rates

There are several aggressive malignancies with high rates of recurrence (>23%), including soft tissue sarcomas, breast cancer, and symptomatic

RCC (69–71). Recurrence in patients with soft tissue sarcomas is based on the tumor grade; those transplant recipients who suffered tumor recurrences all had high-grade sarcomas. The overall incidence of recurrence among recipients with high-grade lesions was 43%. Among the breast cancer survivors, tumor recurrences have been reported to occur many years after the primary disease of the patient has been treated. Individuals with stage I and stage II breast cancers saw limited recurrence, with rates of 6% and 8%, respectively. In stage III patients, the tumor recurrence was a staggering 64%, with a corresponding five-year survival of 14%. Patients with the highest recurrence rates were those with symptomatic lesions (80%) or with bilateral cancers (25%). Transitional cell carcinoma (TCC) of the bladder and non-melanoma skin cancer often occurs as metachronous multi-focal lesions rather than as extensions of a localized primary lesion. While the majority of skin and bladder cancers are considered as nuisance malignancies, a small number were found to present with advanced local disease or with nodal metastasis.

Post transplant cancer screening

Individuals who are at risk for the development of female malignancies, such as breast cancer, should undergo routine screening based on their age and risk factors. The most important risk factors for the development of breast cancer are a history of breast cancer or a first-degree relative that has developed breast cancer. When risk factors exist, mammography should be conducted before the age of 50. Biennial mammography is otherwise recommended after the age of 50. Annual Pap smears should also be obtained as part of routine monitoring for cervical cancer (Table 13.4).

Table 13.4 These are recommended guidelines for malignancy screening in renal transplant recipients published in the *American Journal of Transplantation*

- ◆ Breast
  - – Women > 50 years: mammogram every 1–2 years
  - – Women < 50 years at high risk (family history or prior cancer): mammogram every 1–2 years
- ◆ Cervical
  - – Women > 18 years: Pap smear every year
- ◆ Prostrate
  - – Men > 40 years: Rectal exam and PSA every year
- ◆ Colorectal
  - – Recipients > 50 years: fecal blood test yearly and flexible sigmoidoscopy every 5 years
- ◆ Skin
  - – Annual self exam and biopsy of all suspicious lesions

Reproduced with permission from Zafar SY, Howell DN, Gockerman JP. *The Oncologist*, 2008; **13**: 769–778. Copyright ALPHAMED PRESS, INC.

Table 13.5 Current guidelines for cancer screening in the general population and after transplantation

Cancer site	Current guidelines and recommendations		Randomized trial evidence for screening	
	General population	Transplant population	General population	Transplant population
Breast	Biennial mammography for all women older than 50 years (32)	Biennial mammography for all women older than 50 years	Cancer-specific mortality reduction by 20–24% (33)	Nil
Colorectal	Annual or biennial FOBT at age >50 years, combination of FOBT and flexible sigmoidoscopy at age ≥ 50 years (34)	Annual FOBT and/or 5-yearly flexible sigmoidoscopy for individuals older than 50 years	Cancer-specific mortality reduction by 15–23% (35)	Nil
Cervical	Cytological screening to commence at age ≥ 21 years, or within 3 months of first sexual intercourse (biennially or triennially) (36)	Annual cytological cervical cancer screening and pelvic examination once sexually active	No RCT evidence, but historical evidence have shown significant reduction in cancer incidence and mortality since the introduction of population cervical cancer screening	Nil
Lung	Not recommended	Not recommended	Nil	Nil
Prostate	No general consensus			
	USPSTF found no evidence to recommend for or against routine screening using PSA or DRA. (37)	Annual DRE and PSA measurement in men older than 50 years	Nil	Hepatocellular

Table 13.5 (*continued*) Current guidelines for cancer screening in the general population and after transplantation

General population	Transplant recipients			Cancer
No firm recommendations, but screening using abdominal ultrasound and α-fetoprotein testing should be considered in high-risk individuals (38)	No firm recommendation, but abdominal ultrasound and α-fetoprotein every 6 months in high-risk recipients	Nil	Nil	Renal tract
No firm recommendations	No firm recommendation, some suggested regular imaging of the native kidneys	Nil	Nil	Skin
Insufficient evidence to recommend for or against total body skin examination	Monthly self-skin exam, total body skin exam, every 6–12 months by expert physician or dermatologists	Nil		FOBT = Fecal occult blood testing; DRE = digital rectal examination; PSA = prostate-specific antigen From Webster et al. (72)

TFN-FOBT = Fecal occult blood testing; DRE = digital rectal examination; PSA = prostate-specific antigen

TS-From Webster et al.

Males of over 50 years of age may be routinely screened for prostate cancer. Serum testing for prostate-specific antigen (PSA) could be incorporated as part of routine screening, although this is now controversial in the general population. Colorectal screening may begin at the age of 50 in all transplant recipients, unless the patient has a history of familial colon cancer, polyps, or inflammatory bowel disease, in which case, it should begin earlier. Fecal occult blood testing may be performed annually, with flexible sigmoidoscopy or full colonoscopic examination being performed every five years. Screening for skin cancer should include an annual self-examination, followed by a routine examination by the patient's primary care physician or dermatologist, with early biopsies being performed on all suspicious lesions. Current guidelines for cancer screening in the general population versus the transplanted patients are compared in Table 13.5 (72) along with the evidence in literature.

References

1 Penn I (2000). Cancers in renal transplant recipients. *Adv Ren Replace Ther* **7**: 147–56.

2 Penn I (1998). Occurrence of cancers in immunosuppressed organ transplant recipients. *Clin Transpl* **12**: 147–58.

3 Adams PL (2006). Long-term patient survival: strategies to improve overall health. *Am J Kidney Dis* **47**: S65–85.

4 Buell JF, Gross TG, Woodle ES (2005). Malignancy after transplantation. *Transplantation* **80**: S254–64.

5 Pedotti P, Cardillo M, Rossini G, et al. (2003). Incidence of cancer after kidney transplant: results from the North Italy transplant program. *Transplantation* **76**: 1448–51.

6 Webster AC, Craig JC, Simpson JM, Jones MP, Chapman JR (2007). Identifying high risk groups and quantifying absolute risk of cancer after kidney transplantation: a cohort study of 15,183 recipients. *Am J Transplant* **7**: 2140–51.

7 Baccarani U, Adani GL, Montanaro D, et al. (2006). De novo malignancies after kidney and liver transplantations: experience on 582 consecutive cases. *Transplant Proc* **38**: 1135–7.

8 Dreno B, Mansat E, Legoux B, Litoux P (1998). Skin cancers in transplant patients. *Nephrol Dial Transplant* **13**: 1374–9.

9 Gupta AK, Cardella CJ, Haberman HF (1986). Cutaneous malignant neoplasms in patients with renal transplants. *Arch Dermatol* **122**: 1288–93.

10 Agraharkar ML, Cinclair RD, Kuo YF, Daller JA, Shahinian VB (2004). Risk of malignancy with long-term immunosuppression in renal transplant recipients. *Kidney Int* **66**: 383–9.

11 Penn I (1980). Immunosuppression and skin cancer. *Clin Plast Surg* **7**: 361–8.

12 Kapoor A (2008). Malignancy in kidney transplant recipients. *Drugs* **68**: 11–9.

13 Kirkwood J (2002). Cancer immunotherapy: the interferon-alpha experience. *Semin Oncol* **29**: 18–26.

14 Paya CV, Fung JJ, Nalesnik MA, et al. (1999). Epstein-Barr virus-induced posttransplant lymphoproliferative disorders. ASTS/ASTP EBV-PTLD Task Force and The Mayo Clinic Organized International Consensus Development Meeting. *Transplantation* **68**: 1517–25.

15 Hojo M, Morimoto T, Maluccio M, et al. (1999). Cyclosporine induces cancer progression by a cell-autonomous mechanism. *Nature* **397**: 530–4.

16 Crum CP, Abbott DW, Quade BJ (2003). Cervical cancer screening: from the Papanicolaou smear to the vaccine era. *J Clin Oncol* **21**: 224s–30s.

17 Koutsky LA, Ault KA, Wheeler CM, et al. (2002). A controlled trial of a human papillomavirus type 16 vaccine. *N Engl J Med* **347**: 1645–51.

18 Brown MR, Noffsinger A, First MR, Penn I, Husseinzadeh N (2000). HPV subtype analysis in lower genital tract neoplasms of female renal transplant recipients. *Gynecol Oncol* **79**: 220–4.

19 Frances C (1998). Kaposi's sarcoma after renal transplantation. *Nephrol Dial Transplant* **13**: 2768–73.

20 Penn I (1997). Kaposi's sarcoma in transplant recipients. *Transplantation* **64**: 669–73.

21 Shihab FS, Bennett WM, Isaac J, Yi H, Andoh TF (2003). Nitric oxide modulates vascular endothelial growth factor and receptors in chronic cyclosporine nephrotoxicity. *Kidney Int* **63**: 522–33.

22 Walz G, Zanker B, Melton LB, Suthanthiran M, Strom TB (1990). Possible association of the immunosuppressive and B cell lymphoma-promoting properties of cyclosporine. *Transplantation* **49**: 191–4.

23 Sorensen HT, Mellemkjaer L, Nielsen GL, Baron JA, Olsen JH, Karagas MR (2004). Skin cancers and non-hodgkin lymphoma among users of systemic glucocorticoids: a population-based cohort study. *J Natl Cancer Inst* **96**: 709–11.

24 Penn I (1991). The changing pattern of posttransplant malignancies. *Transplant Proc* **23**: 1101–3.

25 Pirsch JD (1999). Cytomegalovirus infection and posttransplant lymphoproliferative disease in renal transplant recipients: results of the US multicenter FK506 Kidney Transplant Study Group. *Transplantation* **68**: 1203–5.

26 Browne BJ (1996). The tricontinental mycophenolate mofetil trial. *Transplantation* **62**: 1697.

27 Mathew TH (1998). A blinded, long-term, randomized multicenter study of mycophenolate mofetil in cadaveric renal transplantation: results at three years. Tricontinental Mycophenolate Mofetil Renal Transplantation Study Group. *Transplantation* **65**: 1450–4.

28 Blaheta RA, Bogossian H, Beecken WD, et al. (2003). Mycophenolate mofetil increases adhesion capacity of tumor cells in vitro. *Transplantation* **76**: 1735–41.

29 Engl T, Makarevic J, Relja B, et al. (2005). Mycophenolate mofetil modulates adhesion receptors of the beta1 integrin family on tumor cells: impact on tumor recurrence and malignancy. *BMC Cancer* **5**: 4.

30 Kreis H, Cisterne JM, Land W, et al. (2000). Sirolimus in association with mycophenolate mofetil induction for the prevention of acute graft rejection in renal allograft recipients. *Transplantation* **69**: 1252–60.

31 Stallone G, Schena A, Infante B, et al. (2005). Sirolimus for Kaposi's sarcoma in renal-transplant recipients. *N Engl J Med* **352**: 1317–23.

32 Campistol JM, Eris J, Oberbauer R, et al. (2006). Sirolimus therapy after early cyclosporine withdrawal reduces the risk for cancer in adult renal transplantation. *J Am Soc Nephrol* **17**: 581–9.

33 Penn I (1991). Donor transmitted disease: cancer. *Transplant Proc* **23**: 2629–31.

34 Kauffman HM, McBride MA, Cherikh WS, Spain PC, Delmonico FL (2002). Transplant tumor registry: donors with central nervous system tumors1. *Transplantation* **73**: 579–82.

35 Kauffman HM, McBride MA, Delmonico FL (2000). First report of the United Network for Organ Sharing Transplant Tumor Registry: donors with a history of cancer. *Transplantation* **70**: 1747–51.

36 Chui AK, Herbertt K, Wang LS, et al. (1999). Risk of tumor transmission in transplantation from donors with primary brain tumors: an Australian and New Zealand registry report. *Transplant Proc* **31**: 1266–7.

37 Buell JF, Trofe J, Sethuraman G, et al. (2003). Donors with central nervous system malignancies: are they truly safe? *Transplantation* **76**: 340–3.

38 Penn I (1997). Transmission of cancer from organ donors. *Ann Transplant* **2**: 7–12.

39 Feng S, Buell JF, Chari RS, DiMaio JM, Hanto DW (2003). Tumors and transplantation: The 2003 Third Annual ASTS State-of-the-Art Winter Symposium. *Am J Transplant* **3**: 1481–7.

40 Buell JF, Hanaway MJ, Thomas M, et al. (2005). Donor kidneys with small renal cell cancers: can they be transplanted? *Transplant Proc* **37**: 581–2.

41 Penn I (1995). Primary kidney tumors before and after renal transplantation. *Transplantation* **59**: 480–5.

42 Penn I (1997). Evaluation of transplant candidates with pre-existing malignances. *Ann Transplant* **2**: 14–7.

43 Hartevelt MM, Bavinck JN, Kootte AM, Vermeer BJ, Vandenbroucke JP (1990). Incidence of skin cancer after renal transplantation in The Netherlands. *Transplantation* **49**: 506–9.

44 Penn I (1997). Skin disorders in organ transplant recipients. External anogenital lesions. *Arch Dermatol* **133**: 221–3.

45 Sheil AG (1995). Malignancy following liver transplantation: a report from the Australian Combined Liver Transplant Registry. *Transplant Proc* **27**: 1247.

46 Buell JF, Trofe J, Hanaway MJ, et al. (2002). Immunosuppression and Merkel cell cancer. *Transplant Proc* **34**: 1780–1.

47 Kovach BT, Sams HH, Stasko T (2005). Systemic strategies for chemoprevention of skin cancers in transplant recipients. *Clin Transplant* **19**: 726–34.

48 Opelz G, Henderson R (1993). Incidence of non-Hodgkin lymphoma in kidney and heart transplant recipients. *Lancet* **342**: 1514–16.

49 Taylor AL, Watson CJ, Bradley JA (2005). Immunosuppressive agents in solid organ transplantation: Mechanisms of action and therapeutic efficacy. *Crit Rev Oncol Hematol* **56**: 23–46.

50 Buell JF, Gross TG, Thomas MJ, et al. (2006). Malignancy in pediatric transplant recipients. *Semin Pediatr Surg* **15**: 179–87.

51 Trofe J, Buell JF, Beebe TM, et al. (2005). Analysis of factors that influence survival with post-transplant lymphoproliferative disorder in renal transplant recipients: the Israel Penn International Transplant Tumor Registry experience. *Am J Transplant* **5**: 775–80.

52 Buell JF, Brock GN (2008). Risk of cancer in liver transplant recipients: a look into the mirror. *Liver Transpl* **14**: 1561–3.

53 Lee TC, Savoldo B, Rooney CM, et al. (2005). Quantitative EBV viral loads and immunosuppression alterations can decrease PTLD incidence in pediatric liver transplant recipients. *Am J Transplant* **5**: 2222–8.

54 Funch DP, Walker AM, Schneider G, Ziyadeh NJ, Pescovitz MD (2005). Ganciclovir and acyclovir reduce the risk of post-transplant lymphoproliferative disorder in renal transplant recipients. *Am J Transplant* **5**: 2894–900.

55 Opelz G, Daniel V, Naujokat C, Fickenscher H, Dohler B (2007). Effect of cytomegalovirus prophylaxis with immunoglobulin or with antiviral drugs on post-transplant non-Hodgkin lymphoma: a multicentre retrospective analysis. *Lancet Oncol* **8**: 212–8.

56 Green M, Michaels MG, Katz BZ, et al. (2006). CMV-IVIG for prevention of Epstein Barr virus disease and posttransplant lymphoproliferative disease in pediatric liver transplant recipients. *Am J Transplant* **6**: 1906–12.

57 Cullis B, D'Souza R, McCullagh P, et al. (2006). Sirolimus-induced remission of posttransplantation lymphoproliferative disorder. *Am J Kidney Dis* **47**: e67–72.

58 Choquet S, Trappe R, Leblond V, Jager U, Davi F, Oertel S (2007). CHOP–21 for the treatment of post-transplant lymphoproliferative disorders (PTLD) following solid organ transplantation. *Haematologica* **92**: 273–4.

59 Blaes AH, Peterson BA, Bartlett N, Dunn DL, Morrison VA (2005). Rituximab therapy is effective for posttransplant lymphoproliferative disorders after solid organ transplantation: results of a phase II trial. *Cancer* **104**: 1661–7.

60 Haque T, Wilkie GM, Jones MM, et al. (2007). Allogeneic cytotoxic T-cell therapy for EBV-positive posttransplantation lymphoproliferative disease: results of a phase 2 multicenter clinical trial. *Blood* **110**: 1123–31.

61 Zafar SY, Howell DN, Gockerman JP (2008). Malignancy after solid organ transplantation: an overview. *Oncologist* **13**: 769–78.

62 Brunson ME, Balakrishnan K, Penn I (1990). HLA and Kaposi's sarcoma in solid organ transplantation. *Hum Immunol* **29**: 56–63.

63 Mbulaiteye SM, Engels EA (2006). Kaposi's sarcoma risk among transplant recipients in the United States (1993–2003). *Int J Cancer* **119**: 2685–91.

64 Berber I, Altaca G, Aydin C, et al. (2005). Kaposi's sarcoma in renal transplant patients: predisposing factors and prognosis. *Transplant Proc* **37**: 967–8.

65 Gill PS, Wernz J, Scadden DT, et al. (1996). Randomized phase III trial of liposomal daunorubicin versus doxorubicin, bleomycin, and vincristine in AIDS-related Kaposi's sarcoma. *J Clin Oncol* **14**: 2353–64.

66 Gill PS, Tulpule A, Espina BM, et al. (1999). Paclitaxel is safe and effective in the treatment of advanced AIDS-related Kaposi's sarcoma. *J Clin Oncol* **17**: 1876–83.

67 Stewart T, Tsai SC, Grayson H, Henderson R, Opelz G (1995). Incidence of de-novo breast cancer in women chronically immunosuppressed after organ transplantation. *Lancet* **346**: 796–8.

68 Neuzillet Y, Lay F, Luccioni A, et al. (2005). De novo renal cell carcinoma of native kidney in renal transplant recipients. *Cancer* **103**: 251–7.

69 Penn I (1996). Evaluation of the candidate with a previous malignancy. *Liver Transpl Surg* **2**: 109–13.

70 Kasiske BL, Cangro CB, Hariharan S, et al. (2001). The evaluation of renal transplantation candidates: clinical practice guidelines. *Am J Transplant* **1**: 3–95.

71 Goldfarb DA, Neumann HP, Penn I, Novick AC (1997). Results of renal transplantation in patients with renal cell carcinoma and von Hippel-Lindau disease. *Transplantation* **64**: 1726–9.

72 Webster AC, Wong G, Craig JC, Chapman JR (2008). Managing cancer risk and decision making after kidney transplantation. *Am J Transplant* **8**: 2185–91.

Index